Health, Illness, and Well-being

PERSPECTIVES AND SOCIAL DETERMINANTS

Health, Illness, and Well-being

PERSPECTIVES AND SOCIAL DETERMINANTS

Edited by
Pranee Liamputtong,
Rebecca Fanany, and
Glenda Verrinder

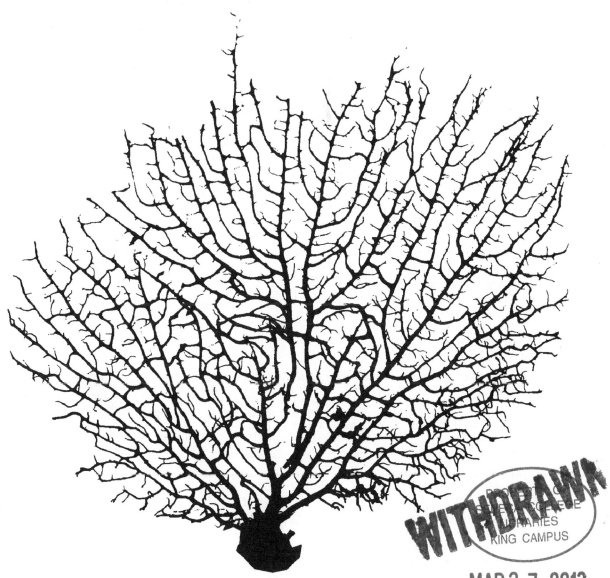

OXFORD
UNIVERSITY PRESS
AUSTRALIA & NEW ZEALAND

OXFORD
UNIVERSITY PRESS

Oxford University Press is a department of the University of Oxford.
It furthers the University's objective of excellence in research,
scholarship, and education by publishing worldwide. Oxford is a registered
trademark of Oxford University Press in the UK and in certain other
countries.

Published in Australia by
Oxford University Press
253 Normanby Road, South Melbourne, Victoria 3205, Australia

National Library of Australia Cataloguing-in-Publication data

Liamputtong, Pranee, 1955–

Health, illness and wellbeing: perspectives and social determinants/Pranee Liamputtong;
Rebecca Fanany; Glenda Verrinder.

978 0 19 557612 2 (pbk.)

Includes bibliographical references and index.

Health.
Heredity, Human.
Familial diseases.
Human beings—Effect of environment on.
Fanany, Rebecca.
Verrinder, Glenda.

613

Reproduction and communication for educational purposes
The Australian *Copyright Act 1968* (the Act) allows a maximum of one chapter
or 10% of the pages of this work, whichever is the greater, to be reproduced
and/or communicated by any educational institution for its educational purposes
provided that the educational institution (or the body that administers it) has
given a remuneration notice to Copyright Agency Limited (CAL) under the Act.

For details of the CAL licence for educational institutions contact:

Copyright Agency Limited
Level 15, 233 Castlereagh Street
Sydney NSW 2000
Telephone: (02) 9394 7600
Facsimile: (02) 9394 7601
Email: info@copyright.com.au

Edited by Venetia Somerset
Typeset by diacriTech, Chennai, India
Proofread by Anne Mulvaney
Indexed by Jeanne Rudd
Printed by Sheck Wah Tong Printing Press Ltd

To my daughters Zoe Sanipreeya and Emma Inturatana Rice – *Pranee*

To David and Runa Fanany – *Rebecca*

To my colleagues in the Department of Health and Environment – *Glenda*

Contents

Expanded Contents   *ix*

Lists of Figures and Tables   *xiv*

List of Case Studies   *xvi*

Preface   *xviii*

About the Editors   *xx*

About the Contributors   *xxi*

About the Book   *xxv*

1   Health, illness, and well-being: An introduction   1
        Pranee Liamputtong, Rebecca Fanany, and Glenda Verrinder

Part 1

Perspectives of Health, Illness, and Well-being   19

2   Introduction to pathogens and impacts on health and illness   21
        Elizabeth Brown

3   Introduction to epidemiology   44
        Rebecca Fanany

4   Human genetics and inheritance: Biological, social,
        cultural, and environmental perspectives   57
        Sandra Taylor

5   Chronic illness and the genome   76
        Chris L. Peterson and Evan Willis

6   Ageing and health: Biological, social, and environmental perspectives 92
        Colette Browning and Chyrisse Heine

7   Introduction to health promotion   107
        Alana Hulme Chambers and Rae Walker

8   Anthropogenic change and human health   125
        Rebecca Fanany

9   Climate change: Drivers and health impacts, mitigation, and
        adaptation strategies for the health sector   136
        Glenda Verrinder and Adrian Verrinder

10 Health and the living environment   154
        Cameron Earl, Jaco Terblanche, and Emma Patten

Part 2

Social Determinants of Health, Illness, and Well-being   175

11	Social determinants of health: Historical developments and global implications Bruce Rumbold and Virginia Dickson-Swift	177
12	Health as a social construct Claire Henderson-Wilson	197
13	Health throughout the life course Christopher Fox	213
14	Language, culture, and health Rebecca Fanany	229
15	Deviance, difference, and stigma as social determinants of health Pranee Liamputtong and Somsri Kitisriworapan	242
16	Health and the media Linda Portsmouth	257
17	Health and social justice Ann Taket	278
18	The economics of health and disease Rob Carter	302
19	The social determinants and the healthcare system Yvonne Parry and Eileen Willis	326
Glossary		344
References		359
Index		407

Expanded Contents

Lists of Figures and Tables   xiv

List of Case Studies   xvi

Preface   xviii

About the Editors   xx

About the Contributors   xxi

About the Book   xxv

1   Health, illness, and well-being: An introduction   1
         Pranee Liamputtong, Rebecca Fanany, and Glenda Verrinder

         Introduction   2
         Conceptualising health   2
         Disease, illness, health, and well-being   4
         Health, illness, well-being, and culture   5
         Determinants of health   8
         The intersections of biological, environmental, and social determinants of health   11

Part 1

Perspectives of Health, Illness, and Well-being   19

2   Introduction to pathogens and impacts on health and illness   21
         Elizabeth Brown

         Introduction   22
         Background to the biology of infectious diseases   22
         What makes a disease an infectious disease?   23
         Pathogens and parasites: What are they?   23
         What is the size of the problem?   24
         The nature of pathogens, and how they make us sick   25
         The nature of parasites, and how they make us sick   31
         Infectious diseases: What are the body's defences?   33
         Can infectious diseases be treated?   36
         Infectious diseases: What factors affect our susceptibility?   37
         Can infectious diseases be prevented?   37

3   Introduction to epidemiology   44
         Rebecca Fanany

         Introduction   45
         A brief history of epidemiology   45
         Epidemiological concepts   46
         The epidemiology of influenza and diabetes   51

4   Human genetics and inheritance: Biological, social,
cultural, and environmental perspectives   57
Sandra Taylor

    Introduction   58
    Human genetics and inheritance: Biological determinants of health   58
    Genes and chromosomes: The mechanisms of heredity   60
    Genetic factors in interaction with cultural, psychological,
    social, and political factors   67

5   Chronic illness and the genome   76
Chris L. Peterson and Evan Willis

    Introduction   77
    Dimensions of chronic disease   77
    What are chronic diseases?   78
    Determinants of chronic illness   78
    The social context of genetic biotechnologies   87

6   Ageing and health: Biological, social, and environmental perspectives   92
Colette Browning and Chyrisse Heine

    Introduction   93
    The biomedical approach to ageing and health   95
    Psychological, social, and environmental approaches to ageing and health   96
    Stereotyping and successful ageing   98
    Determinants of ageing well   100
    Policies for ageing populations   102

7   Introduction to health promotion   107
Alana Hulme Chambers and Rae Walker

    Introduction   108
    Defining health promotion   108
    The determinants of health   109
    Determinants of health: Population health   111
    A conceptual framework for health promotion: The Ottawa Charter   112
    Evidence-based health promotion   115
    Improving equity   116
    Social determinants of health and equity   116
    Community enablement   120
    Working collaboratively   121

8   Anthropogenic change and human health   125
Rebecca Fanany

    Introduction   126
    Anthropogenic change   126
    Changes to the physical environment   127
    Changes to the social environment   129

	Changes to personal behaviour	130
	Anthropogenic change and human health	132

9 Climate change: Drivers and health impacts, mitigation,
and adaptation strategies for the health sector   136
Glenda Verrinder and Adrian Verrinder

	Introduction	137
	Planetary climate change and human adaptation	137
	Environmental determinants of human health	141
	Mitigation and adaptation	145
	Health sector adaptation	148

10 Health and the living environment   154
Cameron Earl, Jaco Terblanche, and Emma Patten

	Introduction	155
	Local government	156
	Environmental health responses	157
	Town planning responses	159
	Emergency management responses	165
	Health promotion response	168

Part 2

Social Determinants of Health, Illness, and Well-being   175

11 Social determinants of health: Historical developments
and global implications   177
Bruce Rumbold and Virginia Dickson-Swift

	Introduction	178
	Social factors in illness	181
	Social factors in health	182
	Health promotion as a response to the emerging evidence	183
	Individual risk factors and social determinants	185
	The social gradient	186
	Social inequality and social exclusion	189
	Health as a global concern	192
	Getting the balance right	194

12 Health as a social construct   197
Claire Henderson-Wilson

	Introduction	198
	Social model of health	198
	Health sociology	201
	Social Skeleton: Health, illness and structure-agency	203
	Ecological models	206

13   Health throughout the life course   213
Christopher Fox

    Introduction   214
    Defining the life course perspective   214
    Basic concepts   216
    Elder's four themes of the life course   219
    Health effects and the life course   223
    The social gradient and the life course   224
    Policy implications   225

14   Language, culture, and health   229
Rebecca Fanany

    Introduction   230
    Culture   230
    Language   231
    Language and culture in health   232
    Indigenous health in Australia and New Zealand   234
    Cultural competency   235
    Illness behaviour and culture   237
    Culture-bound syndromes   238

15   Deviance, difference, and stigma as social determinants of health   242
Pranee Liamputtong and Somsri Kitisriworapan

    Introduction   243
    Deviance and difference   243
    Stigma, stigmatisation, and discrimination   247
    The impact of deviance and stigma on health   248
    Stigma, discrimination, and HIV/AIDS   250
    What has been done to manage stigma   252

16   Health and the media   257
Linda Portsmouth

    Introduction   258
    The mass media   258
    Mass media impact on health   259
    Utilising the mass media for health promotion   264
    Developing media materials to communicate health messages   272

17   Health and social justice   278
Ann Taket

    Introduction   279
    What are our human rights?   281
    Human rights and the social and cultural determinants of health   287
    To respect, protect, and fulfil...the responsibilities of governments in
    respect of human rights   291

Tools for public health advocacy and action—human rights
approaches to seeking social justice and health equity   293
The importance of human rights for public health practice: Rhetoric or reality?   297

18   The economics of health and disease   302
Rob Carter

Introduction   303
Why health economics is relevant to public health   304
'Positive economics' and 'normative economics'   306
Description in health economics   308
Prediction in health economics   315
Evaluation in health economics   317
Explanation in health economics   320

19   The social determinants and the healthcare system   326
Yvonne Parry and Eileen Willis

Introduction   327
The social determinants of health   327
The healthcare system as a structural determinant of health   329
Types of healthcare systems and impact on access   330
Health access as an intermediary determinant of health   332
The Australian healthcare system   334
The limits of access to primary care   338
Distance, supply, and access   339
Health access reform   340

Glossary   344
References   359
Index   407

Lists of Figures and Tables

Figures

Figure 1.1	Determinants of health	10
Figure 7.1	Determinants of health	110
Figure 7.2	Links between the determinants of health and the risk factors for NCD	118
Figure 10.1	Big-box retail centre in Griffith NSW—a design that can be seen anywhere in North America or Australia, that bears no relation to place	160
Figure 10.2	Urban sprawl in a curvilinear layout (left) and New Urbanism in a modified grid layout (right)	161
Figure 10.3	Section of an urban sprawl residential street (top) and a New Urbanist street (below)	162
Figure 10.4	Urban sprawl in Griffith (NSW) with wide roads and large setbacks, and the streetscape dominated by driveways and garages	162
Figure 10.5	New Urbanism in Mawson Lakes, Adelaide, with narrow roads and small setbacks	163
Figure 10.6	Town centre in Mawson Lakes, Adelaide	165
Figure 10.7	A laneway in Griffith NSW (left) compared to a laneway in a New Urbanist development in Adelaide	166
Figure 10.8	Aspects of our living environment that impact on food security	169
Figure 11.1	The WHO social determinants semi-circle diagram	178
Figure 11.2	The iceberg	186
Figure 11.3	Health and social problems are worse in more unequal countries	189
Figure 11.4	Life expectancy is longer in more equal rich countries	190
Figure 11.5	Bristol Exclusion Matrix	191
Figure 11.6	Preston curve	193
Figure 12.1	Social Skeleton: Health, illness and structure agency model	204
Figure 12.2	Adapted social ecological model	208
Figure 16.1	The stages in the health communication process	273
Figure 17.1	Multiple paths for human rights-based accountability and action	294
Figure 18.1	Disease burden attributable to 14 risk factors by sex, Australia 2003	309
Figure 18.2	Breakdown by cost driver of projected change in total health and residential aged care expenditure, 2012–13 to 2032–33	316
Figure 18.3	Premature deaths at ages 15–64 years, by sex and socio-economic status, 2002–06	321

Figure 19.1   The structural and intermediary social determinants of health   328

Figure 19.2   Separations per 1000 population for public and private
elective surgery, by remoteness of area of usual residence   336

Figure 19.3   Percentage of persons with private health insurance by
quintile for Adelaide, South Australia   337

Tables

Table 3.1   Basic concepts of descriptive epidemiology   48

Table 6.1   Summary of the predictor variables for poor or good
outcomes in old age   101

Table 7.1   Health promotion interventions and methods for managing NCDs   119

Table 10.1   Environmental health factors associated with the living environment   156

Table 11.1   Men's life expectancy at birth in 2008   187

Table 11.2   Life expectancy by social class 1972–76 and 1992–96,
England and Wales   187

Table 17.1   Linking human rights and the social and cultural
determinants of health   288

Table 18.1   Leading causes of burden by sex, Australia 2003   309

Table 18.2   Total health burden and total recurrent direct healthcare
expenditure for adults in selected diseases causally
related to overweight/obesity (Steps 1 and 2)   312

Table 18.3   The health burden attributable to overweight and obesity (Step 3)   313

Table 18.4   Healthcare expenditure attributable to overweight/obesity (Step 3)   314

Table 18.5   Projected total health expenditure (2002–03 dollars)
by cause, Australia, 2002–03 to 2032–33   316

Table 18.6   Prevalence of selected health measures by socio-economic
status, 2007–08 (%)   321

Table 19.1   Models of healthcare access   331

Table 19.2   Ratio of GP to population; selected SLA, South Australia   339

List of Case Studies

Case Study 1.1	Childbirth and soul loss	6
Case Study 1.2	Samantha	9
Case Study 2.1	Carriers of disease: The presence of pathogens in healthy individuals	27
Case Study 2.2	Hydatid disease in a child	32
Case Study 2.3	Epidemic of whooping cough (*pertussis*) in Victoria, 2011	39
Case Study 3.1	An unusual outbreak of salmonella	53
Case Study 4.1	Belinda	60
Case Study 4.2	Brian	64
Case Study 4.3	Kylie	70
Case Study 5.1	Ischaemic heart disease	83
Case Study 5.2	Type 2 diabetes	84
Case Study 5.3	Cystic fibrosis	87
Case Study 6.1	Women living in different social and cultural environments	99
Case Study 6.2	Health and successful ageing	102
Case Study 7.1	A health promotion approach to climate change	114
Case Study 7.2	Minimising the impact of non-communicable diseases on populations	118
Case Study 7.3	A health promotion approach to communicable disease	121
Case Study 8.1	The conquest (and re-emergence) of tuberculosis	133
Case Study 9.1	Unexpected results	140
Case Study 9.2	Healthcare organisations reduce greenhouse gases	148
Case Study 9.3	Monitoring arbovirus	149
Case Study 9.4	Climate Change and Primary Healthcare Intervention Framework	151
Case Study 10.1	EHPs and a food-borne illness outbreak investigation	158
Case Study 10.2	New Urbanism in action, Mawson Lakes, Adelaide	164
Case Study 10.3	Heatwave planning in Victoria	168
Case Study 10.4	Addressing food insecurity: Manatunga community garden, Swan Hill Rural City Council	171
Case Study 11.1	The problem with tobacco	184
Case Study 11.2	The health of 2000 San Francisco bus drivers	188
Case Study 12.1	Social Skeleton: Health, illness and structure agency model	204
Case Study 12.2	Adapted social ecological model	207

Case Study 13.1	Micro transitions and macro transitions: Markers of adulthood	217
Case Study 13.2	Life transitions	217
Case Study 13.3	Understanding age: How old are you?	221
Case Study 13.4	The social gradient and mortality	224
Case Study 14.1	Being sick in Indonesia	238
Case Study 15.1	Breast and bottle-feeding: Moral and deviant mothers	245
Case Study 15.2	Stigma and Thai women living with HIV/AIDS	252
Case Study 15.3	AIDS support group and women living with HIV/AIDS in Thailand	253
Case Study 16.1	Television food advertising and children	263
Case Study 16.2	The 'Go for 2 & 5®' Campaign	265
Case Study 16.3	Anti-tobacco media advocacy	268
Case Study 16.4	The Harvard Alcohol Project, USA	270
Case Study 16.5	Soul City, South Africa	271
Case Study 17.1	HIV/AIDS: Origins of the human rights approach to health	280
Case Study 17.2	How well is Australia doing in relation to its indigenous population?	282
Case Study 17.3	Restricting activities of persons who are HIV-positive	285
Case Study 17.4	The UN system helps effect positive change: An example from Australia	292
Case Study 17.5	Indigenous health: NGO advocacy	294
Case Study 17.6	Use of national litigation to support the right to health: The case of India	295
Case Study 17.7	CARE International, a human rights-based organisation	296
Case Study 17.8	Domestic violence, a major public health and human rights issue	299
Case Study 18.1	Ideology versus economic theory	306
Case Study 18.2	Government involvement in health	307
Case Study 18.3	Is obesity an important public health problem: What is its health and cost impact?	311
Case Study 18.4	Is our healthcare system sustainable?	315
Case Study 18.5	The ACE-Prevention study	318
Case Study 19.1	Access to healthcare by different social groups in Australia	333
Case Study 19.2	GP Plus and GP Super Clinics: Policy futures	340

Preface

This book provides an introduction to some of the important ideas that underlie the field of public health today. The conceptual framework is international even though the examples and case studies are often (although not exclusively) Victorian. It is intended for beginning students who want to understand the forces and trends that combine to shape the health of individuals, communities, and populations. As such, this book provides the basis for a career in any of the health sciences where insight into the meaning of health will allow for the development of effective practice and greater sensitivity to the needs of the community.

This book introduces a range of topics related to health and well-being in the context of a conceptual framework of determinants of health. An examination of biological, environmental, social, cultural, and economic determinants of health allows a number of current issues in public health to be understood in terms of their causes and interrelationships. The first part of the book focuses on perspectives of health and well-being and highlights the way in which people think about how health is informed by biological, environmental, and social factors that affect whole populations. The second part of the book centres on social, cultural, and economic determinants of health specifically to show the ways in which the experience of health is coloured by the characteristics of the society in which people live. Each chapter is free-standing, but all are linked through the framework of determinants that gives the reader an understanding of the causes of health, rather than just the effects of health status in society.

A determinants approach was chosen because it allows the reader to comprehend better the many factors that impact on health and to see the relationships between these factors. The chapters refer to global determinants of health and introduce readers to principles of evidence and practice that can be applied at the local level. The evidence base, upon which our understanding of the contributions of the various determinants is based, is presented in an introductory manner that will allow readers to further their study at higher levels. An understanding of the biological, environmental, social, and cultural determinants of health supports the more nuanced conception of health required of health professionals in order to practise effectively in the modern healthcare context. It also provides the background against which best practice must be determined. The chapters presented here are intended to supply some of the building blocks for the development of professional skills, abilities, and attributes in the understanding of health, in minimising disease, and promoting health across populations.

This book is intended to support the first year of university study of public health. It will be useful as an introduction to the field for students who intend to enter other branches of the health sciences and who may undertake no further study of public health. It will be equally beneficial as a starting point for those students who intend to concentrate on public health as a career and who need a strong foundation of knowledge on which to build. Further, it will serve as a reference for any interested reader who requires a brief but in-depth introduction to any of its topics and wishes to understand the nature of health and well-being in modern society.

In bringing this book to life, we owe gratitude to many people. We thank Debra James, the senior acquisition editor of Oxford University Press, who believes in the value of this book, contracted us to edit it, and provided ongoing support throughout our journey. We are grateful to all contributors who worked hard to make this book possible. We express our utmost thanks to our families who put up with our busy work and provided support throughout the period of the production of this book.

Pranee Liamputtong, Rebecca Fanany, and Glenda Verrinder
March 2011

About the Editors

Pranee Liamputtong holds a position of Personal Chair in Public Health at the School of Public Health, La Trobe University, Melbourne, Australia. Pranee has a particular interest in issues related to cultural and social influences on childbearing, childrearing, and women's reproductive and sexual health. She has published numerous books and a large number of papers in these areas. Her recent books in the health area include: *Community, health and population* (with Sansnee Jirojwong, Oxford University Press, 2008), and *Infant feeding practices: A cross-cultural perspective* (Springer 2011). She is editing a series of books on HIV/AIDS for Springer including two upcoming books: *Motherhood and HIV/AIDS: A cross-cultural perspective*, and *Stigma, discrimination and HIV/AIDS: A cross-cultural perspective*. Pranee is a qualitative researcher and has also published several method books. Her most recent method books include: *Researching the vulnerable: A guide to sensitive research methods* (Sage, 2007), *Performing qualitative cross-cultural research* (Cambridge University Press, 2010), *Research methods in health: Foundations for evidence-based practice* (Oxford University Press, 2010), and *Focus group methodology: Principles and practice* (Sage, 2011).

Rebecca Fanany is a lecturer in the School of Public Health, La Trobe University, Australia. Her background is in the area of environmental and occupational health, and she has worked in compliance and management in the USA and Australia. Her research interests include the ways in which health is conceptualised; the interaction between language, culture, religion, and health practices; and health status in the context of social and cultural change. She has published numerous articles, two books, and several textbooks on a wide range of topics related to language, culture, and health.

Glenda Verrinder is a Senior Lecturer in the La Trobe Rural Health School, La Trobe University, Australia. Before this she worked in various roles in the health sector in metropolitan and rural Victoria. Her current teaching, research, and publications reflect her interest in population health with respect to health promotion and ecological sustainability. Her recent publications include *Promoting health: The primary healthcare approach* 4th edn (Elsevier, 2009, with Lyn Talbot), co-editor, *Sustainability and health: Supporting global ecological integrity in public health* (Earthscan, 2005), and 'Health and quality of life' in *Understanding environmental and social policy* (Policy Press, 2011).

About the Contributors

Elizabeth Brown has a particular interest in teaching human physiology, along with its relevant applications, such as education as a means for the promotion of health and well-being. She has extensive experience as a teacher, especially to students in the health sciences at La Trobe University. She has had continuing academic appointments since 1974, and retired from La Trobe University in 2010. Elizabeth also has a research interest in human fertility and the factors that affect it. Currently she is an Honorary Associate of the School of Human Biosciences, Faculty of Health Sciences, La Trobe University.

Colette Browning is Professor of Healthy Ageing at Monash University and Director of Monash Research for an Ageing Society. Her research focuses on biopsychosocial approaches to ageing, culture and ageing, health behaviours, and chronic illness management. She is a Co-Director of the Melbourne Longitudinal Studies on Healthy Ageing Program, a longitudinal study of older people living in Melbourne that commenced in 1994. She is recognised as a national and international leader in psychology and health with a special focus on healthy ageing and chronic illness. Her recent book includes *Behavioural change: An evidence-based handbook for social and public health* (Elsevier, 2006). Colette is also an associate editor of *Australian Psychologist*.

Rob Carter is Head of Deakin Health Economics and Deputy Director of the Deakin University Strategic Research Centre in Population Health. Rob has taught health economics and economic evaluation to Master of Public Health students for many years and is an active researcher. His track record includes over $20.6 million in competitive research income and over 230 publications. Rob is widely recognised for his expertise in economic appraisal, both nationally and internationally, and he has been appointed by health ministers to serve on a range of key government committees.

Chyrisse Heine is a speech pathologist and audiologist. She is a Senior Research Fellow at Monash University, School of Primary HealthCare, and a Lecturer at La Trobe University, School of Human Communication Sciences. Chyrisse is a Fellow of Speech Pathology Australia. Her research focuses on healthy ageing and the assessment and management of communication and quality of life issues in older adults with vision and/or hearing loss. Chyrisse also has a special interest in (Central) Auditory Processing Disorder.

Alana Hulme Chambers is the Manager of Health Promotion at Gateway Community Health, Wodonga, Victoria. Alana's background is in health promotion and she has worked in a variety of roles including strategy and policy development, social research, and program management. Her research interests include evaluation, ethics, sexual health promotion, and collaboration between health promotion and other health disciplines.

Virginia Dickson-Swift is a Senior Lecturer in the Department of Health and Environment, La Trobe Rural Health School, La Trobe University, Australia. Virginia has taught across a range of units within both the undergraduate and postgraduate programs. Virginia has particular interest in the role of emotion in qualitative research and the use of qualitative methodologies in health research. She has published papers based on this work internationally and presented her work at a number of conferences. She has published several papers in the areas of undertaking sensitive research and other health-related issues. Her recent book is *Undertaking sensitive research in the* *health and social sciences: Managing boundaries, emotions and risks* (with Erica James and Pranee Liamputtong, Cambridge University Press, 2008).

Cameron Earl is a lecturer within the Department of Health and Environment, La Trobe Rural Health School. He has extensive experience working in environmental health within the local government and tertiary sectors and is particularly interested in environmental health management systems and their implementation, and the implementation of ecological sustainable development through the use of regulatory and strategic systems. Cameron has an undergraduate environmental health qualification, a Masters from Griffith University, and a Professional Doctorate from Queensland University of Technology.

Christopher Fox is a Fellow-Licentiate of the Royal Society for Public Health. He has extensive teaching experience in public health, sociology, and psychology. Before his current position, Christopher was a lecturer in the La Trobe Rural Health School, La Trobe University, where he taught a number of subjects relevant to health, illness, and well-being. He has consulted on a number of research projects on gender, health, and sexuality and with community organisations on development and evaluation, management, policy, and public health/health promotion. He is currently completing his doctoral thesis on men's body image.

Claire Henderson-Wilson is a lecturer in health promotion and ecological health and an Early Career Researcher within the School of Health and Social Development at Deakin University, Melbourne. Claire has a background in public health/health promotion and psychology and is involved in research that investigates people–environment relationships, in particular the links between housing, neighbourhoods, and residents' health.

Somsri Kitisriworapan is an Associate Professor at the Kasetsart University's Demonstration School, Thailand. Somsri teaches social science, history, and Thai language at both primary and secondary levels at the Demonstration School as well as in the Faculty of Education of Kasetsart University. Her main interest is in the health and psychology of children and her research has involved children's understanding of social and health issues. She has published several book chapters, journal articles, and textbooks in Thai and English.

Yvonne Parry has a research interest in the area of health access and the influence of the structural and intermediary social determinants on health supply and access. She actively promotes the inclusion of consumer experiences into the development and assessment of health access and service provision.

Emma Patten is a lecturer within the Department of Health and Environment, La Trobe Rural Health School, and has considerable experience in health promotion and community development. Emma has an interest in the creation of conditions for living without jeopardising the environment and has conducted research into the links between knowledge of environmental sustainability, attitudes, and behaviour change, as well as exploring the psychosocial health benefits of living sustainably. Emma has a degree in Public and Environmental Health (Honours) from La Trobe University.

Chris Peterson works in the School of Social Sciences at La Trobe University and conducts research in the Youth Research Centre, University of Melbourne. He previously worked in the School of Public Health at La Trobe, and together with his work at the National Centre for Epidemiology and Population Health at the Australian National University has developed an epidemiological focus to his sociological research into health and illness and particularly chronic diseases. He has a jointly edited book on chronic illness and has published widely in local and international journals on chronic disease. He has also focused on chronic disease as an occupational health and safety concern. He works on chronic illness projects both in Australia and as part of an international group of health writers and researchers.

Linda Portsmouth is a lecturer in health communication, media, and advocacy in the health promotion program of the School of Public Health at Curtin University. She has a Masters in Health Communication and is currently completing a PhD in Social Marketing. Her areas of interest include the social determinants of health, behaviour change communication, and communication campaigns in public health. Her background includes many years of community-based work, both internationally and in Australia, as a speech pathologist, health promotion professional, and health filmmaker. She still works as a freelance filmmaker communicating health messages via film.

Bruce Rumbold is a senior lecturer at La Trobe University and also Director of the Palliative Care Unit in the School of Public Health. Before taking up this appointment he was Professor of Pastoral Studies at Whitley College, an associated teaching institution of the Melbourne College of Divinity. He holds a PhD in Physics (Monash University 1971), a PhD in Social and Pastoral Theology (Manchester University 1976), and an MA in Health Studies (La Trobe University 1996), and has published articles and chapters in all three fields. His research interests are in social dimensions of end of life care, with spirituality as a particular lens upon the topic. Currently, he and two co-editors are nearing completion of a major handbook, *Spirituality and healthcare*, for Oxford University Press, Oxford.

Ann Taket is Chair in Health and Social Exclusion and Director of the Centre for Health through Action on Social Exclusion (CHASE) at Deakin University. She has over thirty years' experience in public health-related research, with particular interests in research directed at understanding the complex interactions between social exclusion and health, the design and evaluation of interventions to reduce health inequalities, the use of action research, participatory methods and experiential learning, and prevention and intervention in violence and abuse. She has a long-term interest in ethics and human rights issues. Her most recent books include *Health equity, social justice and human rights* (Routledge, 2011), *Domestic and sexual violence and abuse: Tackling the health and mental health effects* (Routledge, 2010, with Itzin and Barter-Godfrey), and *Theorising social exclusion* (Routledge, 2009, with Crisp, Nevill, Lamaro, Graham, and Barter-Godfrey).

Sandra Taylor is Professor and Head of Social Work at the University of Tasmania. She has extensive social work experience in healthcare services including clinical genetics, acute and community health, mental health, disability, aged care, and rehabilitation. Recent projects funded by the Australia Research Council include a national study of genetic discrimination in Australia and research relating to gender and genetic risk. Sandra has published widely in the area of healthcare and genetics. Recent publications relate to community attitudes about genetic risk and predictive genetic testing and implications for primary care, and consumer experiences of genetic discrimination. Her recent books include *Healthcare practices in Australia* (Oxford University Press, 2008).

Jaco Terblanche is a town planner based in Adelaide. He has extensive experience in town and regional planning in rural areas, working in the private as well as public sectors in regional South Africa and regional New South Wales. He has an interest in sustainable development models for regional areas, and is currently doing a doctoral thesis on new urbanism in regional Australian cities at Flinders University. Jaco has a Bachelors degree in Geography and Anthropology as well as a Masters degree in Town and Regional Planning from the University of Stellenbosch.

Adrian Verrinder has a particular interest in physiology and human ecology and health. He recently retired from La Trobe University after 20 years. Before that, he designed and built ecologically sensitive housing in remote locations, pioneering the use of solar cells, biomass, and water self-sufficiency. He is also a musician and has arranged and produced gold and platinum albums. During his time at La Trobe University, he taught students from public health, nursing, dentistry, pharmacy, engineering, arts, and education. He has been following the climate change debate since the 1970s.

Rae Walker is Associate Professor in the School of Public Health, La Trobe University. Initially she was trained as a nutritionist and worked in hospital and community settings, including a marginal Aboriginal community in southern Western Australia, before a major career shift into the field of providing social and community services. She completed an undergraduate degree in the social sciences, a postgraduate degree in education, and a PhD that explored a multi-scale perspective on the development and implementation of IT policy in education. The policy and program threads were applied to the development of health promotion in Australia and its implementation in the community based sector to achieve population level health outcomes. Rae is the Editor of the *Australian Journal of Primary Health*.

Eileen Willis is Associate Professor and Assistant Dean: Medical and Health Programs in the School of Medicine, Flinders University. Her research interests are in Indigenous health and in the impact of health reform on the work of health professionals. Her most recent publications include *Understanding the Australian healthcare system* (Elsevier, 2009, with Reynolds and Keleher), *Purgatorial time in hospitals* (Lambert Academic Publishing, 2009), and *Workplace reform in the healthcare system: The Australian experience* (Palgrave Macmillan, 2005, with Stanton and Young).

Evan Willis is Professor of Sociology and Associate Dean (Regions) at La Trobe University. Over a long career, primarily as a medical sociologist, he has worked on a variety of topics including the division of labour in healthcare, occupational health and safety, complementary and alternative healthcare, RSI, evidence-based healthcare, genomics, the social relations of medical technology, and most recently the health impacts of climate change. His 1989 book *Medical dominance* was in 2003 voted by peers one of the ten most influential books in Australian sociology. He has served on a number of both federal and state inquiries, including a national inquiry into Medicare, the Australia Health Technology Advisory Committee of the NHMRC, and the future of Chinese medicine in Victoria.

About the Book

This book comprises two parts and 19 chapters. **Chapter 1** is written by Pranee Liamputtong, Rebecca Fanany, and Glenda Verrinder. The concepts of health, illness, and well-being are introduced. Discussions on how individuals understand health, illness, and well-being as well as how different cultures perceive these concepts differently are also provided. Health determinants include biological, environmental, social, cultural, and economic factors. The authors point out that these determinants do not operate in their own space but intersect to produce health and illness in individuals and populations.

Part 1 of this text focuses on perspectives of health, illness, and well-being and is composed of nine chapters. **Chapter 2**, by Elizabeth Brown, is an introduction to pathogens and their impact on health. We live in a world populated by a remarkable variety of organisms with a wide range of complexity. Some of these organisms use our bodies for their survival, and some of them—pathogens—make us sick in the process. Organisms that rely on infecting us for their own survival do so in a variety of ways—but our bodies have various defences against infection, and assist us to survive should we become infected. However, these defences are not always successful: prevention of infection is therefore a priority. Knowledge about the ways that organisms infect us and make us sick, and the mechanisms that our bodies use to survive infectious disease help us to develop measures that will prevent infection in the first place. And what of the person who is infected and sick? The consequences of infectious diseases continue to influence the course of human history. Human societies have developed a wide variety of treatments for the consequences of infectious disease. Some of these are very effective in curing the disease, some treat only the symptoms of the disease, some may have no beneficial effect at all. There are some infectious diseases for which there is no effective treatment. Such diseases are likely to have a very high mortality rate. In order to understand the impacts of pathogens on health and illness we need to have some understanding of what our body's defences against infection are, and the consequences to our health if we develop an infection, or infestation with a parasite. Knowledge and management to prevent infection includes clean water supply, safe food handling, sanitation, control of vermin; improving nutritional status; immunisation programs; notification of certain diseases/contact tracing, isolation of infected persons, education and legislation.

Chapter 3 introduces epidemiology. Rebecca Fanany points out that epidemiology is one of the basic tools of public health and can provide important information about the appearance of disease in society, the way in which disease spreads, and the particular population subgroups that are most at risk. While the principles of epidemiology have traditionally been applied most often to the study of infectious disease, epidemiological principles are now often used to study a wide range of health and social conditions. This chapter will introduce readers to the meaning and use of rates in epidemiology; provide an understanding of incidence and prevalence; and illustrate how epidemiological data can be used to assess the health of populations as well as offer insight into the nature of disease in a given population. The concept of risk will be discussed in some detail with respect to both individuals and populations as the basis for public health interventions. The chapter assumes no knowledge of epidemiology and will not contain problems requiring calculation. Examples will include infectious disease (influenza), and chronic disease (diabetes).

In **Chapter 4** Sandra Taylor writes about human genetics and inheritance from biological, social, cultural, and environmental perspectives. This chapter introduces students to human genetics and inheritance as one of the potential factors that can interrelate with social, cultural, and environmental determinants to influence health and well-being. First, key genetic concepts are introduced; these include genes and chromosomes, patterns of inheritance, interactions of genes with other factors such as environment, genetic conditions and genetic tests for screening, and risk prediction. A brief overview of recent human genetic science is given including the discovery by Watson and Crick of the double helix in 1953 and the completion of the Human Genome Project in 2001. Second, the relationships between genes as biological determinants of health and the cultural, social, and environmental contexts within which people operate are introduced and examined. People's subjective beliefs about their genetic risks, for example, may be very different from the Mendelian or statistical risk that has been calculated based on their family history; subjective beliefs or risk perceptions can in turn significantly impact on a person's understanding of their risk or their behaviour in response to it. People's beliefs can be affected by factors like cultural understanding of inheritance, education, or gender. The limitations of simplistic thinking about genes totally determining people's health outcomes (notions of genetic determinism and reductionism) are examined. The final section of the chapter introduces some of the social, ethical, and political implications for individuals and groups who have information about genetic risks or genetic disorders. These implications include concerns about potential loss of privacy and even discrimination on the basis of genetic information. In spite of continuing advances in genetic developments, these concerns remain, as a result of which governments, including the Australian government, have undertaken comprehensive reviews of these issues and concerns, with many introducing targeted policies or laws to pre-empt genetic discrimination.

Issues concerning chronic illness are discussed in **Chapter 5** by Chris Peterson and Evan Willis. They suggest that in most developed countries, the trend for the near future is the continued growth of older populations and difficulties associated with supporting the needs of this group. Together with this there is a large growth in chronic illnesses in the population, particularly as older populations continue to expand. This chapter will look at major chronic diseases occurring over time, including the increase in diabetes as well as cardiovascular disease, asthma, and a number of other conditions. The chapter examines a range of factors associated with the development and spread of chronic diseases. These include investigating biological determinants on the development and spread of chronic disease; the influence of social factors such as socio-economic status and gender on prevalence. Further, cultural influences such as the impacts of different cultural and lifestyle factors will be examined; and finally, environmental factors found to be conducive to the development and growth of chronic diseases are presented. In the later stages of the chapter, a case study approach is adopted to review the impact of the Human Genome Project on the incidence and treatment of chronic diseases. The genome has ushered in new medical ways to develop potential cures for a number of diseases and in the future is seen as empowering patients with information about treatment and cures. Yet, how many conditions have cures been found for, and have they met expectations of success? The authors examine the effects of the Human Genome Project on four chronic illnesses in order to see the impact of the project on conditions—what impact has the project had on offering cures, and what different treatment regimens has it offered? Has the project offered hope and empowerment to the large populations suffering chronic conditions?

Chapter 6 dedicates its discussion to health and ageing. Colette Browning and Chyrisse Heine examine the phenomena of population ageing and the heterogeneity of the ageing process.

They argue that ageing is not solely driven by our biology and that many of the factors associated with ageing can be modified. The chapter also examines the concepts of successful, healthy, and active ageing as alternatives to inevitable age-related decline in health and well-being. The authors contend that our challenge is to create environments and programs for older people that support optimal well-being as we age while supporting vulnerable older citizens.

Chapter 7, by Alana Chambers and Rae Walker, provides an introduction to health promotion and the definition of health promotion. The authors outline the determinants of health and population health and introduce a conceptual framework for health promotion, the Ottawa Charter. They explore the common elements in best-practice approaches to health promotion: evidence-based health promotion, improving equity, community enablement, and working collaboratively. Three case studies are presented to bring together the various elements involved in a comprehensive approach to health promotion, demonstrating that health promotion can take various forms to address diverse issues.

Rebecca Fanany writes about the health impacts of anthropogenic change to the environment in **Chapter 8**. She argues that human beings have attempted to change their environment since prehistoric times in an effort to provide themselves with adequate shelter, a stable source of food and water, and protection from threats. In addition to achieving these ends, anthropogenic change of this kind has also created new opportunities for illness, conditions that are conducive or detrimental to health, and new risks and opportunities for individuals as well as populations. The pace of anthropogenic change has increased over the course of human history, especially in the latter half of the 20th century and beginning of the 21st, with the result that the current health situation faced by human populations is extremely complex. This chapter contains an overview of how human activity since the earliest times has had the effect of altering the environment in which human beings live and, as a result, has continued to change the health risks people are exposed to. The main focus of the chapter is on anthropogenic change in the 20th and 21st centuries, including changes in the living environment, work environment, chemical use, and the effects of expanding human populations. A case on the re-emergence of tuberculosis is presented to demonstrate how anthropogenic change can affect a disease in human populations. Examples in the text describe the appearance of West Nile Virus in the USA, workplace rage, and measles as the effects of different kinds of change created by people.

In **Chapter 9**, climate change and its health impacts are discussed by Adrian and Glenda Verrinder. They propose that the mounting evidence of the impact of climate change is transforming our views of what determines health. They argue that a healthy ecosystem is a prerequisite for human health, and that all species fundamentally depend on adequate shelter, food, and water, freedom from excess disease, and the safety and comfort conferred by climate stability. Anthropogenic climate change is having, and will increasingly have, an impact on human health. The authors propose that health professionals will be affected individually, as family members, as community members, and as professionals. Unprecedented events in Australia such as heat waves, cyclones, floods, and drought have stretched health services to the limit and beyond in recent times. These events have highlighted the need for health professionals to have a firm understanding of the evidence and implications of climate change as they will continue to be at the front line of professionals responding to the health impacts.

The authors argue that climate change literacy is important for health professionals. The chapter is presented in two parts. In the first part, the science of climate change is outlined. In the second part, some of the known impacts of climate change on human health are presented along with case studies to illustrate the roles that some health agencies are already playing. They conclude that health is determined by the relationship between humans and the environment in which they live. When the relationship between humans and their environment changes, particularly when the change is rapid, health is fundamentally affected. The health implications of climate change are extensive. The health sector will be required to work in partnership with other sectors to implement mitigation and adaptation responses to protect the health of humans.

Chapter 10 has its focus on health and the living environment and is written by Cameron Earl, Jaco Terblanche, and Emma Patten. The aim of this chapter is to identify and explore traditional, current, and emerging environmental health issues in relation to the built environment, and discuss current practice examples that manage these issues, such as urban planning, health protection, and health improvement. The chapter provides detailed discussions about the responses of society over time. For example, how is the living environment changing? As the impacts of suburban sprawl are becoming apparent, alternatives are being sought and developed. These include Traditional Neighbourhoods, New Urbanism, Sustainable Development, Liveable Neighbourhoods, and Smart Growth. The authors introduce the enforced regulation of human behaviour to protect the health of the individual and fellow human beings. Health protection includes the prevention and control of infectious diseases as well as response to emergencies and engages with the regulation for clean air, water, and food as well as preventing or dealing with environmental health hazards. The health improvement domain covers key aspects of activity to reduce inequalities, working with partners such as education and workplaces. It involves engagement with structural determinants such as housing and employment, as well as individuals and their families to improve health and prevent disease by adopting healthier lifestyles.

Part 2 is dedicated to the social determinants of health, illness, and well-being and comprises nine chapters. **Chapter 11** discusses the social determinants in the context of history and on a global scale. Bruce Rumbold and Virginia Dickson-Swift contend that today it is clear that health in every society is fundamentally determined by social and cultural factors. But national healthcare systems, particularly in developed nations, have been built to deliver clinical services that respond to immediate health problems confronting individual citizens. The underlying social and cultural determinants, the causes of these health problems, have been neglected as secondary to meeting immediate needs or as raising issues that are too difficult to address through the short-term policy agendas that reflect the priorities of governments driven by election cycles. These clinical models have also influenced the healthcare systems of most developing nations through the types of programs provided through overseas aid programs and the developed-world training given to their healthcare workforce. Nevertheless, as healthcare costs escalate, and as the burden of disease shifts from acute, remediable illnesses to chronic and degenerative conditions, the need for more fundamental action in developing health as well as in combating illness has become obvious. At the same time, the evidence for social determinants of health has become compelling. Any failure to act on these findings can no longer be attributed to a lack of evidence; it is now a matter of social and political will.

This chapter traces the growth in understanding of the role played by social factors in health, and the development of a body of evidence that identifies these factors and the strategies through which they might be addressed. The findings and recommendations of the World Health Organization Commission on Social Determinants of Health, currently the most comprehensive repository of global information on social determinants, are outlined. Discussion of these findings and recommendations are applied particularly to Australian society and current debates about reforming the health system.

Health as a social construct is discussed in **Chapter 12** by Claire Henderson-Wilson. It argues that individuals' perceptions of health and illness are subjective and are understood to be influenced by a range of social and cultural contexts and determinants. This chapter explores how constructions of 'health', 'illness', and 'well-being' have moved beyond traditional biomedical interpretations that focused on an individual's medically defined pathology, to an awareness of how they are influenced by a range of social and cultural contexts and determinants. The first section of this chapter defines and discusses the social model of health. Relevant examples are used to explore how valuable this model is for understanding the social construction of health, illness, and well-being. The next section discusses how health sociology can be used to understand the construction of health, illness, and well-being. Drawing on Germov's (2005) Social Skeleton Model, which represents the social structures individuals are part of, this section explores how social groups, social institutions, and the wider culture influence perceptions of health, illness, and well-being. A final proposed section of this chapter is a focus on how ecological models can be used to explore social constructions of health, illness, and well-being. Human ecologists contend that an individual's health is part of a structure of relationships (contexts and determinants) and is altered by changes in that structure. They are interested in the relationships between humans and the physical, natural, cultural, and social dimensions of their environment. Urie Bronfenbrenner, a renowned human ecologist, argued that an individual's health and well-being is dependent on their interaction with the environment and developed an ecological model to depict this. Bronfenbrenner's (1979) Social Ecological Model depicts the contexts and determinants impacting on an individual's health and well-being, both directly and indirectly, from the wider, macrosystem layer to the inner, microsystem layer. A case study using an adapted version of Bronfenbrenner's model is used to explore how health and well-being is socially constructed. Throughout the chapter, recognition of the relevant program and/ or policy responses to changing perspectives and understandings of health is explored via a critical examination and analysis of key literature.

In **Chapter 13**, Christopher Fox introduces the concept of life course determinants to health. He suggests that this is one of the social determinants that is often forgotten. Life course determinants can account for some of the chronic disease experienced in later life. Often, people are placed in a position to take responsibility for the causes of chronic disease. With a life course approach, we can see that the 'causes' are not always a result of the individual but a function of experiences earlier in life. Readers are introduced to ideas of how experiences in the womb and from birth can have a major impact much later in life. Through the chapter, readers learn of key concepts and ideas that underpin life course determinants and learn how to apply the ideas in practice. In this chapter, readers will undertake a life mapping process to explore the impacts of their life on their health in later adulthood.

Rebecca Fanany writes about language, culture, and health in **Chapter 14**. She suggests that the language people speak and their cultural background are singularly important in forming their understanding of health and illness. Ideas and information are categorised according to the structures available in a given language, and cultural practices tend to develop in accordance with the worldview described by language and experience. While the linguistic and cultural aspects of perception are often studied in the context of sociolinguistics and semiotics, consideration of this aspect of human experience is very appropriate in the field of health because the perception of illness can affect whether an individual sees themselves as healthy or ill, the prognosis of diagnosed disease, the outcome of treatment, and even whether such treatment is sought. Today the health sector is very much aware that different language and cultural groups have differing perceptions about health and illness, and efforts are made to ensure that healthcare professionals are aware of the need for cultural competence in working with groups and individuals with different backgrounds.

This chapter describes the ways in which language and cultural background can influence the ways in which individuals and groups understand health, deal with the experience of illness, and make use of healthcare services. A general introduction to the principles of sociolinguistics is included, and the issue of cultural appropriateness is discussed in the context of cultural competence among healthcare professionals. A set of examples comparing how health and illness are conceptualised in various languages is used to demonstrate the different ways in which health is experienced by groups of speakers. Additionally, a case study showing expected health behaviour in a Western, Anglo-Saxon culture as compared to expected health behaviour in Indonesia is used to illustrate the effects cultural practices can have on the experience of illness.

Chapter 15 introduces deviance, discrimination, and stigma as social determinants of health. Pranee Liamputtong and Somsri Kitisriworapan discuss health issues and behaviour that are seen as 'difference'. The main focus is on deviance, difference, stigma, and discrimination. They first introduce notions of deviance, difference, and stigma, then discuss the impact of deviance and stigma on the health and well-being of those who are stigmatised. The chapter also discusses stigma and HIV/AIDS and what has been done to combat HIV-related stigma as a case example. It suggests that stigma is associated with stereotyping and prejudice. It is employed by individuals to define certain attributes of others as unworthy and as such these people are seen as 'tainted'. Stigma is socially constructed and is attributable to cultural, social, historical, and situational factors. Stigmatised individuals are subject to feelings of shame and guilt. A major consequence of stigmatisation is discrimination and it occurs when an individual is treated unfairly and unjustly due to the perception that the individual is deviant from others. As such, many health issues such as HIV and AIDS are perceived as deviance. Individuals living with HIV/AIDS are socially constructed as the 'other'. The chapter also points out that health and illness conditions which tend to produce stigma are those that are connected with negative characteristics, have uncertain or unknown causes and limited treatment, and produce intense reactions such as fear and disgust. Individually, the effects of stigma and social exclusion can be destructive. They can result in isolation, low self-esteem, depression, self-harm, poor academic achievement and social relationships, and poor physical and mental health. The impact of stigma on the public health of the stigmatised individuals and groups is huge. In the area of HIV/AIDS, for example, it is now clear that the stigmatisation of certain groups such as commercial sex workers, injecting drug users, and gay men would only make them more susceptible to HIV infection and push them out of reach of those who attempt to help them modify the behaviours that put them and others at risk.

In **Chapter 16** Linda Portsmouth suggests that the mass media are a social determinant of health. It is one of the many features of a society that impacts on people's knowledge, attitudes, and beliefs about health—and thus on their health behaviours. The mass media that people are exposed to, and interact with, have had a measurable impact on their health choices and outcomes. Many people gain much of their understanding of health from what they see and hear on television, the internet, radio, newspapers, and magazines. The mass media are pervasive and persuasive, reaching population-wide with health information in a way that promotes and normalises the health concepts portrayed. The mass media play a role in the socialisation of children and adolescents—influencing them as to what to expect and what is expected of them in their society. News and current affairs, entertainment, the internet—and the advertising that pays for most of it—often contain messages of significance to public health. Public health professionals seek to explore the impact of the mass media—aiming to describe, quantify, and counter any negative influence on population health. We also study the effective techniques utilised by media professionals and learn to work in partnership with media professionals. This enables public health professionals to successfully communicate health messages via the mass media in a way that promotes population health. We seek to influence news and current affairs content to increase people's awareness of health issues—often advocating for a change in policy or legislation. We also seek to influence existing entertainment and develop entertainment-education media. We have also successfully developed advertising (among other social marketing activities) to promote health. Working closely with members of population groups at risk allows us to develop concepts, messages, and media materials that will communicate most effectively with that particular group.

Health and social justice are discussed by Ann Taket in **Chapter 17**. It is suggested that the achievement of social justice is closely connected to progress on human rights and the achievement of health equity. Australia, along with most member states of the UN, has ratified the Universal Declaration on Human Rights and the other covenants and conventions covering human rights, thereby acquiring obligations to respect, protect, and fulfil human rights. This chapter examines the role of human rights in the social and cultural determinants of health. Using a series of case studies on domestic violence, Indigenous health, and HIV/AIDS this chapter explores the relationships between health and human rights and introduces readers to a wide range of resources relevant to their application in policy and practice. Issues covered in this chapter include: How progress in meeting obligations to respect, protect, and fulfil rights relates to progress in achieving the social and cultural determinants of health and progress towards health equity; how human rights-based argumentation can provide a strong grounding for public health and health promotion advocacy; and how health and social policy can be scrutinised for its human rights implications.

The economic impact of health and disease is discussed by Rob Carter in **Chapter 18**. This chapter provides an introduction to how the discipline of health economics is relevant to the field of public health. The starting point is to appreciate that the discipline carries out three separate but related tasks, 'description', 'prediction', and 'evaluation'. Researchers often confuse what task is appropriate to answer what research question. Related confusions involve seeing the aims of 'efficiency' and 'affordability' as the same thing and not distinguishing between the tasks of 'prioritising problems' and 'prioritising solutions'. The economics discipline also distinguishes between 'positive economics' and 'normative economics', with the former covering 'what is' and the latter 'what ought to be'. Positive economics is meant to be as value-free as possible and is dominated by the task of description. Normative economics, on the other hand, is consciously based on value judgments that underlie suggested change. The failure of some economists to make these value judgments transparent can lead to confusion as to whether recommendations are based on economic theory or on ideology. The reliance on the free market by economic rationalists, for example, embodies the ethical judgment that it is acceptable for access to healthcare to be determined by the consumer's ability and willingness to pay. Alternative notions of social justice embody the judgment that access should be based on need and give rise to government involvement through health insurance. When governments choose to intervene in markets, then the task of economic evaluation has a role to play in guarding against 'government failure'. The basic questions that markets have to answer (or governments when they intervene) are: 'what to produce', 'how to produce it', and 'who gets access'?

The author invites readers to consider what rationales are appropriate for answering what questions. The role of markets and what arguments provide the justification for government intervention are considered. The notion of market failure and its counterpart, government failure, are explained. The aims of efficiency, equity, and affordability, among others are considered, and they are located in the context of three broader questions: how is economic circumstance a determinant of good health or illness for individuals, communities, and the nation; what is the economic impact of exposure to risk factors and illness; and what role should efficiency play in what we as a nation want from our healthcare system? The material presented in this chapter is intended to give readers an introduction to health economics as a way of thinking and problem-solving. It provides the economic perspective on how best practice can be determined and funding priorities set. It is intended to give students the building blocks for understanding why and when you need to consult health economists—or indeed why you may want to become one!

In the last chapter, **Chapter 19**, written by Yvonne Parry and Eileen Willis, the social determinants and the healthcare system are discussed. The authors suggest that social factors are major determinants of health for individuals and populations. In previous chapters, these social and cultural factors, along with biological and life system factors, have been identified and their impact on health status analysed. Overcoming the negative impact of these social determinants requires innovative interventions that address the power and socio-political structures within society and within the health system. This chapter explores the impact of health access as a specific social determinant of health. The authors argue that even where health access is free and universal, specific disadvantaged groups such as those of low socio-economic status, people with disabilities, Indigenous groups, or the geographically isolated do not enjoy equal access to healthcare services. Differences in access include variable access to timely and appropriate services, and quality of community care.

This chapter outlines a conceptual framework for understanding the impact of health access as a social determinant of health (SDH). The discussions draw on work done by the World Health Organization (WHO). The WHO (2007) divides the SDH into two groups: those that are structurally determined or 'upstream' from the individual, for example socio-economic status, gender, employment, or race, and those that are intermediary or 'downstream', thus nearer to the individual and more amendable to community intervention through policy intervention. The development of the two categories evolved from an extensive review of the current SDH frameworks and models by WHO researchers Solar and Irwin (2007). The two categories are necessary to explain which determinants of health are influenced by governments and the socio-political constructs (structural) of a society. Access to appropriate healthcare services is an intermediary SDH. Access is shaped by the nation's healthcare system, but also by a range of policies that enhance equity of access to existing social and welfare services. This chapter uses a case study of variable and unequal access to pediatric emergency care to illustrate the impact of the structural determinants of health on health access for various population groups. It illustrates that even where healthcare is free and universal, access to quality healthcare is still determined by socio-economic status and other forms of disadvantage that can be overcome to some extent through more refined policy.

1

Health, illness, and well-being: An introduction

Pranee Liamputtong, Rebecca Fanany, and Glenda Verrinder

TOPICS COVERED

This chapter covers the following topics:
- an introduction to health, illness, well-being, and disease
- cultural understanding of health, illness, and well-being
- determinants of health
- biological determinants
- environmental determinants
- social determinants of health
- gender, ethnicity, and social class
- health inequality

KEY TERMS

Biological determinants
Culture
Determinants of health
Disease
Environmental determinants
Ethnicity

Gender
Health
Illness
Social class
Social determinants
Well-being

Introduction

Health There is no definite meaning of health. Its meaning can be different depending on individuals, social groups, and cultures and can differ at different times. However, the World Health Organization (1978, p. 2) defines health as 'a state of complete physical, mental and social well-being and not merely the absence of disease or infirmity'.

See Chapter 16 *for more about health and the media.*

The concept of **health** has different meanings to different people (Jirojwong & Liamputtong 2009). Each individual has a different perception and experience of health, illness, and well-being. For some people, health may mean being active and fit. For others, health means having a balance in their lives, being productive or able to fulfil their responsibilities (Blaxter 2004; Levin & Browner 2005; Taylor 2008a; Jirojwong & Liamputtong 2009; AIHW 2010a). Additionally, members of one cultural group may see health, illness, and well-being differently.

In Australia, the notion that health is of primary importance is pervasive. This is reflected in the fact that health and illness are featured in all kinds of media. Often, there are reports or stories about health issues, health-related behaviours and experiences, the importance of fitness and health, new medical and scientific discoveries, healthcare services and government policies (Taylor 2008a; Germov & Freij 2009).

There are many things that can determine our health, illness, and well-being. These range from societal influences to individual aspects such as genetic makeup as well as the healthcare to which we have access. These are referred to as 'the determinants of health' since they 'determine how likely we are to stay healthy or become ill' (AIHW 2010a, p. 63; see section below on determinants of health). According to the Australian Institute of Health and Welfare (AIHW) (2010a, p. 63), the health, illness, and well-being of an individual comprise many aspects: 'They result from complex interplay between societal, environmental, socioeconomic, biological and lifestyle factors.'

This chapter will take you through several important concepts. First, the meaning of health, illness, well-being, and disease is introduced. Then these meanings are discussed within a cultural context. The determinants of health are then introduced. Last, the relationships between health determinants are discussed, in particular the intersection of gender, ethnicity, and social class.

Conceptualising health

See Chapter 12 for more on health as a social construct.

According to Keleher and MacDougall (2009), it is impossible to find a universal definition of health which can be applied to all individuals, locations, and time. The meanings of health are 'embedded in the unique individual, family, social and cultural contexts in which the term is used'. Hence, health is 'socially and culturally constructed' (Taylor 2008a, p. 5). The AIHW (2010a, p. 3) defines health as an essential component of well-being. It is about how we 'feel and function'. Health is not simply about the non-existence of injury or illness but about degrees of wellness and illness in health. Health is situated within broad social and cultural contexts. The state of health of individuals in the society also contributes to the social and economic well-being of that particular society. The following quotes suggest that health is defined differently according to the contexts within which the definition is located.

Health is a personal and social state of balance and well-being in which a woman feels strong, active, creative, wise and worthwhile: where her body's vital power of functioning and healing is intact; where her diverse capacities and rhythms are valued; where she may decide and choose, express herself and move about freely. (Centre for Health Education, Training and Nutrition Awareness 2011)

Health is a social, economic and political issue and above all a fundamental human right. Inequality, poverty, exploitation, violence and injustice are at the root of ill-health and the deaths of poor and marginalised people. (People's Health Movement 2011, p. 2)

Health is 'a sustainable state of wellbeing, within sustainable ecosystems, within a sustainable biosphere'. (Honari 1993, p. 23)

Keleher and MacDougall (2009, pp. 5–6) outline different perspectives which can be used to conceptualise health. Several perspectives are relevant to this textbook. The lay or cultural perspective suggests that health is understood and interpreted differently by individuals depending on their experiences, life situations, and cultural backgrounds. The biological perspective examines the role of genes and risk factors as well as their interactions with other health determinants (see later section on these determinants). Closely related to the biological approach is the biomedical perspective. Within this approach, health and illness are perceived in terms of a person's 'medically defined pathology'.

See also Chapters 4 & 14 for the cultural implications of health.

The behavioural perspective advocates that superior quality of life results from having good health, which is founded on risk factors and lifestyle behaviours. Health education is often the response to improving these determinants. The health promotion approach includes all of these perspectives and in addition pays attention to the powerful impact of a 'place' or location in determining health. Hence, we see projects such as 'Healthy Schools', 'Healthy Workplace', and 'Healthy Cities' (Baum 2008, p. 13). Research suggests that disadvantaged individuals such as poor people may have poorer health because they reside in places which are damaging to health (Macintyre & Ellaway 2000; Baum 2008). The influence of location on health can be clearly seen in remote indigenous communities in Australia and other parts of the world where important health facilities such as healthy food, clean water, good sewerage system, suitable accommodation, and access to healthcare are insufficient or absent (Baum 2008). This also applies to poor people living in slums in many parts of the globe.

See also Chapter 6 on the various physical aspects of health and illness.

See Chapter 10 for a discussion of the living environment as it affects health.

The Ottawa Charter for Health Promotion (WHO 1986) is considered the formal beginning of the new public health, which has its focus on the social causes of illness and disease, health equity, and social justice (Baum 2008). It suggests that social inequalities and health are situated within the complex connection between social, economic, political, and environmental determinants (see also the section below in this chapter). As such, health is perceived as 'a complex outcome' which is influenced by factors including genetic, environmental, economic, social, and political circumstances (Baum 2008, p. 16). This perspective is the focus of this book.

See Chapters 7, 12, 13, & 16-19 for the social determinants of health.

Disease, illness, health, and well-being

Disease A condition adversely affecting health that has measurable (clinical) symptoms.

Illness A condition adversely affecting health as perceived by the individual in question.

When an individual experiences ill symptoms, two terms tend to be used to describe the sickness: 'disease' and 'illness'. The term **disease** refers to as 'medically defined pathology' (Blaxter 2004, p. 20). It is a malfunctioning of biological mechanisms (Jirojwong & Liamputtong 2009). The word incorporates 'a set of signs and symptoms and medically diagnosed pathological abnormalities' (Baum 2008, p. 4). On the other hand, **illness** involves the subjective experience of ill health of an individual (Blaxter 2004; Baum 2008; Taylor 2008a). Primarily, it is about how a person lives through the disease (Baum 2008). Often, it involves personal, social, and cultural reactions to a disease. Illnesses can disrupt people's lives, which may lead individuals to seek medical care. An ailing person may have to rely on others for their basic needs in daily living (Spector 2009; Suwankhong 2011).

Health, when situated within a biomedical framework of biological determinants, can be seen as 'the absence of disease or pathology' in a person (Taylor 2008a, p. 10). It suggests that if the person does not have a disease, he or she is healthy. Taylor (2008a, p. 10) contends that this view implies two main assumptions. First, there are two opposite states of being: an individual is either healthy or ill. In this view, health and illness are seen as uniform and permanent concepts. Second, it implies that having good health is the norm and being ill is deviant. Thus, illness connotes 'abnormality, deficiency or impairment' (see also Scambler 2003; Blaxter 2004). As Blaxter

See also Chapter 15 for a discussion of illness as deviance.

(2004, p. 7) contends, 'the objective observation of a lack of "normality" meets a very ancient and universal tendency to see the sick person as in some way morally tainted or bewitched. Possibly, they are responsible for their own condition.'

The concept of health as the absence of disease has been perceived as being 'too narrow' (Taylor 2008a, p. 11). Health should be seen as a more credible and holistic condition (Blaxter 2004; Levin & Browner 2005; Taylor 2008a). This is reflected in the definition of health proposed by the World Health Organization (WHO 1978, p. 2), which advocates that health is 'a state of complete physical, mental and social well-being and not merely the absence of disease or infirmity'. This definition suggests that it is not only the biological functioning of individuals that determines the state of their health, but also their social and psychological conditions. These components do not function separately but interact with each other in complicated processes (Taylor 2008a; see the section below on determinants of health).

Well-being A positive conceptualisation of health: feeling healthy, happy, or doing well in life. It can be completely separated from the objectively measured health or disease status of an individual.

This view of health is also reflected in the mental health area. There has been an attempt to define mental health in a way that moves beyond the focus on biological factors (Baum 2008). The Victorian Health Promotion Foundation (VicHealth 1999, p. 4) developed the following positive definition: 'Mental health is the embodiment of social, emotional and spiritual well-being. Mental health provides individuals with the vitality necessary for active living, to achieve goals and to interact with one another in ways that are respectful and just.'

The WHO definition of health also incorporates the concept of **well-being**. This concept is seen as more expansive than that of health because it signifies an individual's sense of general contentment with life (Eckersley 2001; Taylor 2008a).

Well-being is used in a subjective sense in that there is nothing wrong, and can be completely separated from the objectively measured health or disease status of an individual (Jirojwong & Liamputtong 2009). People may possess a sense of personal well-being even when they are in very deprived situations, for example during stressful life events or confronted with acute or chronic disease. In a way, according to Jones and Creedy (2008), it could be said that well-being symbolises the opposite of illness.

Stop and Think

- What does health mean to you?
- What does illness mean to you?
- What does well-being mean to you?
- How do you know if someone is healthy or not?

Stop and Think

Sophie is a 78-year-old woman who has experienced a range of symptoms in the last few years. She suffers from severe tinnitus (ringing in the ear) in both ears. She has also suffered from hearing loss in one ear. Additionally, she has high blood pressure which is being controlled by prescribed medication. Although she is slower with everyday activities and often has aches and pains, she still eats and sleeps well. She is poor but she has good support from her children. She thinks what she has been experiencing is part of growing old. She does not think she is ill.

- What do you think about Sophie's idea of her health?
- In your view, should Sophie's conditions be categorised as illness? Discuss.

Health, illness, well-being, and culture

All human beings have to deal with good health, illness, disease, sickness, and death. In all human groups, no matter how small or large, whether technologically primitive or advanced, there exists a set of beliefs about the nature of health and illness, its cause and cures, and its relations to other aspects of life. These are conditions that shape an aspect of social experience and cultural knowledge. As such, concepts of health, illness, and well-being are likely to reflect a marked cultural influence (Mackenzie et al. 2003; Helman 2007; Jones & Creedy 2008). What is seen as health or illness in one location, or by the members of one group, is not always perceived the same way in another (Jones & Creedy 2008). Because health and illness are socially constructed, different **cultures** would have different perceptions of health and illness. It has been shown that cultural understandings of health and illness operate as an important aspect in determining the health and illness of individuals (Julian 2009).

While health is well understood by most people in mainstream Australian society, within Indigenous Australian cultures there is no one single word that stands for

Culture A system of shared ideas, attitudes, and practices that defines the social system of its members.

See also Chapters 4, 12 & 14 for different ways in which culture impacts on health.

health (O'Connor-Fleming & Parker 2001). Concepts of health and well-being entail 'relationship with family, community and connectedness with traditional land or country rather than referring to an individual as a separate entity' (Taylor 2008a, p. 6). These collective approaches of health are held by many Indigenous people (Levin & Browner 2005). In the Indigenous context, the concept of 'well-being' has a broader meaning than 'health' since it embraces the wider relationship and connection of people with their environment and community (O'Connor-Fleming & Parker 2001; Taylor 2008a).

For Thai people, being in good health is understood as being normal and strong, and free of illness and disease. In the Thai worldview, this understanding symbolises the characteristics of people's capability and is related to traditional understanding of *me ar-kaan crop sam-sib-song pra-garn* (having the complete 32 components of the body) in order to fulfil a person's normal routine such as eating, sleeping, and working (Suwankhong 2011). Thai people also have their own cultural knowledge about causes of good health and illness which has been part of the culture for centuries. These include *kam* (bad karma), loss of soul, imbalance of bodily elements, and supernatural beings (Muecke 1979; Liamputtong 2007; Lundberg & Kerdonfag 2010).

Hmong people, including the Hmong ethnic community in Australia, have a number of beliefs concerning supernatural beings that can cause illness and death to humans. Although they believe the primary cause of such misfortune is the loss of soul (see Case Study 1.1), they also see that some illnesses are due to natural or organic factors. The Hmong are conscious of the influence of natural forces on a person's good health or illness. When a woman has just given birth, her body is believed to be in a state of disequilibrium with nature. She is therefore prohibited from participating in daily work for 30 days. During this period, she needs to rest and be mindful of 'cold' and 'wrong' food. Hot food, mainly chicken cooked with herbal medicines, is consumed for the entire period of 30 days. Failure to do this is believed to result in ill health later in life (Liamputtong Rice 2000).

Traditional healers, referred to as shamans, are an important part of Hmong life (Cha 2003; Symonds 2004; Liamputtong 2009a). In Australia, there is at least one shaman in each state, and there are at least four shamans in Melbourne. The rituals of a shaman are mainly concerned with fertility, protection, and curing (Cha 2003; Culhane-Pera et al. 2004; Liamputtong 2009a). The majority of Hmong in Australia continue to seek help from their traditional healers despite the availability of care within the Australian healthcare system. This is most obvious when the Hmong are confronted with severe illnesses and health-related issues which are seen to be closely related to the Hmong cosmos (such as in the case of childhood illnesses, burns, bone fractures, infertility, and childbirth).

Case Study 1.1   Childbirth and soul loss

The Story of Mai

This case study is from Pranee's research with women from the Hmong ethnic community in Melbourne (see Liamputtong Rice et al. 1994; Liamputtong 2010a). Mai was 34 years old, married, and had six children. Four children were born in a refugee camp in Thailand and two in Australia. Five of her children were born naturally. However, when Mai had her last child she was advised that she needed a caesarean operation since the baby was in a transverse lie.

Mai refused the operation and insisted that she could give birth naturally. She was told that if she attempted a vaginal birth the baby might not survive. Because of the concern about the survival of her baby, Mai agreed to a caesarean. However, the caesarean was done under a general anaesthetic and she was alone in the operating theatre as her husband was not allowed to stay with her. Since the birth of her last child Mai had been physically unwell. She had seen a number of specialists about her health, but they could find nothing wrong with her.

Mai believed that while she was unconscious under the general anaesthetic, one of her souls, which takes care of her well-being, left her body and was unable to re-enter. Because she was moved out of the operating theatre and regained consciousness in a recovery room, she believed that her soul was left in the operating theatre. She strongly believed that the departure of this soul was the main cause of her ill health because she had frequent bad dreams in the next ten months, occurring two or three times a week. Each time, after the dream, she felt very ill and experienced bad pains. In her dreams, she wandered to faraway places. She did not know where she was going since she had never seen those places before. It was as if she just had to keep walking and there was no ending. Mai believed this was the sign that her lost soul was wandering in another world.

In order to regain her health, she believed that she must undergo a soul-calling ceremony and that this must be performed at the theatre in which the caesarean was done, where the soul would still be waiting to be called back. Pranee asked her if she had considered a soul-calling ceremony at the operating theatre but she thought this would not be possible as the hospital staff would not understand her customs and would refuse the request since the ceremony involves taking a live chicken into the theatre and burning an incense stick there. Her husband commented that since he was not able to accompany his wife into the operating theatre, it would be impossible to be granted permission to perform a ceremony that is alien to Western healthcare providers. Because Mai was unable to perform a soul-calling ceremony at the operating theatre, the family believed that the soul had left her body for a lengthy period and transformed into another living thing. As a consequence, her health continued to deteriorate.

Concerned about Mai's well-being, Pranee and her colleagues discussed the possibility of taking Mai back to the hospital to perform the ceremony. They contacted one of the hospital staff. Through this person, the deputy CEO of the hospital agreed to the request. Her positive response was that 'the hospital is more than happy to do anything for the woman if this can help her'. She left the name of a person to contact for making the arrangements.

Pranee approached the operating theatre manager to arrange the ceremony. She was told the theatre would be quite busy during the week so she suggested that Mai have it done on the weekend. Since the date was not important, Mai agreed to have the ceremony performed on a Sunday morning. At eight o'clock one Sunday morning, Mai, her husband, and a shaman met Pranee and her bi-cultural research assistant at the ground floor of the hospital with the essential ingredients including a live chicken in a cardboard box. They reached the theatre where the charge nurses were expecting them. The nurses were very helpful and supportive. They showed Mai where she was put to sleep and where she regained consciousness. They also showed her the path along which she was carried to the operating theatre because they wanted to ensure that the ceremony was performed appropriately. At 8.30 a.m. the shaman performed a soul-calling ritual in the operating theatre. There, it took him about 20 minutes to persuade Mai's soul to come home with her. However, to ensure the soul would not be confused with the body and where it belonged, the shaman performed the same ritual at the spot where Mai regained consciousness in the recovery room. This took him only 10 minutes. Then they all went back to Mai's house to perform another ceremony. This was to welcome the soul back to its home.

Stop and Think

» Could this situation have been prevented? In your view, how could it be prevented?

The positive aspect of this ceremony was the agreement of the hospital to allow Mai and her family to perform a soul-calling ceremony in the operating theatre in addition to the concerns about her well-being by hospital staff. This illustrates how mainstream health services can provide culturally sensitive care to consumers from different cultural backgrounds, if informed of these cultural beliefs and practices.

» If you are a healthcare provider where Mai gave birth, how would you respond to her case? What would you do to accommodate for cultural differences among your clients?

Cross-cultural studies have shown that people's experience of health can be usefully organised under the following categories:

- feeling vital, full of energy
- having good social relationships
- experiencing a sense of control over one's life and living conditions
- being able to do things one enjoys
- having a sense of purpose in life
- experiencing connectedness to 'community' (Labonte 1997, p. 15).

This positive cross-cultural perspective on health enables us to plan different healthcare systems from the current dominance of the focus in Australia on illness care.

Determinants of health

Situated within the new public health perspective, the health, illness, and well-being of individual persons, groups, and communities are determined by a diverse range of complex individual, social, cultural, environmental, and economic factors and healthcare systems (AIHW 2010a). This is referred to as the determinants of health (Marmot & Wilkinson 1999; Taylor 2008a). Conceptually, the focus of this perspective is on factors that could influence and determine the health of people, instead of on the state and outcomes of their health. It also underscores the prevention of ill health, rather than the measurement of illness (Keleher & Murphy 2004; Taylor 2008a).

Case Study 1.2   Samantha

Samantha, a 3-year-old child, was born into a poor family and lived in a remote part of the country. One day, while running around in the street with her older brother, she was pierced by a nail that was discarded on the ground. Her mother bandaged the wound for her. Several days later, the wound became infected. Samantha began to feel pain in her groin and had fever. Her mother tried to manage her pain and fever with whatever she could within her capacity. However, Samantha became very unwell and this prompted her mother to take her to a hospital, which was many kilometres away. Tragically, Samantha died a few days after being admitted to the hospital (adapted from Werner 1997).

Stop and Think

- What do you think contributed to Samantha's tragic death?
- Could her death have been prevented? How?
- Who or what should be blamed for her death?
- Would her death have occurred if she had been born into a better-off family and lived in an urban area like Melbourne or Perth?

The **determinants of health** are characteristics or factors which can bring about a change in the health and illness of individuals and populations, for better or worse (Reidpath 2004; Taylor 2008a). Determinants of health include biological and genetic factors; health behaviours (such as risky lifestyles, abuse of alcohol, and cigarette smoking); socio-cultural and socio-economic factors (such as gender, ethnicity, education, income, and occupation); and environment factors (such as housing, social support, social connection, geographical position, and climate). Resources and systems also have effects on the health and well-being of individuals and populations. These include access to health services, healthcare policy, and the healthcare system (Najman 2001; AIHW 2010a).

Essentially, these determinants are connected with conditions that can either improve or hinder individuals' possibilities of having and sustaining good health. Some conditions have a direct impact on the health and illness of individuals, for example direct contact with heat or asbestos in their environment, cigarette smoking, or lack of physical activities. Other conditions have an indirect impact on individuals. They can increase or reduce the influences of other factors, for example when people are poor and cannot access suitable healthcare (Cashmore 2001). These conditions can interact and function in complex ways. For instance, when people do not have good health, they may not be able to work or take exercise. And this in turn will have further impact on their health (Taylor 2008a).

According to the AIHW (2010a, p. 64), health determinants can be perceived as 'a web of causes', but they can also be described as part of broad causal pathways that can influence health. Figure 1.1 presents a conceptual framework that shows

Determinants of health A range of individual, social, economic, environmental, and cultural conditions that have the potential to contribute to or detract from the health of individuals, communities, or whole populations.

See also Chapters 4, 5, 6, 7, 9 & 12 on the social aspects of health.

See also Chapter 19 on the healthcare system as a social determinant of health.

Figure 1.1   Determinants of health

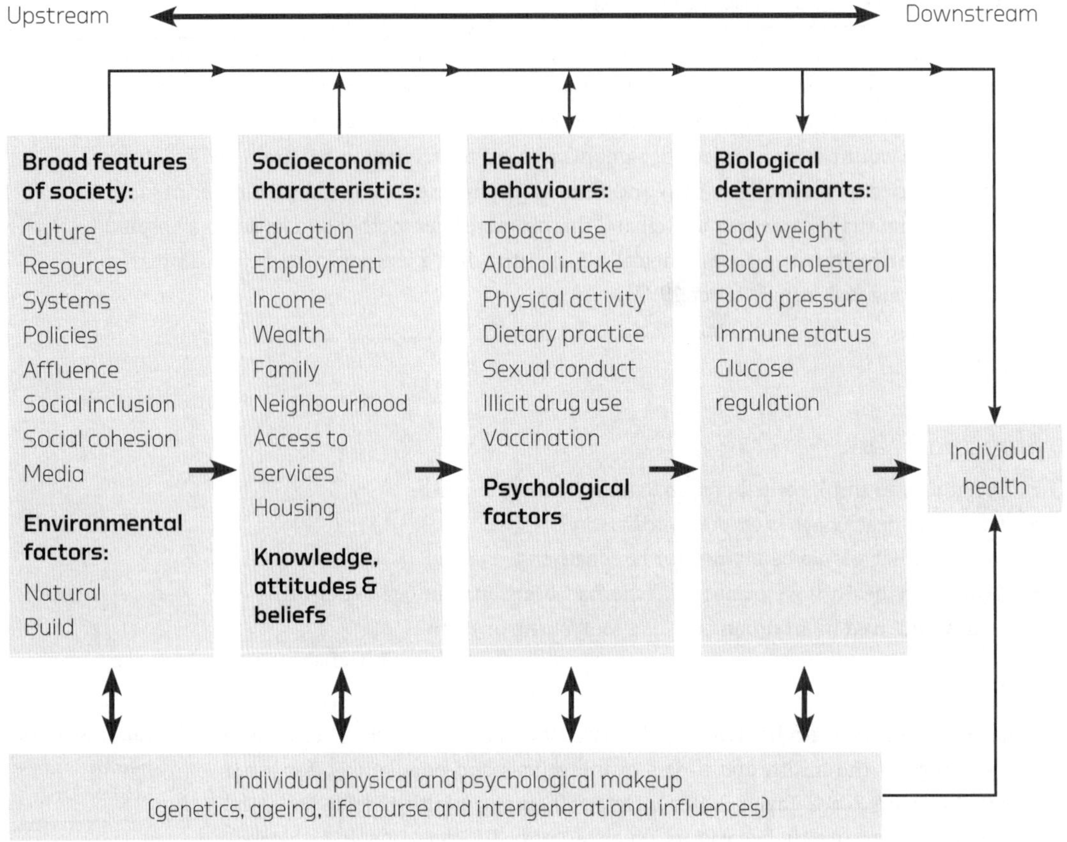

Upstream ←————————————————————————————→ Downstream

Broad features of society:
Culture
Resources
Systems
Policies
Affluence
Social inclusion
Social cohesion
Media

Environmental factors:
Natural
Build

Socioeconomic characteristics:
Education
Employment
Income
Wealth
Family
Neighbourhood
Access to services
Housing

Knowledge, attitudes & beliefs

Health behaviours:
Tobacco use
Alcohol intake
Physical activity
Dietary practice
Sexual conduct
Illicit drug use
Vaccination

Psychological factors

Biological determinants:
Body weight
Blood cholesterol
Blood pressure
Immune status
Glucose regulation

Individual health

Individual physical and psychological makeup
(genetics, ageing, life course and intergenerational influences)

Source: Adapted from AIHW 2010a, p. 64

the complex relationships of health determinants. The determinants are divided into four main categories. The direction of influence moves from left to right: from the 'upstream' factors (such as culture, resources, and affluence) to more 'downstream' or direct influences (such as body weight and blood pressure). The figure illustrates how one broad category (the broad features of society and environmental factors) can determine the nature of another main group (individuals' socio-economic characteristics such as their level of education and employment). Both these broad categories in turn have an impact on individuals' health behaviours, their psychological state and safety. These can then affect biomedical components, such as body weight and blood pressure, which would have further health effects through different pathways. Along the different paths and states, these various factors interact with the genetic composition of the individuals. It should also be noted that the direction of these influences can occur in reverse. For instance, an individual's health can also have an impact on his or her levels of physical activity, employment status, and wealth.

Health-promoting conditions can also be divided into four main categories from the upstream factors such as ecosystem viability, equitable public policies, and convivial communities, through to health-promoting mediating structures, for example caring relationships, and service to others, through to health lifestyles such as town planning to promote physical fitness and on to community-managed health services (Labonte 1997). It is argued that equitable public policies, for example, do much to promote healthy lifestyle choices.

See also Chapter 7 on health promotion and population health.

The intersections of biological, environmental, and social determinants of health

As discussed in the previous section, health determinants interact in a complex way; it is important to examine some of the relationships between the three major determinants of health that play an important part in the health, illness, and well-being of individuals: biological, environmental, and social determinants.

Biological determinants

The **biological determinants** of health and disease indicate a diverse range of 'heterogeneous, intra-individual factors' which push, intervene, or mitigate the passage of an individual towards health or disease (Swinburn & Cameron-Smith 2009, p. 248). Fundamentally, genes play a crucial role in underlying biological differences between individuals, but genes also interact with other social and environmental components that influence health and disease (see examples below) (Bortz 2005; Swinburn & Cameron-Smith 2009). According to Swinburn and Cameron-Smith (2009, p. 248), 'the genetic and physiological systems within the body are dynamic, complex, and highly interconnected, with whole systems balancing and competing against each other' to achieve homeostasis. This is very similar to the complex processes of the social and environmental system outside the physical body of the individual.

Biological determinants The inner physiological aspect of health and disease. Genes play a crucial role in underlying biological differences between individuals.

This can be seen in the case of HIV. HIV is dispersed in three ways: through sexual intercourse, blood transfusions (also through the use of needles and syringes), and from mother to child (Vaughan 2009). While everyone can be infected with HIV, there are biological factors that increase an individual's susceptibility to infection. For instance, if an individual has another sexually transmitted infection (STI) such as *Chlamydia* or gonorrhoea, the risk of becoming infected with HIV during sex is higher. If someone has a blood disorder (which indicates that they need regular blood transfusions), that person is also at higher risk of contracting HIV. If a woman who is infected with HIV has health problems during pregnancy and also breastfeeds her baby, there is a greater chance that the infection will be transmitted to the baby. According to Vaughan (2009, p. 176), the risk of HIV infection is also connected with the behaviours of individuals, for instance having multiple sexual partners and having sex without a condom. Sharing equipment used for injecting drugs is also a high-risk behaviour among certain groups of people. Hence, although the biological factors are important, a focus on biological risk factors only will not stop the spread of HIV epidemic in populations (Vaughan 2009).

See also Chapters 4, 5 & 6 on the biological determinants of health.

See also discussion of HIV/AIDS in Chapter 2.

Three biological determinants that play a part in health and illness are race, sex, and age. However, these three are also intertwined with social and environmental determinants. Sometimes it can be difficult to differentiate between biological or other social or environmental conditions that determine people's health and illness.

Age is a clear biological determinant of the health of human beings (Miller 2009; West & Bergman 2009). According to Keleher and Joss (2009, p. 370), genes may have some impact on the causation of disease. However, for many diseases the causes are environmental. For example, cognitive functioning decline among older people is not only the result of being old but may also be affected by lack of exercise, illness (such as depression), behaviours (such as the use of medications), psychological components (such as lack of confidence, motivation, and low expectations), and social aspects (such as isolation and loneliness). Some aspects of race and gender will be covered under the social determinants of health in a section below.

See also Chapter 6 on ageing and health.

Environmental determinants

Environmental determinants Physical environmental factors such as climate and location, which can affect the health of people.

The important connection between the **environment** in which individuals live and their health and well-being has long been observed (Hancock 1985; WHO 1986; McMichael 1993, 2001; Nicholson & Stephenson 2009; Griffith et al. 2010). Historically, environmental dangers to people's health tended to be related to issues of underdevelopment such as inadequate water quality, the absence of sanitation, and poor housing. Although these traditional threats have been managed successfully in the more affluent areas within the developed countries, there are still problems among socially disadvantaged and vulnerable groups of developed nations, and also in the poorer countries of the globe (Nicholson & Stephenson 2009). This can be seen clearly in the environmental threats some indigenous people have to deal with in Australia and elsewhere. Nowadays, we see 'modern' threats, which have emerged because of overconsumption and overdevelopment in developed nations (WHO 1997a). These modern threats, including climate change, have now become global hazards (McMichael 1993, 2001; Eisenberg et al. 2007; Baum 2008; Nicholson & Stephenson 2009). Australia is one developed nation that is highly susceptible to the impacts of climate changes (Diamond 2004; Garnaut 2008; Kennedy et al. 2010).

See also Chapters 5, 8, 9 & 10 on various environmental impacts on health.

Global climate changes can impact on many aspects of human life and health (Goldsworthy et al. 2009). Thermal extremes, such as heatwaves, can cause difficulty for many people, in particular the very young, very old, very poor, and very sick (Baum 2008; Goldsworthy et al. 2009; Nicholson & Stephenson 2009; Talbot & Verrinder 2009). In 1959, a fourfold increase from the normal mortality was the result of a long period of heatwave in Melbourne (McMichael 1993). Climate change and global warming are also directly connected with the dispersion of infectious disease vectors and pests as well as with reduced food production (Nicholson & Stephenson 2009; Talbot & Verrinder 2009). And this of course will affect people from poor areas and nations more than those from rich areas and locations with better resources (Hancock 1994; Baum 2008). Poor people who live in poor nations are disproportionately burdened by environmental problems and their related health impacts (Hancock 1994; Agyeman & Evans 2002; Baum 2008).

Mythbuster

Consider whether you see the following as questionable. What does this tell you about your own values?

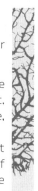

- Your government wishes to develop a plan for a more sustainable environment for the city and country as a whole. But this necessitates commitment and a huge budget, which means more tax levies on local people. This has created anger among some people, particularly those with high incomes.
- There has been an extensive drought in your country for a number of years. The government has developed a plan to save more water and this means certain cuts in the use of water in some sectors of the country, particularly farmers. Those who are affected blame people who live in the city for an unequal access to water.

The World Health Organization (1997a, p. 198) puts it clearly: 'Impoverished populations...are at greater risk from degraded environmental conditions. The cumulative effects of inadequate and hazardous shelter, overcrowding, lack of water supply and sanitation, unsafe food, air and water pollution and high accident rates impact heavily on the health of these vulnerable groups.'

Increasingly and globally, we have witnessed more environmental hazards and the health impacts of climate change resulting from human behaviours. Severe drought, flooding, storms, and extreme temperatures have become very common in recent years (Nicholson & Stephenson 2009, p. 122; Verrinder 2011). This is what we have recently experienced in Australia—the Black Saturday bushfires in Victoria in February 2009, the widespread floods in Queensland, New South Wales, and Victoria in January 2011, the Yasi cyclone in north Queensland, and the Carlos cyclone in Darwin in February 2011.

See also Chapter 9 on climate change.

Social determinants

Not all illnesses are caused by biological and environmental agents. The health and well-being of individuals is also influenced by a number of **social determinants**. According to Lawn (2008, p. 36), there are a number of factors, including social, cultural, economic, and political, which can impact health. This position goes beyond the restricted view of biological and genetic aspects of health (Marmot & Wilkinson 1999; Kelly et al. 2007; Keleher & MacDougall 2009). Social determinants of health are also seen as determinants that are 'attributable to the structure and functioning of society' (Reidpath 2004, p. 22). For example, transportation can be seen as one social determinant of health since it can impact on individuals' physical activities, and this in turn can influence their nutritional intake and cardiovascular condition. Social expectations regarding sexual behaviours are also social determinants of health as they can influence individuals' approaches to risky sexual conducts, and this can lead to marginalisation, stigma, and discrimination (Reidpath 2004).

Important social determinants of health are related to the positions of social life including gender, ethnicity, and social class (Reidpath 2004).

Social determinants
A number of factors, including social, cultural, economic, and political, which can impact on the health of individuals.

See also Chapters 5, 6, 11, 12, 18 & 19 on the social determinants of health.

See also Chapter 15 on stigma and discrimination.

See also Chapters 4, 5, 6 & 12 on the various social aspects of health.

Stop and Think

» Have you ever looked at the homeless men who sleep on the local park bench with a blanket to cover their bodies, while their possessions are kept in some plastic bags next to them? When they wake, they tend to talk to themselves and do not seem to care about others around them. Have you ever thought about how they came to be like this? Have you been curious enough about what type of journey they have been through in their lives and what it would have been like for them before this misfortune, such as when they were somebody's son, father, husband, or colleague?

To develop an understanding of the life of these men necessitates some understanding of the social determinants of health (adapted from Lawn 2008, p. 36).

Gender Socially and culturally constructed categories reflecting what it means to be 'masculine' and 'feminine' and associated expectations of roles and behaviours of men and women.

Ethnicity Refers to a shared cultural background which is a characteristic of a group within a society.

Social class The position of a person in a system of structured inequality; it is grounded in unequal distribution of income, wealth, status, and power.

See also Chapter 18 on the impact on health of economic circumstances.

Gender is understood as a social construct, referring to the distinguishing characteristics of being female or male. Gender can be seen as the full range of personality traits, attitudes, feelings, values, behaviours, and activities that 'society ascribes to the two sexes on a differential basis' (Keleher & MacDougall 2009, p. 56). It is different from sex, which is a 'biological construct premised upon biological characteristics enabling sexual reproduction' (Krieger 2003, p. 653). **Ethnicity** refers to 'a shared cultural background'; it is a characteristic of a group within a society (Julian 2009, p. 177). Ethnicity includes other dimensions than biological determinants (which are referred to as race). These are social, cultural, and economic factors. Ethnicity is now accepted as the more appropriate determinant of health than race (Jones & Creedy 2008; Swinburn & Cameron-Smith 2009). **Social class** (also termed socio-economic status or SES) refers to the position of a person in 'a system of structured inequality' which is grounded in the unequal distribution of income, wealth, status, and power (Germov 2009, p. 86). Income, poverty, and wealth are closely connected with health; people who live in poverty are likely to have worse health status than those who are better-off (Marmot & Wilkinson 1999; Reidpath 2004; Baum 2008; Germov 2009). The Australian Institute of Health and Welfare (AIHW 2006a, p. 232) states that 'people who are poorer or socioeconomically disadvantaged in other ways generally live shorter lives and suffer more illness and reduced quality of life than those who are well-off'.

None of these social determinants exists in isolation (Reidpath 2004). They intersect in a way that can create inequalities in health among people. For example, women from a low socio-economic background are likely to be in poorer health than those from a higher social class (Baum 2008; Germov 2009). Men from ethnic minority groups and lower social classes are also likely to be disadvantaged in terms of health and well-being in comparison to white Anglo-Celtic men with a higher income (Jones & Creedy 2008; Julian 2009). We have witnessed examples of such relationships. Saggers and colleagues (2011) suggest that the most influential indicator of health inequalities is life expectancy at birth. From 2005 to 2007, the life expectancy of Indigenous males was 67.2 years and 72.9 for Indigenous females. They live 11.5 and 9.7 years less than their non-Indigenous counterparts (ABS 2009b, p. 7). Indigenous Australians also fare worse in health issues. For example, they are three times more likely than non-Indigenous Australians to suffer heart attacks, more than twice as likely to die from them and, even if admitted to hospital, likely to receive different treatment from their non-Indigenous counterparts (Mathur et al. 2006). The health inequalities of Indigenous Australians are the consequences of 'poorer socio-economic status, long-standing marginalisation from mainstream society and healthcare and, in many instances, geographical location and isolation' (Taylor 2008a, p. 18; see also Genat & Cripps 2009; Gray & Saggers 2009; MacDonald 2010; Saggers et al. 2011).

We have also seen that there are a number of circumstances and conditions which have created basic inequalities that not only contribute to the ill health of people, but also establish a recurrence of adverse physical and mental health consequences for many individuals and groups within the current socio-cultural, economic, and political contexts around the globe including in Australia (Lawn 2008). As such, there exists health inequality among populations. Health inequality, according to Kawachi and colleagues (2002, p. 647), is a term that is employed 'to designate the differences, variations, and disparities in the health achievements of individuals and groups'. Inequalities are the consequence of inequitable societies and are addressed through social justice. As such, it has been suggested that social justice approaches to health are crucial for any healthcare system that aims to fulfil individuals' rights to good health (Marmot 2000; Keleher & MacDougall 2009; Wilkinson & Pickett 2009).

See Chapters 17 & 18 on social justice and the economics of health.

See also Chapters 7, 17 & 18 on health promotion, social justice, and the economics of health.

Stop and Think

» Consider the following examples. What do they tell you about our society and our own values?

- Rachel is an old woman who has been widowed for more than ten years. She has little education and has always been poor. She does not have her own house to live in and has been renting a house in a suburb in Sydney. Recently, she was told to leave the house because the owner wishes to renovate it and increase the rent. Rachel does not have another place to move into and it has been very difficult to find rental accommodation in Sydney.

- Due to some difficulties in his life, Jack has become an alcoholic. He has been drinking heavily recently and as a result he was asked to leave his job. He is separated from his wife and two young children, and has been living on his own in a small flat. Because of his drinking problem and the difficulty he has caused to his family, his colleagues and social network do not wish to have anything to do with him. Virtually, he has lost all of his social support.

🔖 Summary

Health, illness, and well-being are inevitable aspects of our lives and have always played a part in the life of all human beings. However, the concepts of health, illness, and well-being are socially and culturally constructed because individuals and cultures see them differently. Diverse factors can have an impact on the health, illness, and well-being of individuals, groups, and populations. These are known as determinants of health and include biological, environmental, social, cultural, and economic determinants. These determinants can affect how healthy or sick an individual can be. Additionally, within the social determinants of health, there are three crucial social structures that can affect the health and well-being of people: gender, ethnicity, and social class. These three factors do not operate in isolation, but rather interrelate to the extent that they create inequality in health among people.

🔖 Tutorial exercises

1   Form a group of five with your peers in the class. Each of you needs to write down as many definitions of health as you can. Then compare your answers with your peers in the group. Are there similarities in your definitions? Are they different? Discuss the similarities and differences that you have noted in the group and how they have come about.

2   After finishing this chapter, have a tour around the university campus and take note of any determinants that can make you healthy or ill. What have you noticed?

3   It has been suggested that women live longer and men die sooner. What is your view about this suggestion? Is it true? What would be the determinants of this difference?

4   As a group, watch the documentary *The Shape of Water* (2006) (available online: www.theshapeofwatermovie.com). Discuss the possible determinants that can create inequalities and social justice in different groups of people.

Further reading

Annandale, E., & Hunt, K. (eds) (2000). *Gender inequalities and health.* Buckingham, UK: Open University Press.

Australian Institute of Health and Welfare (2010a). *Australia's health 2010.* Canberra: AIHW. <www.aihw.gov.au>.

Baum, F. (2008). *The new public health: An Australian perspective,* 2nd edn. Melbourne: Oxford University Press.

Bergholt, K. (2008). *Wellbeing: A cultural history of healthy living,* translated by Jane Dewhurst. Cambridge: Polity Press.

Blaxter, M. (2004). *Health.* Cambridge: Polity Press.

Cockerham, W.C. (2007). *Social causes of health and disease.* Cambridge: Polity Press.

Fadiman, A. (1997). *The spirit catches you and you fall down: A Hmong child, her American doctors, and the collision of two cultures.* New York: Farrar, Straus & Giroux.

Germov, J. (ed.) (2009). *Second opinion: An introduction to health sociology,* 4th edn. Melbourne: Oxford University Press.

Keleher, H., & MacDougall, C. (eds) (2009). *Understanding health: A determinants approach,* 2nd edn. Melbourne: Oxford University Press.

Kennedy, D., Stocker, L., & Burke, G. (2010). Australian local government action on climate change adaptation: Some critical reflections to assist decision-making. *Local Environment*, 15(9–10), 805–16.

MacDonald, J.J. (2010). Health equity and the social determinants of health in Australia. *Social Alternatives*, 29(2), 34–40.

Marmot, M., & Wilkinson, R.G. (eds) (2006). *Social determinants of health*, 2nd edn. Oxford: Oxford University Press.

Robertson, S. (2007). *Understanding men and health: Masculinities, identity and well-being*. Berkshire: Open University Press/McGraw Hill.

Taylor, S. (2008a). The concept of health. In S. Taylor, M. Foster & J. Fleming (eds), *Healthcare practice in Australia*. Melbourne: Oxford University Press, 3–21.

Thackrah, R., & Scott, K. (eds) (2011). *Indigenous Australian health and cultures: An introduction for health professionals*. Sydney: Pearson.

Websites

<www.unep.org>

This is the website of the United Nations Environment Program (UNEP). It gives a number of resources regarding environmental issues, for example urban issues, waste, water quality, sanitation, air quality, climate change, and ozone depletion.

<www.who.int/social_determinants/en>

This is the website of the World Health Organization's Commission on Social Determinants of Health. It is a good source of discussions on social determinants and provides crucial background papers and reports as well as examples of actions in relation to social determinants.

<http://phmovement.org/cms>

The website of the People's Health Movement (PHM) provides discussions about health and inequalities in health. It contains information about health networks and activists who have their concerns about the inequalities and inequities in health.

Part 1
Perspectives of Health, Illness, and Well-being

2 | Introduction to pathogens and impacts on health and illness

Elizabeth Brown

TOPICS COVERED

This chapter covers the following topics:
- definitions of infection and infectious disease
- criteria to establish the cause of infectious disease
- definition of the terms pathogen and parasite
- characteristics of pathogens and parasites
- examples of infections due to specific organisms
- defences against infection, innate and adaptive
- treatment of infectious diseases
- factors affecting susceptibility to infectious diseases
- environmental factors and the prevention of infectious disease
- the role of immunisation in the prevention of infectious disease

KEY TERMS

Communicable disease, contagious disease
Defences against infection, innate and adaptive
Immunisation
Infection

Infectious disease
Morbidity
Normal flora
Parasite
Pathogen
Vaccination

Introduction

> To understand infectious diseases, one must consider the infecting organism, the host and the environment. It is the interplay between these elements that determines the likelihood of disease, the manifestations and outcome. (Yung et al. 2010, p. xxix)

Infectious diseases can be life-threatening. Existing infectious diseases, such as influenza and tuberculosis, tend to keep changing, and new diseases such as H1N1 influenza ('swine flu') emerge. The consequences of infectious diseases continue to influence the course of human history: consider the outcome of bovine spongiform encephalopathy (BSE, also known as 'mad cow disease') in Europe (1986–2002) (WHO 2011a). Smallpox was an untreatable, dreaded disease with a high mortality (death) rate. The global eradication program conducted by the World Health Organization means that smallpox no longer occurs. Eradication was achieved in 1980 by a program of vaccination, education, isolation of infected individuals, and other measures (WHO 2011b).

Our bodies have defences against infection, but pathogens have various ways of breaching these defences. Prevention *is* better than cure—in fact, cure is not always possible. Prevention of infection can be achieved in a number of ways, but this requires knowledge about both the pathogen, or parasite, and body defences. Treatments for established infectious diseases vary in their availability and effectiveness. This is why it is important to understand pathogens and their impacts on health and illness.

This chapter will define what is meant by 'communicable disease' (also known as infectious disease), 'pathogens' and 'parasites', and describe body defences against them. It will consider aspects of treatment and prevention of infectious diseases, including some discussion of drugs that are available for treatment, individual differences in response to infectious diseases, and the significance of environmental factors. Finally, the chapter will discuss immunisation as an effective means of prevention of vaccine-preventable diseases.

Infection The presence of pathogens or parasites on or in body tissues and/or fluids with the result that they cause disease.

Infectious disease Any disease transmitted from one person or animal to another either directly or indirectly.

Communicable disease, contagious disease Alternative terms for *infectious disease*.

Background to the biology of infectious diseases

Infection can be defined as the presence of pathogens or parasites on or in body tissues and/or fluids with the result that they cause disease.

Infectious disease is defined as **communicable disease** (Harris et al. 2010, p. 895): the terms can be used interchangeably. Mosby's Dictionary (Harris et al. 2010, p. 403) defines communicable disease as 'any disease transmitted from one person or animal to another: directly, by contact with excreta or other discharges from the body; indirectly, via substances or inanimate objects such as contaminated drinking glasses, toys or water; or via vectors such as flies, mosquitoes, ticks or other insects.... [It is] also called **contagious disease**'.

Mythbuster

'Don't get cold, or you will catch a cold!'

Is there a causal link between cold and the common cold? What is the evidence?

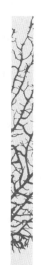

- A group of healthy volunteers each had equivalent doses of a virus that causes the common cold introduced into their nasal passages.
- Approximately half of them—the experimental group—were then exposed to unpleasantly cold conditions for several hours.
- The remainder—the control group—were not exposed to the cold conditions.
- Approximately half of ALL of the volunteers developed a cold after these events. That is, the numbers of participants who developed the common cold were approximately equal in both the experimental and the control groups.
- It was therefore concluded that exposure to a cold environment was *not* a contributor to the likelihood of developing a cold in individuals who had been given an intranasal dose of a common cold-causing virus that was adequate to cause a cold.
- People are more likely to catch the common cold in winter than in summer, in temperate (cool) climates. Is this due to a direct effect of the cold weather? Or could winter weather have some indirect effect that predisposes us to catching a cold?

» *What do you think causes the common cold?*

» *How does this experiment help you to decide?*

» *What causes infectious diseases?*

What makes a disease an infectious disease?

The main criteria are that, for a particular infectious disease, the microorganism responsible must be present in all cases of the disease, and that transmission of the microorganism to an uninfected person can cause the disease. Robert Koch was a physician and bacteriologist who first proposed criteria necessary to establish the relationship between a particular microorganism and the disease it causes. His original criteria were modified as more was learnt about the nature of infectious disease. These ideas were first published in 1890, and are known as 'Koch's postulates' (Harris et al. 2010).

Pathogens and parasites: What are they?

Pathogen is defined variously, for example as 'a disease causing organism' (Marieb & Hoehn 2010, p. G-17) or 'any microorganism capable of producing disease' (Harris et al. 2010, p. 1302).

Pathogen A microorganism that can cause disease.

These definitions can cause confusion because there are bacteria that are beneficial in one body location but can cause disease if they are in the 'wrong' place. For example, *Escherichia coli* (*E. coli*) is a common bacterium that colonises the large intestine of the healthy human digestive tract, and produces vitamin K (a factor necessary for normal blood clotting). But it can cause serious illness if it contaminates other body regions, such as pneumonia if it is in the lungs.

Many parts of the body are colonised by bacteria and fungi, with the type of organisms varying with the part, for example the mouth, nose, digestive tract, respiratory tract, urethra, vagina, and different regions of the skin. These are the parts of the body that interact, directly or indirectly, with the external environment. These microorganisms are known as the **normal flora**, and are acquired during and after birth. The normal flora live on or in the body, but not at its expense; they are also referred to as commensal organisms. The normal flora keep overgrowth of pathogens under control. Disease may occur if the balance between numbers of the normal flora is disturbed: for example, a vaginal thrush infection (*Candida albicans*) can result from a course of antibiotics, due to loss of bacteria that are usually present. Microorganisms are not normally found in the internal viscera (organs) that do not communicate with the external environment.

A **parasite** is defined as any organism that obtains nourishment from the host that it lives on or in (Dunne & Ledeboer 2009; Harris et al. 2010). The relationship between parasite and host is usually beneficial for the parasite, but results in pathology (disease or harm) for the host. The parasite is provided with nutrients and shelter, while the host is deprived of nutrients, and may suffer other harm such as chronic (long-term) blood loss. It is interesting to note, however, that there is some evidence that an *absence* of contact with parasites may contribute to disorders of the immune system such as allergy.

Normal flora The microorganisms that live, without detriment, on or in regions of the body that communicate with the external environment; they help to control populations of potential pathogens; also known as commensal organisms.

Parasite Any single- or multi-cellular organism that obtains nourishment from the host that it lives on or in.

Parasites typically have a life cycle in which different forms of the animal live in different hosts. The term 'parasite' is commonly used to refer to protozoa and metazoa that cause disease. Protozoa that cause disease are single-celled organisms or 'microparasites', such as the ones that cause malaria. Metazoa that cause disease are multicellular organisms or 'macroparasites' such as worms (helminths), including tapeworms, and insects (arthropods) such as lice.

It is clear that there is overlap between the meanings of the terms *pathogen* and *parasite*. Both can act as parasites, and both can act as pathogens. For simplicity, pathogens will be referred to as disease-causing microorganisms, and parasites as disease-causing protozoa and metazoa.

Certain fungi, bacteria, and viruses are human pathogens; this chapter will describe selected examples of each, and also make brief mention of prions. Certain worms and protozoa are human parasites; selected examples of these will also be described. These descriptions will illustrate not only how each class of organism can make a person sick, but how the person can become infected. Such information enables deduction of ways to prevent infection.

What is the size of the problem?

Sizes of human pathogens and parasites cross a number of orders of magnitude from the macroscopic (visible to the naked eye), to the microscopic, to the molecular. Tapeworms are large parasites that can exceed several metres ($>1 \times 10^1$) in length; ticks, lice, and fleas are also readily visible (1×10^{-3}m).

Microorganisms such as fungi and bacteria require a light microscope to observe them (1×10^{-6}m), while viruses are smaller still (1×10^{-9}m), and require an electron microscope for visualisation. Prions are protein molecules, probably with particular structural modification, potentially 'visible' only with a very powerful electron microscope.

The nature of pathogens, and how they make us sick

Bacteria

Bacteria are organisms found almost everywhere on earth, including the most extreme environments. Bacteria are known as prokaryotes because their genetic material is not contained within a nucleus, in contrast to the metazoa (macroparasites), protozoa (microparasites), and fungi, which are eukaryotes, with their genetic material located within the nuclei of cells.

Bacteria have a cell wall external to the bacterial cell membrane. The structure of the bacterial wall contributes to the properties of the bacterium, including its response to a Gram stain: bacteria are Gram-positive if they stain, and Gram-negative if they do not. Gram staining contributes to diagnosis of the type of bacteria causing an infection, and to decisions regarding suitable drug treatment for an infection.

Different types of bacteria have characteristic shapes: cocci are spherical; bacilli have an elongated rod shape; and spirilla have a spiral shape. Testing of specimens of tissues or fluids includes microscopic examination: bacterial shape also contributes to the diagnosis. Bacteria are autonomous in that they normally do not require cells of a host in order to reproduce, but they do require nutrients as a source of energy, and obtain these from their immediate environment, including their host.

Transmission of bacteria to a host can occur in a variety of ways including ingestion, inhalation, sexual transmission, transmission via the placenta, and transmission via skin lesions, especially where the integrity of the skin is damaged by injury from surgery or another infection, and injection due to the bite of an arthropod vector. Blood-borne bacterial infections can be transmitted by shared intravenous injecting equipment, or by transfusion of untested blood. Bacterial infections can also be due to a change in the balance of the commensal flora.

Chlamydia trachomatis–Chlamydia

Chlamydia trachomatis (*C. trachomatis*, also known simply as *Chlamydia*) is the bacterium that causes the most prevalent sexually transmissible infection (STI) in Australia. *Chlamydia* is spread by intimate contact with another person, commonly by sexual intercourse, or any other activity that results in the exchange of body fluids such as semen or vaginal secretions. It does not survive readily outside the body. Indeed, *C. trachomatis* is a bacterium that lives within cells of its host.

If untreated, chlamydial infection of the reproductive tracts of men and women can result in inflammation and ultimately blockages of ducts of systems of both the male and, especially, the female. Infection is commonly asymptomatic, that is, the infected person may have no idea that they have this infection (Better Health Channel 2010a). In a woman, infection may involve the uterine cervix initially; in time the infection can ascend, ultimately involving the uterus, uterine (Fallopian) tubes, and beyond, causing pelvic inflammatory disease (PID). PID usually causes pain and malaise (feeling unwell). Inflammation of the uterine tubes can result in partial or complete blockage, with repeated episodes increasing the chance of this occurring. Partial or complete blockage of the uterine tubes causes ectopic pregnancy or infertility respectively. Infertility can be a devastating diagnosis for many people.

Chlamydia can cause inflammation at sites other than the reproductive system. *C. trachomatis* conjunctivitis is a severe eye infection that can occur following infection of a baby during birth; this is an example of transmission of infection from mother to child, or vertical transmission. Chlamydial conjunctivitis can also occur in adults.

Relatively recent developments in testing for *Chlamydia* allow for accurate diagnosis of the condition when it is present. Chlamydial infections can be treated effectively with antibiotics. The partner should also be tested, and treated if infected. Any person who has any concern that they may have contracted an STI is well advised to seek testing. The incidence of chlamydial infection is increasing in Australia. Persons of any age can become infected, but young people 15 to 25 years of age are most likely to.

Notification of chlamydial infection in an individual, to a government agency, is mandatory in Australia. Tracing and follow-up of the contacts of a person who is diagnosed with a *Chlamydia* infection help to limit the spread of the disease in the community. Follow-up includes treatment, if necessary. Notification of disease is a process that preserves the privacy of the individuals involved. Infection with *Chlamydia*, and indeed any STI, can have a profound negative effect on the self-esteem of the individuals involved, and on the relationship between a couple, in addition to the physical consequences of the infection.

Clostridium tetani–tetanus

Tetanus is a potentially life-threatening disease caused by *Clostridium tetani* (*C. tetani*). *C. tetani* is a bacterium that has worldwide distribution. The bacteria live in the digestive tracts of domestic animals, including horses, and form spores that survive indefinitely in the soil.

A person develops the disease following wounding that permits entry of dirt contaminated by *C. tetani* spores—the wound can be anything from an unnoticed scratch acquired during gardening, to a major wound from a car accident, or injury of war. In resource-poor countries, newborn babies are particularly vulnerable to tetanus infection via the stump of their umbilical cords. In these circumstances, there may be no childbirth attendant, equipment or bedding used during the birth may not clean, and contamination with dirt or dust may occur.

C. tetani is an anaerobic bacterium that therefore functions in the absence of oxygen, in a 'tetanus-prone wound': a deep wound that is closed to the air. The bacteria release a powerful neurotoxin that affects the functioning of the nervous system. This neurotoxin causes skeletal muscle contraction to be overactive by blocking the release of inhibitory agents that normally contribute to the control of skeletal muscle contraction.

One of the first signs and symptoms of tetanus infection may be 'lockjaw', that is, the persistent contraction of the muscles that close the jaw. The muscle spasms of tetanus can cause injury. The increasing muscle contractions cause rigidity that interferes with breathing. The toxin can also cause disturbances in the functioning of the autonomic nervous system as well as control of skeletal muscle function.

Management of the infection includes administration of antibodies to the toxin (human tetanus immunoglobulin), muscle-relaxant drugs (which necessitate artificial ventilation), and care of the

Case Study 2.1   Carriers of disease: The presence of pathogens in healthy individuals

Typhoid (typhoid fever) is a serious infectious disease caused by *Salmonella typhi* (*S. typhi*). It is spread by the faecal-oral route, including faecal contamination of drinking water and food. Typhoid causes not only diarrhoea, but also systemic complications due to lesions in the gastrointestinal tract, and to widespread infection of body tissues and organs; before the development of antibiotic therapy approximately 15% of people infected died from complications. A person who is recovering from typhoid may shed the bacterium for months after the illness has subsided.

Some individuals acquire *S. typhi*, and continue to shed the bacterium without ever developing signs or symptoms of the illness; such a person is called a carrier of the disease.

More than a century ago, the story of 'Typhoid Mary' alerted us to this. She was a healthy woman who worked as a cook for a number of families, in the early 1900s. Unfortunately, more than 50 of the people that she worked for developed typhoid, with three fatalities, so that Mary was forcibly placed in quarantine. After her death (which was not related to typhoid) it was found that *S. typhi* were present in her gall bladder, and ultimately in her faeces. Mary was an asymptomatic carrier of the infectious disease, typhoid fever. She had never been ill with the disease herself. It is possible that she had been infected before birth because her mother had typhoid during her pregnancy.

People can be carriers for other infectious diseases, for example, carrier of the virus that causes hepatitis B.

» *Can you suggest one measure that could have helped to reduce the spread of typhoid via Mary's cooking?*

infected wound. In general, the outcome of tetanus infection is likely to be good in a resource-rich country; however, the very young and very old may do less well.

Tetanus is a vaccine-preventable disease that occurs rarely in Australia now, with 2 to 5 cases reported each year. When it does occur it is likely to be in an older person who is inadequately immunised (Newton-John & Eisen 2010). The annual incidence of tetanus infection globally is declining as rates of vaccination increase (WHO 2010c).

Viruses

Virus particles are not regarded as living organisms because they require the functions of host cells in order to reproduce. A virus is little more than some hereditary material within a coating—but it is still a pathogen. Viruses are classified on the basis of the type of hereditary material present (DNA or RNA), the shape of the particle, and the nature of its coatings. Knowledge of these features is important in the development of drugs for treatment of certain viral infections.

Infection of cells of the host is required in order for a virus to reproduce. Viral replication occurs by a sequence of events including entry of the virus into the host cell, followed by formation of many new viruses that are then released, often causing death of the host cell. Attachment to the host cell requires a receptor for the virus on the host cell membrane. Depending on the nature of the virus, formation of the new viruses will use cellular machinery either of the host cell or of the virus itself. Specific steps in this sequence of events have been targeted in the development of anti-viral drugs that have become available over the last 15 or so years.

Viruses can be transmitted to a host by inhalation, especially of droplets from a sneeze or cough, ingestion, sexual transmission, and injection, especially by an arthropod vector. Blood-borne viral infections can be transmitted by shared intravenous injecting equipment, or by transfusion of untested blood.

Some viruses cause transformation of cellular genetic material, contributing to the development of cancer, for example certain strains of the wart virus can cause cancer of the cervix of the uterus, and sometimes of the external genitalia and anus.

Influenza

Influenza ('the flu') is due to an infection with one of several viruses. It is a potentially serious disease that affects the upper respiratory tract—the nose and throat—with cough, and also causes fever, headache, sore throat, muscle and joint pain, and general malaise. Influenza varies in its severity. It commonly has more serious effects in older persons and babies than in young adults, and also in people who have pre-existing respiratory or cardiovascular disease, or who are immunocompromised (that is, people who have suppression of function of the body's normal defences against infection).

Influenza viruses are spread readily by droplet infection due to sneezing, coughing, and speaking, beginning in the 1–2 days before the infected person experiences symptoms, and continuing for about a week afterwards. Most people feel better after about a week. However, the infection damages respiratory epithelium, predisposing them to other respiratory infections such as secondary bacterial infections.

Drug treatments such as aspirin or paracetamol can provide relief for the symptoms, but use of aspirin is contraindicated for children because of potential complications. However, see 'innate defences' below for discussion of benefits and risks of treatment of fever. Rest, and water intake adequate to prevent dehydration and drying of the respiratory epithelium, are important.

Prevention of spread of the infection includes hygiene practices such as covering the nose and mouth during coughing and sneezing, frequent handwashing, and cleaning of surfaces and items such as drinking vessels and cutlery that may be contaminated by the virus. Antiviral drugs are of debatable benefit in the treatment of influenza, but may have a place in prevention of the infection in immunocompromised individuals (Dwyer 2010).

Influenza occurs worldwide, especially now with the high frequency of international travel (Goldsworthy et al. 2009). Outbreaks or epidemics occur seasonally, typically in winter in cool climates.

As noted previously, several different types of virus cause influenza. Minor changes ('antigenic drift') in the influenza virus occur from year to year and are the reason for annual outbreaks. Major changes ('antigenic shift') in the virus cause a worldwide pandemic of influenza. There were three influenza pandemics in the 20th century: the 'Spanish flu' in 1918–19 at the end of the First World War, which caused the death of 20–40 million people, the 'Asian flu' in 1957, and the 'Hong Kong flu' in 1968. As has been noted previously, H1N1 (also known as 'swine flu') is a new type of influenza that emerged in 2009 as an influenza pandemic (Dwyer 2010).

The World Health Organization meets annually to decide the composition of the next current influenza vaccine that will meet the immunisation requirements of the predicted influenza season of each hemisphere (Dwyer 2010). Vaccination for influenza is the most effective way of preventing the spread of the disease.

The Human Immunodeficiency Virus

The Human Immunodeficiency Virus (HIV) is a virus that specifically infects cells of the immune system, especially T cells (T lymphocytes), causing their destruction when they rupture during the release of new viruses into the circulation. T cells are also known as CD4 cells because they possess CD4 receptors, that is, receptors for the HIV.

If a person infected with HIV remains untreated, their 'viral load' (that is, the concentration of the virus in the blood) is likely to be very high, while the concentration of T cells in the blood declines. Eventually, the T cells are likely to reach such a critically low concentration (less than 200 T cells per microlitre of plasma) that the person will probably experience severe immunodeficiency, and is likely to die as a consequence of opportunistic infection. This condition is called the Acquired Immunodeficiency Syndrome, or AIDS. Opportunistic infections, such as *Pneumocystis carinii* pneumonia (PCP), are known as AIDS-related conditions (Vujovic et al. 2010).

HIV/AIDS was first recognised in the early 1980s in the Western world, but was probably in existence for many years before this. Patterns of infection with HIV vary from country to country, with the infection being common in the heterosexual population in resource-poor countries, and common in the male gay (homosexual) communities and/or injecting drug using communities in resource-rich countries. It was estimated that in 2009 there were approximately 33 million people worldwide living with HIV/AIDS, and that it caused about 1.5 to 2 million deaths (WHO 2010c). Unfortunately, HIV infection is often complicated by simultaneous infection with tuberculosis in resource-poor countries.

> See also Chapter 15, which discusses HIV/AIDS in the context of stigmatisation.

HIV is a retrovirus. This means that it is able to copy the Ribonucleic acid (RNA) of its hereditary material into the genetic material of the host cells it infects, ensuring the synthesis of the proteins required to form multiple new copies of the virus from each infected cell. The process begins when HIV attaches to receptors of target cells, including T cells.

A person who becomes infected with HIV may experience flu-like symptoms, including fever, chills, and headache, usually in the first three to six weeks, but it can take up to six months. This is known as seroconversion illness, and is the time when the person begins to form antibodies against HIV. With the exception of the seroconversion illness (which may not occur), an infected person may have no indication at all that they are infected, but unfortunately they can transmit the virus, for example sexually.

When HIV was first recognised, tests and treatment for it were understandably not available. Tests were developed quite rapidly, and treatments followed. Highly active anti-retroviral therapy (HAART) became available in the mid-1990s; these drugs target various features of HIV. Use of these drugs has transformed infection with HIV from a disease that caused almost certain death within about ten years, and due to AIDS, to a chronic illness—but only in countries where the drugs are readily available to infected people. These drugs continue to be developed so that nowadays combination antiretroviral therapy (cART) results in the development of less drug resistance by the virus. Unfortunately, drug toxicity and side-effects continue to present problems.

HIV is a blood-borne virus, and so it can be transmitted by infected blood and blood products, other body fluids such as semen and vaginal secretions, and across the placenta or by breast milk from mother to child. The most common mode of transmission of the virus is sexual transmission, both heterosexual and homosexual. Prevention of transmission of HIV includes avoidance of spills or contact with infected tissues or secretions on mucous membranes or broken skin. Safer sex practices that reduce the risk of exchange of body fluids are crucial in reducing the spread of this disease, as is the use of uncontaminated equipment for injection. The potential for transmission of HIV infection in the workplace is an occupational health and safety issue for healthcare workers, who should practise the Standard (or Universal) Precautions (Hoy & Richmond 2008). Standard Precautions have the aim of reducing the risk of transmission of HIV and other blood-borne infections, and contribute to the protection of both the healthcare worker and the client.

Where one of a couple is infected with HIV, and the person apparently has a chronic illness rather than a threat to life, they may wish to have children. In this case there are interventions that can reduce the risk of transmission of HIV from a positive man to the woman, and from a positive woman to her partner and/or fetus/child.

Early diagnosis and treatment of HIV infection constitutes a benefit to the HIV-positive person and to the community. Previously undiagnosed, untreated HIV-positive individuals are likely to seek medical advice when they are very sick with AIDS-related illnesses (certain opportunistic infections or cancer). It has been noted previously that a person who is unaware of their HIV status can transmit the infection, for example during sexual activity.

When a person has their infection with HIV confirmed, counselling and support should be provided, and management should include vaccinations (for hepatitis A and B and pneumonia), along with education about HIV and strategies for minimisation of its spread. Combination antiviral therapy and prophylactic medication for opportunistic infections should be considered on the basis of the person's level of immune system function, and treatment of any existing conditions should occur (Vujovic et al. 2010).

Prions

Prions are protein molecules, and have the capacity to cause transmissible degenerative disease of nervous tissue by a mechanism that remains incompletely understood (Dunne & Ledeboer 2009). Prion disease is inevitably fatal.

Creutzfeld-Jakob disease (CJD) is a rare prion disease that affects humans. Bovine spongiform encephalopathy (BSE, or mad cow disease) is a disease that affects cattle and potentially humans. Both CJD and BSE are neurodegenerative diseases (WHO 2011a). Exposure to prions occurs either by ingestion or other direct contact. Prevention of exposure to prions is currently the only known way of preventing infection. Prions are very resistant to the normal means of sterilising equipment.

Fungi

Fungi differ from bacteria and viruses in that they do not require a host for their survival. They are free-living organisms that are found in wide-ranging types of habitats on earth. Certain fungi form part of the flora of humans. Fungal infections are usually limited to local skin infections, but serious systemic (whole-body) fungal infections can occur in persons who are immunocompromised, or who have experienced instrumentation, or both. Instrumentation is use of instruments for treatment or diagnosis, and includes the insertion of instruments such as endoscopes or catheters into body structures such as the urethra, or a blood vessel, potentially causing or permitting future entry of microorganisms, including fungi. The fungi that infect humans are usually endogenous, that is, a part of the normal flora. Treatments are available to cure fungal infections.

Candida albicans

The yeast *Candida albicans* (*C. albicans*) forms part of the normal flora of the skin, digestive tract, and female genital tract. Infection due to *C. albicans* can occur locally in the mouth or vagina due to the endogenous organisms rather than ones from an external source. As noted previously, a woman may experience vaginal candidiasis (vaginal candida infection) following a course of treatment with antibiotics. Protective acid secretions of the vagina are due to actions of bacteria that are normally present in the vagina (*Lactobacillus acidophilus*). Unfortunately, antibiotic treatment usually removes these bacteria and their protective function as well as the bacteria for which the antibiotic has been prescribed.

Widely disseminated (spread) infection in the body due to *C. albicans* results in abscesses in organs such as the liver or kidneys, and has a high mortality rate. Such an infection is uncommon, and is most likely to occur in people who are either immunocompromised or are subject to instrumentation, or both. Candidiasis is an important nosocomial (hospital-acquired) infection (Slavin et al. 2010).

The nature of parasites, and how they make us sick

Helminths–worms

Helminthiasis is the parasitic infection (infestation) by worms (helminths). Helminthiasis can have a variety of consequences on the host, depending on the nature of the worm involved. Consequences include liver damage affecting function, obstruction of blood or lymphatic vessels, tissue damage resulting in chronic blood loss from the gut, malnutrition, and blindness. Human populations most affected by worm infections live in resource-poor countries with limited access to adequate sanitation and hygiene, safe food-handling practices, and appropriate animal husbandry (care of farm animals). However, worm infections can and do occur in any population. Worm infections are preventable and treatable. Two types of worms that infect people in Australia will now be considered.

Enterobius vermicularis–pinworms

The most prevalent worm infection in Australia is due to pinworms, commonly known as 'worms' (*Enterobius vermicularis*, *E. vermicularis*). Humans are the host for pinworms. The adult worm lives in the digestive tract and emerges via the anus, commonly at night, to lay eggs on the peri-anal (nearby) skin. A common symptom of pinworm infection is itching around the anus. Eggs are likely to contaminate bed linen and clothing, and may be found under fingernails. Unless hygiene practices are strictly observed, eggs will be ingested, and will mature in the digestive tract, thus perpetuating the cycle. Pinworms do not have serious consequences, but may cause irritability and local itching (Better Health Channel 2010b).

Echinococcus granulosus–the hydatid tapeworm

Dogs are the definitive host for the hydatid tapeworm (*Echinococcus granulosus*, *E. granulosus*): that is, the form of the parasite that infects dogs is the form that produces eggs. Human infection follows ingestion of eggs from dog faeces: the eggs hatch in the human digestive tract, then the embryos

Case Study 2.2   Hydatid disease in a child

In 1956, John, a 4-year-old boy, was taken to the family doctor because he had persistent abdominal pain. Examination revealed that the child had an enlarged liver. John lived with his parents on a farm in country Victoria. The family grew their own vegetables, and they had a number of dogs that the boy played with on most days, in the garden and on the lawn. The farmer regularly killed a sheep for the family to eat, and fed the offal to the dogs.

An X-ray showed the presence of what was probably a cyst in John's liver. The X-ray and history led to a diagnosis of hydatid disease. The surgeon removed the hydatid cyst successfully from the liver, apparently without any spillage of the contents of the cyst, which had a volume of about 500 mL.

Two years later John became persistently confused and drowsy, and examination revealed raised intracranial pressure. X-ray showed extensive hydatid disease in the brain. Although some cysts were removed at operation, it was not possible to remove them all. Unfortunately, John died about eight months after this surgery.

Each of the statements in the case history provides information that is directly relevant to hydatid disease. Link the case history to the information provided about the disease in the text below.

This disease is now rare in Australia. For example, in Queensland approximately ten cases occur annually (Queensland Health 2010); some of these cases may occur in immigrants to Australia.

» *What changes in practice that have occurred since the 1950s are likely to have resulted in a reduction in the incidence of hydatid disease in Australia?*

migrate to viscera (internal organs) such as liver, lungs, or brain where they develop as hydatid cysts, or 'watery blisters' (Better Health Channel 2010c). The cycle continues when a dog (or dingo) ingests hydatid-infected offal of an animal such as a sheep or kangaroo.

Symptoms of hydatid cyst infection vary with the organs involved—these cysts occupy space and can affect function in an organ such as the brain; they can rupture and cause adverse reactions. Hydatid cysts can have serious or even fatal consequences.

Prevention of hydatid cyst infection requires appropriate care of dogs and farm animals, including regular worming, and personal attention to hygiene, including handwashing after handling dogs, and before food preparation and consumption. Inspection of meat at abattoirs also helps to prevent hydatid and other helminth infection.

Plasmodium—malaria

Malaria is estimated to cause about a million deaths per year, and is therefore a major contributor to the global burden of disease. Malaria occurs predominantly in the tropics, especially in parts of Africa and the Asia-Pacific region (WHO 2011d). Should the climate change globally, prevalence patterns of malaria may also change. Malaria is caused by several species of *Plasmodium*, including *P. Falciparum*, which is the species most likely to cause fatal disease. The *Plasmodium* species are protozoa that have a complex life cycle for which humans are host to several stages.

Malaria is likely to begin following the bite of an infected *Anopheles* mosquito, when the infectious organisms are injected while the mosquito feeds on human blood. Liver cells are infected initially, and subsequently red blood cells. The different stages of the *Plasmodium* life cycle proliferate in these cells, eventually bursting from them to infect more and more cells of the host. The host usually experiences marked fever, headache, and muscle pain at the time of red blood cell rupture and parasite release, due to immune system responses to the parasite (Brown et al. 2010).

Red blood cells infected with *Plasmodium* tend to aggregate, potentially causing harm if this occurs in the brain, lung, kidneys, or placenta. Anaemia occurs virtually universally in people with malaria: rupture of red blood cells contributes significantly to this. Aggregation of red blood cells in the brain circulation may be the cause of 'cerebral malaria', the most dangerous form of malaria. Pregnant women and young children are most susceptible to malaria infection.

From time to time, *Plasmodium* sex cells are formed and transported by the blood: should a mosquito bite at this time, these sex cells are taken up and fertilisation occurs within the mosquito, producing new organisms that are ready for injection to another human host. The life cycle of *Plasmodium* can continue for years in its human host, until immunity develops, or a cure occurs, or the person dies.

Any traveller to a region where malaria is endemic should take careful precautions against mosquito bites, and probably take prophylactic (preventive) medication, bearing in mind that some strains of *Plasmodium* are resistant to certain drugs. Should our traveller experience a febrile illness following their return, they should be investigated for malaria. Malaria is both preventable and treatable; however, both prevention and treatment continue to provide challenges, especially in resource-poor countries.

Infectious diseases: What are the body's defences?

Some of the rather daunting variety of organisms that either simply coexist with us, or act as pathogens or parasites that threaten our health and well-being have been discussed. The defences that the body has against infection will now be considered.

We are born with **defences against infection**. The first line of defence is the prevention of infection by prevention of entry of infectious organisms. This is followed by inactivation and removal of organisms that have managed to enter our bodies, and now have the potential to cause disease. Effective body defences against infection, including the functions of the immune system, are essential for survival. Lack of such defences results in overwhelming infection, or cancer, or both.

Innate defences are present from birth, and act immediately to prevent any foreign materials from entering the body, or from establishing an infection should one have already gained entry. Innate defences range from barriers, to physiological functions, to cellular and molecular responses, and can involve some cells or molecules of the immune system.

Adaptive defences act against the unique antigens that are the identifiers of specific pathogens or parasites. These mechanisms result in the destruction and

Defences against infection—innate (also known as non-specific) defences Structures and functions that are present from birth, and that act immediately to prevent any foreign material either from entering the body or from establishing an infectious disease should one have already gained entry.

Defences against infection—adaptive (or specific) defences Antibodies and cells that act against unique antigens, that is, against the identifiers of specific pathogens or parasites, ultimately enabling their destruction and removal. Adaptive defences are acquired in response to exposure to these unique antigens, but depend on our inherited capacity to respond to them.

removal of the pathogens or parasites. Adaptive defences are acquired in response to exposure to these unique antigens, but depend on our inherited capacity to respond to them. Adaptive defences always involve the immune system, and include antibodies and cellular immunity. Body defences also act against cancers, and foreign tissues such as a tissue or organ transplant.

Innate defences

Innate defences include barriers, physiological functions, secretions, and cells. According to Marieb and Hoehn (2010, p. 115), 'epithelia form boundaries between different environments'. The body surfaces that interact with the external environment are barriers to infectious organisms. The epithelia of the skin and conjunctiva of the eyes present protective barriers to the outside world. The mucous membranes that line the digestive and respiratory tracts, and the urethra and vagina of the urinogenital systems, are also barriers that prevent entry of microorganisms from the external environment into the fluids and tissues of the body. Although the interior of the digestive and other tracts are intimately within our bodies, they still communicate with the external environment.

These boundaries are known as 'portals (gateways) of entry' to the body because they are boundaries between the external environment and the fluids and tissues of the body. Tight junctions between adjacent epithelial cells, together with the basement membrane that supports the epithelium, reinforce the barrier that the sheets of epithelial cells form. Skin damage, for example following extensive burning, poses a serious threat to survival, not only from fluid loss, but also from infection: the larger the surface area of the burn, the greater the threat.

Epithelia produce secretions that contain antibacterial agents: lysozyme is found in tears, saliva, and breast milk; antibodies are found in breast milk and digestive tract secretions; acid secretions are produced by the skin, stomach, urinary tract, and vagina; mucus is secreted by the respiratory and digestive tract epithelia. These factors all play a part in controlling microorganism populations and preventing infection. The placenta is a barrier that prevents many substances from entering the fetal circulation, but unfortunately not all, for example HIV and the bacterium that causes syphilis.

Physiological functions that contribute to removal of infectious organisms include sneezing, coughing, vomiting, and diarrhoea. All of these are automatic responses that reduce the likelihood of infection becoming established.

Certain cells and molecules of the immune system are also part of innate body defences. Phagocytes are cells that kill microorganisms by engulfing them; natural killer cells kill virus-infected cells. Various types of molecules contribute to coordination of the functions of the immune system, including inflammation and fever, and responses to bacterial and viral infections.

Infection causes inflammation, which is characterised by an increase in blood flow to the affected area, causing redness, swelling, heat, and pain. The increase in blood flow transports the cells and molecules that will deal with the infection at the site. These include the phagocytic cells that engulf and destroy foreign material.

Fever occurs in response to pyrogens. Pyrogens are molecules that are secreted during the immune response to infection; they are also molecules derived from the infectious microorganisms. Pyrogens act to increase the 'set point' for body temperature, and as a consequence the body responds by decreasing heat loss mechanisms, and increasing heat production by shivering (otherwise known as rigors). These responses are interspersed with episodes of sweating and activation of other heat loss mechanisms. Fever has beneficial effects on the outcome of infectious disease: the treatment of fever tends to prolong the illness; however if the fever is extreme (40°C or more), treatment is necessary because of its adverse effects (Gottlieb et al. 2010).

Unfortunately, despite their benefits, some of these innate responses, such as vomiting, inflammation, and fever, can make us feel ill, and if severe, have adverse consequences of their own.

Adaptive defences

As we have defined, adaptive defences are specific to a particular organism, because they act against the unique antigens that are the identifiers of a specific pathogen (or parasite): for example, against the measles virus, but against no other viruses. The identifying antigens are a part of the pathogen. Adaptive defences include antibodies and cellular immunity.

Antibodies are produced as a part of the adaptive responses to infectious organisms. An antibody has a shape that is complementary to that of the antigen that it targets, thus enabling antibody–antigen binding, with inactivation of the antigen. The antibody–antigen complex can be readily removed by phagocytic cells. Antibodies are referred to as humoral immunity because they are transported by the plasma. Antibodies are plasma proteins; they are also called immunoglobulins.

B cells (also known as B lymphocytes, or plasma cells) respond to foreign antigens by secreting antibodies. Once a foreign antigen, for example of a bacterium, binds to a B cell, the B cell is stimulated to divide. Some of the daughter B cells eventually secrete antibodies that specifically bind to and inactivate the foreign antigen—in this case, the type of bacterium that initiated this process. Other daughter B cells remain as 'memory cells' providing immunological memory. Should the antigen enter the body a second or subsequent time, the B memory cells synthesise more antibodies more rapidly, resulting in a higher concentration in the blood more quickly than following the original exposure (Marieb & Hoehn 2010).

Humoral immunity can be active or passive. Active humoral immunity occurs when a person secretes their own antibodies to a particular antigen. Active immunity is usually long-lasting (years or a lifetime). Passive humoral immunity occurs when the person has antibodies to a particular antigen circulating in their blood, but they do not have B cells that have been stimulated to synthesise these antibodies. Passive immunity is lost over time as the antibodies are degraded and lost from the plasma (Marieb & Hoehn 2010) (see Vaccination and Immunisation below).

Adaptive immunity also includes cell-mediated immune responses. T cells can become cytotoxic T cells. Cytotoxic T cells recognise their specific target cells by their identifying antigens, then bind with them and destroy them. Cytotoxic T cells destroy cells that are infected with a virus, or cancer cells. Infected cells display the antigens of their infectious organism; cancer cells have antigens that are changed and are no longer recognised as 'self' by the body's immune system, therefore they are attacked and destroyed.

T cells form memory cells, providing immunological memory in a way analogous to that of B memory cells. These memory cells respond rapidly to a subsequent exposure to the same type of target cell (Marieb & Hoehn 2010).

The foreign antigens that the immune system can recognise and mount an immune response against are determined by genes. The genetic 'library' of a person provides the basis of the capacity of the immune system to recognise vast numbers of infectious organisms, including the ones that the person is likely to encounter throughout their lifetime. However, in the unlikely event that a person does encounter an infectious organism that immune system cells cannot recognise because it is not in the 'genetic library', an adaptive immune response cannot be mounted. If such an organism establishes an infection, we are likely to die from the infection.

If the organism can 'hide' its antigen, the immune system cannot respond to it. The malaria parasite and the Human Immunodeficiency Virus spend much of their time in the body within cells. This is probably one of the reasons why these organisms cause such a burden of disease, and why there are continuing problems with the development of a vaccine against either infection.

In addition to cytotoxic functions, T cells perform many regulatory functions in the immune system. HIV preferentially attacks T cells and, as we have noted, will cause a marked drop in T cell (CD4 cell) numbers if the infected person remains untreated. If a person has very low T cell count, they will be susceptible to infections and certain cancers, that is, the HIV-positive person now has the Acquired Immune Deficiency Syndrome or AIDS.

Lack of immune system responses results in severe combined immunodeficiency. These conditions are rare, but can be congenital (exist from birth). Severe immunodeficiency means that a person's immune system is unable to respond to infectious organisms, with the result that they are likely to die from overwhelming infection unless extraordinary precautions are taken to protect them from the infectious organisms in the environment (Marieb & Hoehn 2010).

Can infectious diseases be treated?

Morbidity Having to do with disease; the morbidity rate is the rate of a particular disease in a given population during a period of interest; the relative incidence of a particular disease.

See also discussion of morbidity and mortality in Chapter 3.

Possibilities for treatment of infectious disease range from curative, to treatment of symptoms but without cure, to no treatment. The development of antibiotics in the 1940s revolutionised the treatment of bacterial infections, and reduced **morbidity** and mortality considerably. Treatment for HIV with combined anti-retroviral therapy (cART) means that people now live for many years without developing AIDS—but the HIV infection is not cured. Drug treatment of other viral infections continues to be limited; the treatments that are available tend to reduce the severity of the disease, but do not cure the infection, for example *Herpes* infections.

We have seen that organisms that cause infectious diseases differ considerably from each other with respect to the nature of the organism, and their mechanisms and consequences of action. It will be no surprise to learn that there are classes of drugs specific to the different types of organisms: antibacterial, antiviral, antifungal, and antiparasitic. The choice of drug therapy should be based on knowledge of the organism causing the infection, likely effectiveness of the drug, and any particular circumstances of the patient, such as pregnancy or breastfeeding, very young or older age, impairment of function of liver or kidneys (Grayson & Howden 2010).

As readers would expect, drugs known to have no effect should not be used: it is inappropriate to treat a viral infection with an antibacterial agent (an antibiotic). Unfortunately, inappropriate drug use continues to lead to drug resistance of infectious organisms: a drug that an organism is resistant to will no longer have any therapeutic effect on that organism. Inappropriate drug use can include not only poor choice of drug treatment by the doctor, for a particular infection, but failure of the patient to follow the regimen of drug taking for optimal effect.

Stop and Think

Antibiotics are fed to some animals that are produced for food. The stated aim of this practice is to maintain health of the animals. There are regulations regarding both the nature of the chemicals used, and of residues that are permitted to remain in the meat that will be consumed (Food Standards Australia and New Zealand 2011).

» Suggest one reason why the use of antibiotics in the production of food is regulated.

Infectious diseases: What factors affect our susceptibility?

Some of the reasons for individual differences in susceptibility to certain infectious diseases have been noted in previous sections. These will be discussed further here. Increased susceptibility can be due to life stage, where the very young and very old tend to be more susceptible than a young adult, probably because the infant takes time to acquire adaptive immunity, and the older person may suffer from diminished responses of the immune system, or may already be suffering from another disease, or both. Pregnant women are more vulnerable to the effects of some infections, including influenza and malaria, than non-pregnant women. Nutritional status is important: starvation, and deficiency of vitamin A and protein predispose to infectious disease. Co-morbidities, such as infection with certain STIs, increase susceptibility to other STIs because of lesions of the mucous membrane of the reproductive tract. Drug treatment for certain diseases such as inflammatory arthritis can cause immunosuppression. The environment that a person lives in can expose them to pathogens or vectors of pathogens; for example, overcrowded housing fosters the transmission of tuberculosis; lack of sanitation contributes to water-borne diseases such as cholera; and accumulation of rubbish attracts rats and flies that can be vectors of disease.

Can infectious diseases be prevented?

Stop and Think

Advice from government health authorities reported in the local press at the time of writing urges people in Victoria to take precautions against the potentially serious viral infectious diseases Murray Valley Encephalitis and Ross River Fever.

» What is the link between these infectious diseases and the unusually cool, wet summer experienced this year?

» What precautions can be taken?

» Who do you think should be responsible for any precautions necessary?

The organism, the host, and the environment

Knowledge about an infectious organism, its host, and the environment that they share can enable development of powerful strategies to control the infectious diseases caused by the organism. Control of mosquito populations is a key feature for control of malaria in regions where it is endemic; in addition, different stages of the life cycle of the *Plasmodium* that causes malaria are susceptible to different drug therapy. It should be noted that mosquitoes are vectors for many more diseases than just malaria.

> **Stop and Think**
>
> Discuss the ways in which well-designed buildings and associated infrastructure can contribute to the control of infectious diseases.

Before it was recognised that infectious diseases were caused by pathogens and parasites, it was thought that malaria was caused by 'miasms' (putrid-smelling air) from marshes: indeed, the derivation of the word 'malaria' is 'bad air'. People sought to prevent disease by warding off bad smells: priests used incense, and people relied on a posy of flowers to protect them from the Black Death (plague).

Environmental and other factors that affect our susceptibility to infectious diseases are also relevant here (refer to the previous section).

Vaccination and immunisation

Vaccination Administration of substances that will normally induce adaptive immunity in a person, including memory cells.

Immunisation The acquisition of adaptive immunity to an infectious disease, including both humoral and cellular immunity. Humoral immunity (antibodies in plasma and other body fluids) can be active or passive. Immunisation can be naturally acquired following exposure to a pathogen, or artificially acquired as a result of vaccination.

Throughout history, it has been recognised that some people in a community always survived an epidemic of infectious disease, even if it had a high mortality; that a person usually does not get the same infectious disease twice; and that a baby is usually protected against most of the infectious diseases its mother has had, for some months after birth. The body's responses to infectious organisms have already been described.

Vaccination for a particular infectious disease involves the administration of substances that will cause immunisation of the person to that disease: that is, the person develops adaptive immunity, including memory cells. The substances administered can be fragments of the microorganism, or killed or attenuated ('weakened') microorganisms; these stimulate the immune responses, but do *not* cause the disease. Immunisation is a very powerful cost-effective intervention for the control of many infectious diseases: these are known as vaccine-preventable diseases (VPDs).

Immunisation is defined as the acquisition of immunity to an infectious disease, including both humoral and cellular immunity; humoral immunity can be active or passive. Immunisation can be naturally acquired following exposure to a pathogen, or artificially acquired as a result of vaccination. As has been noted, antiviral drugs tend to treat symptoms but do not bring about a cure. Certain bacterial infections can progress, rapidly causing overwhelming disease, such as meningococcoal infection

Case Study 2.3   Epidemic of whooping cough (*pertussis*) in Victoria, 2011

Whooping cough is a highly contagious (highly communicable to others, easily spread) infectious disease, due to a bacterial infection (*Bordetella pertussis*). It is a vaccine-preventable disease.

A baby does not obtain any protection against whooping cough from its mother before birth. Although antibiotics can be used in its treatment, whooping cough can have serious, even fatal, consequences, especially for babies before they begin their standard vaccinations, usually at 2 months of age.

What steps can be taken to prevent whooping cough, especially in young babies? Adults tend to lose protection against whooping cough and can therefore be susceptible to infection with it: vaccination of new parents (and grandparents) is recommended to reduce the risk of a baby becoming exposed to the disease. New parents, and indeed any adult who wishes to reduce their risk of contracting this infection, can choose to have a booster vaccination.

including meningitis. Prevention is a priority. This is now possible for many diseases because of immunisation.

Immunisation of infants has resulted in a marked decrease in the incidence of childhood infectious diseases such as diphtheria, whooping cough (pertussis), tetanus, polio, and a number of others. One hundred or so years ago, these so-called childhood diseases caused hundreds to thousands of deaths annually, but nowadays relatively few incidences of infection are notified. However, there are exceptions: at the time of writing, there was an epidemic of whooping cough in Victoria (Chief Health Officer 2011).

The 'Immunise Australia Program' (Australian Government Department of Health and Ageing 2010) promotes immunisation for common, vaccine-preventable diseases (VPDs). In an unimmunised person, many of these diseases cause only mild illness in childhood, but they have a risk of serious complications: this is why they are included in the immunisation program. We also immunise for VPDs that are rare but that have very serious or fatal outcomes if a person becomes infected, such as meningococcal infection and Rubella. The Rubella virus causes an infection with mild consequences for an adult, but can cause the Rubella syndrome comprising severe defects in heart, brain, eye, and ear development and function if a pregnant woman is infected, especially in the first trimester (the first three months).

Not everyone who is vaccinated becomes immunised. This is one of the reasons for 'booster' vaccinations. High vaccination rates for a particular disease—close to 100% of the population—result in herd immunity, that is, protection of unimmunised individuals against that disease. This can result in complacency regarding a particular infectious disease—it may no longer appear to affect our community. People intending to travel should be aware that the prevalence of infectious diseases varies from country to country, and that it is wise to take precautions in addition to vaccination for disease prevention.

Immunisation against influenza is advised for adults older than 65 years because of their reduced immune responses, and for individuals with respiratory or cardiovascular disease, to reduce morbidity and mortality.

Elizabeth Brown

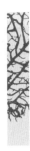

Mythbuster

Some people think that the risk of vaccination outweighs any benefit that may result.

» *Discuss the validity of the following arguments that are sometimes put forward:*

» The childhood diseases that are vaccinated for usually cause only mild illness, so it does not matter if a person gets the disease.

» Australians have a high vaccination rate and so the disease rarely occurs anyway: my children and I will be protected by this 'herd immunity'.

Adverse events following immunisation include minor problems such as a mild fever or some pain at the injection site. Rare adverse events, including an allergic reaction to the vaccine, are well documented. Any person who is considering avoidance of vaccination for themselves, or their children, is advised to first weigh up the risks of the vaccination versus the risks of the disease. This is discussed in the Australian Government's *Australian Immunisation Handbook* (see the 9th edition, 2008).

Antibodies can provide passive immunity. Some of the antibodies that are synthesised by the mother cross the placenta and provide a newborn baby with some passive immunity against

Mythbuster

Does vaccination for measles, mumps, and Rubella (MMR) cause autism?

• The findings of a large population-based study of more that 537,000 children (Madsen et al. 2002) were that (1) there was a similar risk of autism in vaccinated versus unvaccinated children, (2) autism did not occur around the time of vaccination, and (3) there was no association of autism with MMR vaccination. The conclusion of the study was that MMR vaccination does not cause autism.

• A number of other large studies support these findings of no causal association between MMR vaccination and autism.

• The original study that triggered fear that MMR could cause autism was published in *The Lancet* in 1998 (Wakefield et al. 1998). This paper was subsequently found to be flawed, and was retracted by *The Lancet* in February 2010. Flaws included the small sample size of 12 children in the study, the method of subject selection, and the study design, which lacked statistical power to reach the conclusion that MMR vaccination could cause autism. The research was later found to be fraudulent.

• Unfortunately, this flawed 1998 publication caused a fall in vaccination rates, especially for MMR. Vaccination rates fell from 92% to 84% in the UK, and the incidence of measles and mumps both increased.

• Retraction of the paper, and the publication of other research that did not support the original hypothesis, has not resolved all of the heated debate around this topic.

» *Suggest reasons vaccination rates fell, especially for MMR, following the publication of the paper by Wakefield and colleagues (1998).*

» *Discuss reasons why heated debate continues about this topic, with some people remaining concerned that there is a link between MMR vaccination and autism, despite the retraction of the original paper, and the publication of other research that did not support it.*

infectious disease for 6 to 12 months after birth, until the antibodies are degraded. Breast milk also contains antibodies that act within the gut preventing gastrointestinal infection, and systemic infection such as respiratory tract infections.

Summary

Infectious diseases constitute a continuing major cost to human life and health in all communities. We coexist with a remarkable variety of organisms, some of which live on or in our bodies. Infection occurs in a variety of ways but there are also numerous defence mechanisms that prevent infection, and reduce illness and death. Unfortunately, these defences are not always successful. In addition, there continue to be infectious diseases for which there is no cure. Prevention and treatment are therefore important priorities. Knowledge about pathogens and parasites, the host, and the environment are all necessary for the development of strategies for prevention of infectious diseases, and for development of effective treatments.

Immunisation is a safe, cost-effective measure that harnesses aspects of the body's defences to achieve protection against certain infectious diseases—the vaccine-preventable diseases. It therefore protects against the adverse, sometimes life-threatening, consequences of these diseases. Over the last 100 years, immunisation programs have had the combined results of reducing the burden of infectious disease, and significantly increasing average life expectancy. A major reason for the increase in average life expectancy has been the reduction in deaths due to infectious diseases that previously occurred in large numbers of young children. A well-coordinated immunisation program was a key contributor to the global eradication of smallpox that was completed in 1980 by the World Health Organization.

Tutorial exercises

1   List and discuss reasons why it is people in the 15–25-year age group who are most likely to become infected with *Chlamydia trachomatis*, when compared with other age groups.
2   Discuss the validity of the following comment: 'The development of antibiotics is the main reason for the marked decline in the incidence of, and deaths due to, infectious diseases in the Australian community over the last 100 years.'

    Take into account the types of infectious diseases that can occur, their modes of transmission, and factors that affect susceptibility of a person to infection.
3   List and discuss reasons why malaria is difficult to control in resource-poor countries.
4   You are the person providing advice for a Community Health Help Line. An older woman has rung for information about the flu vaccine. She suffers from asthma, but is reluctant to be vaccinated for the flu this year because she is sure that the last vaccination she had caused the flu. What advice is relevant to this person? Can a modern vaccine give someone the flu? Explain.
5   Look up the *National Immunisation Program Schedule* of the *Immunise Australia Program:* go to <www.immunise.health.gov.au>. Note the number of vaccine-preventable diseases, and the ages and groups for which vaccination is scheduled or recommended, and suggest reasons why these ages and groups have been targeted.

    Suggest why a series of vaccinations is scheduled for some infectious diseases, rather than one single vaccination.

Further reading

Australian Government Department of Health and Ageing and NHMRC (2008). *The Australian immunisation handbook*, 9th edn. <http://immunise.health.gov.au/internet/immunise/publishing.nsf/Content/handbook-home>

Marieb, E.N., & Hoehn, K. (2010). *Human anatomy and physiology*, 8th edn. San Francisco: Pearson Education Inc.

World Health Organization (2011e). *Infectious diseases*. <www.who.int/topics/infectious_diseases/en>.

Yung, A., Spelman, D., Street, A., McCormack, J., Sorrell, T., & Johnson, P. (eds) (2010). *Infectious diseases: A clinical approach*, 3rd edn. Melbourne: IP Communications.

Websites

<www.immunise.health.gov.au>

This website and related links are prepared by the Australian Government Department of Health and Ageing (2010). These present information about all aspects of the National Immunisation Program Schedule in Australia for vaccine-preventable diseases.

<http://immunise.health.gov.au/internet/immunise/publishing.nsf/Content/handbook-home>

This website presents the *Australian immunisation handbook*, 9th edition. This publication is written by the Australian Government Department of Health and Ageing and NHMRC (2008). This handbook presents clinical guidelines on the safe and effective use of vaccines.

<www.betterhealth.vic.gov.au/bhcv2/bhcpdf.nsf/ByPDF/Worms_pinworms/$File/Worms_pinworms.pdf>

This website is prepared by the Better Health Channel (Victorian Government) (2010a). It provides information about pinworms, which are the most common type of worm infection in Australia.

<www.betterhealth.vic.gov.au/bhcv2/bhcarticles.nsf/pages/Tapeworms_and_hydatid_disease>

This website is prepared by the Better Health Channel (Victorian Government, 2010b). It provides information about tapeworms and hydatid disease, which occur rarely in Australia, but can have serious or fatal consequences.

<www.betterhealth.vic.gov.au/bhcv2/bhcarticles.nsf/pages/Chlamydia>

This website is prepared by the Better Health Channel (Victorian Government, 2010c). It provides information about the sexually transmissible infection caused by *Chlamydia*.

<www.betterhealth.vic.gov.au/bhcv2/bhcarticles.nsf/pages/Tetanus?open>

This website and related links are prepared by the Better Health Channel (Victorian Government) (2010d). These provide information about tetanus.

<www.health.vic.gov.au/chiefhealthofficer/alerts/alert-2011-01-pertussis.htm>

This website is prepared by the Chief Health Officer, Victoria, Australia (2011). It presents information about the current Pertussis epidemic in Victoria.

<www.foodstandards.gov.au/consumerinformation/antibioticsandfood.cfm>

This website is prepared by Food Standards Australia and New Zealand. It presents information about the use of antibiotics in the production of animals raised for human consumption.

<http://access.health.qld.gov.au/hid/InfectionsandParasites/Parasites/hydatidDisease_fs.asp>

This website is prepared by the Queensland Government (Queensland Health 2010). It presents information about the rare but potentially fatal disease due to hydatids.

<www.who.int/topics/encephalopathy_bovine_spongiform/en>

This website and related links are prepared by the World Health Organization (2011a). These present information about bovine spongiform encephalopathy (BSE) and its significance to human health.

<www.who.int/topics/malaria/en>

This website and related links are prepared by the World Health Organization (2011a). It presents information about malaria.

<www.who.int/immunization_monitoring/diseases/tetanus/en/index.html>

This website and related links are prepared by the World Health Organization (2011c). It presents information about tetanus.

<www.who.int/topics/infectious_diseases/en>

This website and related links are prepared by the World Health Organization (2011e). These provide general information about infectious diseases.

<www.who.int/hiv/data/2010_globalreport_core_en.ppt>

The series of slides (1-11) at this website is prepared by the World Health Organization (2009). It presents a global summary of the AIDS epidemic for the year 2009.

3 Introduction to epidemiology

Rebecca Fanany

TOPICS COVERED

This chapter covers the following topics:
- the historical development of the field of epidemiology
- the difference between endemic and epidemic diseases or conditions
- the concept of the rate and its use in epidemiology
- the nature of incidence and prevalence in epidemiology and the way in which these measures are derived
- the concept of risk and how it applies to population health
- the kind of information epidemiological study can provide about disease

KEY TERMS

Chronic disease
Disease
Endemic
Epidemic
Epidemiology
Incidence
Infectious disease

Morbidity
Mortality
Outbreak
Prevalence
Rate
Risk

Introduction

Epidemiology is the study of the distribution and determinants of **disease** and other health-related conditions in human populations. The principles and analytical techniques of this field are used to study the frequency of different conditions in groups within society and the factors that influence their distribution. Disease is not distributed equally in populations, and the study of epidemiology allows us to understand these inequities and develop better, more effective interventions and programs for their control. Epidemiology also serves as a very important tool when new diseases or previously unrecognised conditions appear in society and have to be addressed by the health sector. This chapter will discuss salient issues relevant to epidemiology.

> **Epidemiology** The study of the distribution and determinants of disease.
>
> **Disease** A condition adversely affecting health that has measurable (clinical) symptoms.

A brief history of epidemiology

The word **epidemic** comes from two ancient Greek words, ε≡ι [epi], meaning 'upon', and δεμοσ [demos] meaning 'people'. An epidemic, then, was seen as something that was 'upon the people', a disease or plague that was unusual in the society's experience. Epidemiology is the study of epidemics: how disease spreads, who is most likely to be affected, and under what circumstances disease might appear in a particular population (Mausner & Kramer 1985). Epidemiology, as a field of study, originally developed to answer questions about **infectious disease** but more recently it has been applied to a wide range of health and social conditions. This reflects the power and flexibility of the analytical techniques of the field as well as their ability to explain many different phenomena that impact on health.

> **Epidemic** A higher than usual number of cases of a disease or condition in a particular geographic area; there are no requirements for number of cases.
>
> **Infectious disease** A disease that can be transmitted from person to person, either directly through the spread of a disease-causing agent or indirectly such as by a vector.

The earliest epidemiological studies come from ancient Greece. They were based on empirical deductions derived from the experience of relatively small populations. Hippocrates (*c.* 470–400 BC), who is sometimes referred to as the Father of Medicine, showed how human health is affected by a set of easily observable environmental factors in his book entitled *Airs, waters and places*. In the following centuries, epidemiology did not receive much attention, but by the 17th century clinical observation was again becoming important in the treatment of disease. John Graunt (1620–74) applied a demographic approach to data on disease and death. Using weekly records of deaths in London, Graunt was the first to take into account the source of information in an effort to eliminate bias and to use frequencies and ratios (instead of absolute figures) that allowed comparison across time and location. Graunt's book, *Natural and political observation on the bills of mortality* (1662), pointed out a number of interesting findings that remain accurate today, such as the fact that mortality rates among male infants were higher than among females and that more people died of chronic conditions than of acute infections. In 1700, Bernardino Ramazzini (1633–1714) published what is considered to be the first formal work on occupational medicine, *De Mortibus Artificum Diatriba*, in which he considered the common characteristics of the work environment of painters in Rome which he believed contributed to diseases that were common among this population.

Modern epidemiology is often dated from the observations by Dr John Snow (1813–58), a physician in London in the mid-19th century. Snow observed major cholera epidemics in London in 1849 and 1854 and realised that the spread of the disease was associated with use of water from certain sources. Microbiology was in its infancy at the time but, even without laboratory analysis, Snow was able to conclude that the epidemics were associated with water contaminated by sewage that was provided by a particular London water company. Households using water from a different supplier had markedly lower rates of cholera, which Snow attributed to the quality of the source from which each company drew its supply.

Many other scientists, doctors, and observers contributed to the development of epidemiology as a field. The examples above are only selected highlights of this history and illustrate that the modern science of epidemiology has had a long history with many innovations that occurred at different times. A number of authors (e.g. Rosen 1998; Morabia 2006; Susser & Stein 2009) have discussed the history and development of the field and describe the many interesting events that have contributed to the knowledge we have today.

Epidemiological concepts

Chronic disease A disease that cannot be transmitted from person to person, is usually long lasting, and may not be amenable to cure. Many chronic diseases are associated with certain lifestyles or behaviours.

See also Chapter 5 on chronic illness.

Epidemiologists study how disease and other health conditions are distributed across society and what the determinants of these conditions might be. Today, this extends beyond infectious disease, as noted above, to include non-infectious **chronic disease** such as diabetes, cancer, and arthritis, and even a wide range of social conditions. These can include drug and alcohol use, family planning, domestic violence, the use of health services, driving behaviour, and many more. Epidemiological methods are often used to identify affected groups based on exposure, rather than by the existence of disease, as a means of anticipating future health needs more accurately. This means that epidemiologists increasingly consider where and how people live, where they work and the jobs they do, what pastimes they enjoy, and what their personal habits are as a way to understand better the interaction of factors that contribute to health status. It is important to remember that epidemiology can be applied not only to infectious disease in epidemic form (as was the case historically) but to any disease, condition, or health-related phenomenon.

Epidemiology provides very powerful information about the nature of disease as well as the people who are likely to be affected by it. However, we should keep in mind that the conclusions of epidemiological analysis apply to whole groups in society that share certain characteristics. What these characteristics are will vary depending on what condition we are interested in, and it is their presence that allows us to identify a number of individuals whose health experience will have some features in common. We base our expectations on the existence of these common features. For example, we know that smoking cigarettes has the potential to cause physiological changes in smokers. From this, we can assume that some people who smoke will experience similar physiological changes that can be predicted and that these changes may lead to disease. It is very important to understand, however, that epidemiological analysis cannot tell us anything about the health status of any individual; it only provides information about what we can expect in a group whose experience (exposure) is the same. That is, epidemiology is based on the probability of a given health condition appearing in the presence of certain exposures. We may be able to predict that 10% of people with a particular experience will have a certain health problem related to that experience, but we do not know which of the people who share the experience will fall into this 10%. Epidemiology, then, allows us to calculate risk to populations, and the larger the population is, the more likely these predictions are to be accurate. This means that epidemiological analysis tells us very little about individual experience but is very accurate when applied to the entire population of a city, region, or nation.

One of the most useful ways to consider the nature of any health-related issue from the perspective of epidemiology is in terms of whether the occurrence of the event in question is usual or not. If a disease or condition is always present in a particular geographic area, that condition is said to be **endemic**. Endemic simply means that the condition (or the agent that causes the condition) exists naturally in the environment in the area we are interested in. For example, the infectious agent that causes chicken pox, a common childhood illness, is endemic in most of the world. This means that the virus that causes this disease, *Varicella zoster*, is always present in human populations and, in fact, most children will get chicken pox at some time (Berenson 1990).

Endemic Always present in a particular environment; often used to refer to a disease or the organism that causes a disease.

By contrast, a disease or condition may be epidemic. This means that its occurrence in a particular population or geographic location is unusually high. There are no set levels of occurrence that indicate whether an epidemic is in progress. Instead, we base this determination on what is usual in the population we are interested in and say that there has been an **outbreak** if the number of cases exceeds what we usually see. We expect a large number of cases of influenza every year in temperate locations such that the number of additional cases required to constitute an outbreak is very large. Alternatively, an unusual number of cases of influenza after the usual season (winter and spring) would be considered an unusual occurrence and may signal the beginning of an epidemic. By contrast, a single case of smallpox would constitute an outbreak and would lead to immediate, emergency public health measures. In the case of smallpox, the last naturally occurring case was observed in 1984, and the disease is considered to have been eradicated. In this context, even one case would be highly unusual and very dangerous.

Outbreak An unusual cluster of cases of a disease or condition in a particular geographic area; there are no requirements for number of cases.

When we talk about epidemic disease, we should remember that there are no constraints on geography or time. That is, an epidemic may exist within a relatively small area, such as one neighbourhood in a particular city or one village in a rural area, or may extend over a very large area such as a whole country or region. It is also possible for an epidemic to reach most of the world. In this case, we might refer to the disease as being *pandemic* in nature (from ≢αν 'all; every' and δεμοσ 'the people' in Greek), an indication that it exists everywhere. The 1918–19 wave of influenza that followed the First World War was pandemic because nearly every part of the world was affected. Similarly, AIDS is pandemic in the world today because it is present in nearly every country. An epidemic may take place over any period of time. This period might be as short as a few hours in the case of acute chemical intoxication that might result from an industrial accident; it might reach several weeks or months, such as is common in the case of influenza or measles, or extend to years as is the case with AIDS or some of the chronic conditions now common around the world. If a disease is present in epidemic or pandemic state for a number of years, it may become endemic. That is, we may cease to view it as an unusual health occurrence and instead treat it as part of the normal environment in which we live.

The major components of descriptive epidemiology are person, place, and time. These concepts allow us to determine the nature of a disease or condition and suggest ways to control it. The relationship between person, place, and time and the characteristics of a health event of interest is shown in Table 3.1.

Table 3.1   Basic concepts of descriptive epidemiology

Concept	Meaning	Examples	Disease or Condition
Person	Who is affected by this disease or condition?	Age, gender, behaviour, immunity, etc.	Outbreak–unusual cluster of cases of a disease or condition in a particular geographic area
Place	Where does the outbreak occur?	Workplace, town, country, climate, etc.	Epidemic–a higher than usual number of cases of a disease or condition in a particular geographic area
Time	When does the outbreak occur?	Season, long-term patterns, etc.	Endemic–always present in a particular environment

Rates

Rate A proportion for which a particular time period is specified.

Rates are the most important tools used in epidemiology to understand the nature of a particular health phenomenon in society. Ratios and proportions are sometimes used as well, so it is important that we understand what each of these terms refers to.

A ratio expresses the relationship between two values expressed as x:y or x/y. We read this ratio as 'x to y', meaning that for every x number of whatever item we are interested in, there are y number of another item. An example of a commonly seen ratio is the number of male births to female births in a given location in a given period. In Australia in 2009, the ratio of male births to female births was 105.8:100. There were 150,807 males and 144,893 females born in this year (ABS 2010a). This means that, for every 100 female babies born, there were about 106 male babies born. It is usual in human populations for there to be slightly more males born than females; the ratio tends to equalise later in life.

A proportion is a ratio, generally expressed as a percentage, where the numerator is included in the denominator. Knowing the number of male and female births above, we might be interested in the proportion of all births that are male. This proportion can be expressed as follows:

Male births/Male + Female births × 100 = 150,807/(150,807 + 144,893) × 100 = 51%

In 2009, 51% of all births were male.

A rate is a proportion in which a period of interest is specified. Rates are extremely useful when considering the occurrence of disease or other health effect because they allow us to see the probability (or risk) of the condition in a given population during a particular period of time. The general form of the rate is:

Mortality Having to do with death; the mortality rate is the rate of death from a particular cause in a given population during a period of interest.

$$\frac{\text{Number of events (cases of disease, injuries, deaths, etc)}}{\text{Population at risk during a specified time period}} \times 1000$$

Epidemiological rates are often expressed per 100,000 population. This standard form allows the rate of particular phenomena of interest to be compared in populations that are different in size. One commonly used rate is the **mortality** rate (how many people are expected to die in a given year in relation to the total population). There were 140,800 deaths in Australia in 2009 in a total population of 21,964,900 (ABS 2010b). We can calculate this as follows:

140,800/21,964,900 = .0064 × 1000 = 6.4

Therefore, in 2009, there were approximately 6 deaths for every 1000 people in Australia.

Incidence and prevalence

In addition to mortality rates, **morbidity** rates are often used in epidemiology and public health. Morbidity rates, or rates of disease, allow us to estimate the risk of specific diseases or conditions for given populations. These can be divided into rates of **incidence** and rates of **prevalence**.

An incidence rate reflects the probability, or likelihood, that healthy people will develop the disease or experience the condition of interest in a specified period (usually a year). The incidence rate, then, is the number of new cases of a disease or condition in a population during the period of interest. An incidence rate can be expressed generally as follows:

$$\text{Incidence} = \frac{\text{Number of new cases of a disease or condition}}{\text{Population at risk}} \text{ over a period of time}$$

By contrast, prevalence rates indicate the number of people in a population who have a particular disease or condition at a given time. They are a measure of the probability, or likelihood, of the disease or condition existing in a population at a particular point in time. Prevalence depends on the number of people who have had the disease or condition in the past (previous incidence) and the duration of their condition. Prevalence can be expressed generally as:

$$\text{Prevalence} = \frac{\text{Number of existing cases of a disease or condition}}{\text{Total population}} \text{ at a point in time}$$

It is important to understand the relation between *incidence* and *prevalence*. Because prevalence depends on the number of people with a particular condition of interest regardless of when the condition began, it is possible for prevalence in a particular population to be high even though incidence is low. This is an indication that, once people contract the condition, they tend to have it for a long time. If the duration of an illness is short, either because people recover quickly or because they die, incidence may be high, while prevalence is low. Generally, prevalence is approximately equal to incidence multiplied by duration.

Incidence and prevalence rates are useful in understanding population health. Incidence rates are a direct indication of risk because they measure the rate at which members of a population develop particular diseases or conditions of interest. We can compare incidence rates for different population subgroups and identify factors specific to each group that may affect their risk. Prevalence measures the presence of a disease or condition in a population and hence is an indication of burden of disease. Rates of prevalence are especially important in relation to chronic disease, which is an increasing problem in populations around the world.

Morbidity Having to do with disease; the morbidity rate is the rate of a particular disease in a given population during a period of interest.

Incidence The occurrence of new cases of a disease or condition in a particular population during a period of interest.

Prevalence The number of all cases of a disease or condition in a particular population during a period of interest.

Risk

Risk The probability or
likelihood of a particular
effect occurring in a
particular population
during a period of
interest.

See also Chapters 4,
5, 9 & 10 on biological,
environmental and
lifestyle factors
affecting health.

Epidemiological calculations allow us to make certain assumptions about **risk** to a population of interest from particular diseases or conditions. Again, it must be stressed that assessment of risk does not provide information about any individual but relates instead to groups or populations that share certain characteristics. These characteristics are often referred to as risk factors. Risk factors come from many different sources, but they must be present before the onset of disease if we are to assume they have had an impact on the condition of interest.

Some examples of risk factors known to be associated with disease are genetic abnormalities; environmental factors (such as pollution); exposure to radiation; exposure to chemicals; diet; personal behaviour including level of physical activity, smoking, use of alcohol and/or drugs; exposure to bacteria and other microorganisms; and many more. The exact relationship between various risk factors and particular diseases or conditions may be difficult to determine because of the number of risk factors, their possible combinations, and the fact that many individuals who make up populations are exposed to multiple risk factors whose effects may be multiplied under certain conditions. For example, risk factors for type 2 diabetes, a common chronic condition affecting many Australians, include increasing age (older individuals are more likely to contract type 2 diabetes); family history (individuals with relatives who have diabetes may be at greater risk); history of cardiovascular disease; a diet high in fat and sugar; low levels of physical activity; being overweight; and having a history of gestational diabetes (women who had diabetes while pregnant) (Murray & Lopez 1997a,b; Cameron et al. 2003). While some of these risk factors are amenable to change (such as diet or engaging in physical activity), others are not (age, family history). Many members of a given population will have one or more of these risk factors. It is these individuals who make up the population of interest, and the combined effect of all their risk factors will contribute to population risk (incidence) of disease.

In considering risk, we may want to know whether there is an association between a disease or condition and particular risk factors. One way to measure this association is to examine the incidence rates for a population exposed to a particular risk factor and for a population that is not exposed to the risk factor. This measure is called relative risk and describes the chance of developing a disease or condition in relation to exposure. Relative risk is a ratio of the probability of the condition occurring in an exposed group as compared to an unexposed group. The general expression for relative risk is as follows:

$$\text{Relative risk} = \frac{\text{Incidence rate among exposed}}{\text{Incidence rate among unexposed}}$$

The related concept of attributable risk is also useful in epidemiological studies. Attributable risk is a calculation of the number of cases of the disease or condition of interest among the exposed population that could be eliminated by removing the exposure to a particular risk factor. If there is a cause-and-effect relationship between the risk factor and the condition, we can use attributable risk to measure the public health impact of exposure.

When we talk about risk of disease or another health-related condition, we are really discussing probabilities that are based on observations of populations and their particular risk factors. The larger the population size, the more accurate these calculations are likely to be. It is for this reason that governments and other organisations concerned with public health collect detailed statistics at the local, national, regional, and even world level that can be used to make assessments of population health and to study the distribution patterns of various diseases and conditions.

Stop and Think

Rates are based on observed events in whole populations. They describe probabilities of certain things occurring in particular groups or populations.

» What do they tell us about individual risk?

» How should the information provided by epidemiological rates be used in planning health strategies for communities?

The epidemiology of influenza and diabetes

Epidemiology has provided important insight into many of the diseases that have the most potential to affect human populations. It has allowed us to understand the important differences between infectious and chronic disease in terms of risk and the ways in which the conditions are distributed. While every disease has specific determinants and patterns of occurrence, we can use influenza as an example of an infectious disease and diabetes as an example of a chronic disease in considering the kind of information epidemiological study can provide.

Influenza is an acute respiratory infection caused by one of a number of related viruses. While an individual can only be infected with a particular virus once (as infection confers immunity), these viruses show a high degree of antigenic variation. This means that changes in the surface proteins of the virus that trigger an immune response in those infected occur rapidly through mutation (Cox & Bender 1995). For this reason, it is possible for one individual to contract influenza repeatedly. The disease has a long history in human populations, and there are influenza viruses that affect other animal species. It is possible for an animal influenza to mutate in such a way that it becomes infectious to humans; this is the basis of the concern with avian influenza in recent years, and in fact many human influenza viruses seem to have developed from viruses that originally infected birds (Cox & Subbarao 2000; Rambaut et al. 2008).

Because influenza has long been known to human beings and because there have been many epidemics of the disease of varying severity, there has been a great deal of epidemiological study of the disease. Colder climates, such as the temperate regions of Australia, experience a 'flu season' every year in the late autumn to early spring (Monto 2008). The methods of epidemiology have been applied to data available on a yearly basis about cases of influenza, and we now know a great deal about how the disease affects populations.

Influenza is associated with increased mortality, either from the disease itself or from pneumonia associated with the disease. Cardiopulmonary disease, as well as other chronic conditions, may be made worse by influenza and also contribute to excess mortality associated with outbreaks (Chowell et al. 2009). In most years, when a seasonal period of influenza occurs but there is no epidemic (inter-pandemic years), mortality from the disease occurs mainly among the elderly (Dushoff et al. 2005). This is one reason yearly flu vaccination programs often target this population subgroup. In a pandemic year (when the number of cases greatly exceeds the number normally expected), mortality in younger people may be very high, even reaching 50%. This situation was observed during the very serious influenza pandemic following the First World War (1918–19) and is now understood to be a characteristic of an influenza epidemic. Interestingly, while the risk to younger people during a pandemic year has been estimated to be 20 times higher than normal, the risk to the elderly is the same as in inter-pandemic years (Simonsen et al. 1998).

When individual outbreaks of influenza are studied from the perspective of epidemiology, we find that there is no predictable pattern with which pandemics occur. Species specificity does not seem to guarantee that human infection will not occur. That is, an outbreak of influenza in another animal species (birds, pigs, and so on) may lead to the emergence of a virus capable of infecting people (Cox & Bender 1995). Most influenza epidemics emerge suddenly, peak in 2–3 weeks, and subside in 5–10 weeks. During an epidemic, the infection rate tends to be between 10% and 20% (10–20% of the exposed population is expected to become ill) but may be as high as 40–50% among schoolchildren, nursing home residents, and other institutionalised population subgroups (Berenson 1990). Although annual influenza is an expected occurrence, we do not know how or why influenza viruses with the potential to cause a pandemic appear and what triggers this kind of event.

In the context of public health, this epidemiological knowledge of influenza allows for planning and prevention. One of the most commonly used preventive measures against influenza, based on experience with this disease, is vaccination of the individuals most likely to be at risk. Generally, influenza vaccination programs focus on the elderly, individuals with chronic conditions, healthcare professionals, and others who share a risk factor for increased morbidity or mortality (Duclos & Hatcher 1993; Simonsen et al. 2005). Because the influenza virus mutates rapidly and it is not possible to predict which strain will be dominant during the next flu season, the pharmaceutical companies that produce flu vaccines must use past experience and complex statistical techniques to determine the kind of vaccine that is most likely to be effective and make it available before the flu season begins (Leroux-Roels & Leroux-Roels 2009; Nicholson 2009). Even if these calculations do not correspond exactly to the dominant influenza viruses once the season begins, it is likely that those vaccinated will benefit from partial immunity, which may lessen the severity of illness, even if it cannot prevent it entirely.

By contrast, diabetes is a chronic disease. It also has a long history in human populations but until recently has been relatively uncommon (King et al. 1998; Zimmet et al. 2001; Amos et al. 2010). There are two forms of diabetes: type 1 which is the result of a genetic condition present at birth and type 2 which is thought to be affected by a range of risk factors associated with diet, behaviour, and lifestyle as well as biological factors. Type I diabetes (sometimes referred to as juvenile diabetes) usually appears in childhood, while type 2 diabetes (adult onset diabetes) generally emerges in middle age (Krolewski et al. 1987; Adeghate et al. 2006). In most cases, type 2 diabetes is associated with a sedentary lifestyle and obesity and represents an increasing burden on healthcare systems around the world (Zimmet 1999; Zhang et al. 2010).

Type 2 diabetes has been associated with impaired glucose tolerance that causes hyperglycemia (unusually high glucose levels in the blood) following ingestion of food. This condition is estimated to affect some 200 million people worldwide and is an intermediate stage in the development of type 2 diabetes. About 40% of individuals with impaired glucose tolerance develop diabetes within 5–10 years, although some revert to normal or remain the same (Zimmet et al. 2001).

One of the most serious aspects of the current rise in type 2 diabetes is the observation that the disease, which has occurred primarily in adults in the past, is now affecting younger age groups. The increasing incidence of type 2 diabetes in children and adolescents has been ascribed to increasing industrialisation and globalisation around the world (Pinhas-Hamiel & Zeitler 2005; Haines et al. 2007). Type 2 diabetes has been reported in children in the USA, Australia, the UK, Hong Kong, the Pacific Islands, and Japan, where it accounts for 80% of diabetes in children (Kitagawa et al. 1998). The incidence of type 2 diabetes is rising in most regions but is most pronounced in non-European populations. In Australia, for example, type 2 diabetes is a very significant contributor to the burden of disease for the Aboriginal and Torres Strait Islander population, with lifetime risk for males estimated to be 50% and about 65% for women (Wang et al. 2010). Diabetes in this population is positively predicted by waist measurement, smoking, and consumption of alcohol among other factors (Burke et al. 2007).

As we can see, influenza, as an example of an infectious disease, and diabetes, as an example of a chronic disease, affect different population subgroups and are associated with different risk factors. Epidemiological study, including rates of incidence and prevalence, has allowed us to understand the distribution of these diseases in society and provide a way to monitor changes in the health of society. This type of epidemiological information is very important in public health planning and in designing programs that will address society's burden of disease.

Case Study 3.1   An unusual outbreak of salmonella

Whenever an outbreak of disease occurs, epidemiologists step in to try to trace connections between those who are sick and look for common elements in their behaviour, activities, and lifestyle to determine how they might have been exposed to the disease-causing agent. This kind of fieldwork is an important part of disease surveillance and contributes greatly to maintaining the health of the public.

In 1981, there was an unusual outbreak of salmonellosis caused by the bacterium *Salmonella muenchen* in the US states of Alabama, Michigan, Ohio, and Georgia. In most cases, outbreaks of this kind of enteritis are linked to a contaminated food source and can be traced by comparing the food recently consumed by those who are sick, where it was purchased, and how it was prepared. In this case, however, it was not possible for epidemiologists to identify a common source for the infection, and it turned out that there were no factors found that could link all the cases. Finally, one of the first individuals to become ill admitted she was a marijuana smoker, as were many of her friends. Tests showed it was, in fact, the marijuana that was contaminated with the microorganism, which was likely spread as users rolled joints, put them in their mouth, and passed them to other people. Because the marijuana proved to be heavily contaminated with other bacteria like *E.coli* and *K. pneumoniae* in addition to *S. muenchen*, epidemiologists concluded that it had been deliberately mixed with dried manure as a way to increase profits.

The fact that the same kind of salmonellosis caused by the same organism had caused outbreaks in several states puzzled investigators as well until they realised that trade in illegal products such as marijuana is conducted in much the same way trade in legal products is. Just as fruits and vegetables, which are common vehicles for the bacteria that cause salmonellosis, are shipped from the place where they are grown to other locations where they are sold, so is marijuana. However, in the case of an illegal substance, it may be very difficult to get people to say where they purchased it or admit that they sold it because an admission of this kind might lead to prosecution for possession of drugs.

This outbreak was covered heavily in the media as well as in the epidemiological literature (see e.g. *Marijuana Linked to Salmonellosis* 1982; Taylor et al. 1982; Rouche 1984; Reingold 1998) because of its unusual nature and because it served as a reminder to epidemiologists that it is not only the things people are willing to talk about that have the potential to affect their health, but also the whole range of private behaviours that may be much more difficult to find out about and compare. Nonetheless, in the case of salmonellosis at least, most outbreaks are associated with contaminated food and are somewhat easily solved.

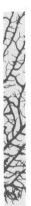

Mythbuster

Many people think that all heavy smokers will get cancer because this is an impression conveyed by the media and other sources. In fact, a large number of people who smoke heavily (or engage in any other behaviour associated with a negative health effect) do not get cancer. When we study the epidemiological relationships between risk factors and disease, we start with people who have the disease and look at risk factors that are common to most of them. It is not practical to study all the people who share a particular behaviour and wait to see whether they develop a disease. It is people who already have a disease who come to the attention of health professionals and whose behaviour and background can be compared to that of people who do not have the disease of interest. Before people are sick, we cannot predict which of them might contract a disease in the future so the strong emphasis on known risk factors we see in the media and elsewhere (such as the association between smoking and cancer) is a precaution that we hope will reach those at risk even though we cannot tell exactly which individuals they are.

Summary

The history of epidemiology begins in ancient times and, for centuries, was based on observations of disease and death. Today, epidemiologists use complex methods of calculation as well as statistical observations. Although originally developed to explain the occurrence of infectious disease, the methods of epidemiology have been effectively applied to many health and social phenomena.

One of the main tools of epidemiology is the rate, which expresses the occurrence of a condition of interest as a proportion with a specified time period. Common rates include morbidity rates and mortality rates and are often standardised to allow comparisons. Incidence and prevalence rates measure the extent to which a population is affected by a disease or condition of interest. Incidence is a direct measure of risk, while prevalence indicates burden of disease.

Epidemiology provides a means for assessing population risk. Risk is a probability calculation relating various risk factors to the emergence of disease. The larger the population size, the more accurate risk assessments tend to be. These estimates of risk relate only to groups and do not provide information about the risk to any one individual that may be part of the group.

The principles of epidemiology have been used to study many diseases, including influenza, which occurs yearly in temperate climates, and diabetes, which is increasing worldwide. An investigation of the patterns and distribution of the disease over time has yielded important information about the nature of the disease as well as groups likely to be at risk.

Tutorial exercises

1   Go to the website of the Australian Bureau of the Census and look at the tables about causes of death. What do the figures suggest about mortality in Australia?
2   What might it mean if a particular condition has high incidence but low prevalence? What about low incidence but high prevalence? What does this suggest about risk?
3   How might knowledge of the epidemiological characteristics of a particular disease help us control that disease? Explain.

Further reading

Merrill, R.M. (2010). *Introduction to epidemiology*. Sudbury, MA: Jones & Bartlett.

Parfrey, P., & Barrett, B. (2009). *Clinical epidemiology: Practice and methods*. Totowa, NJ: Humana; London: Springer.

Susser, M., & Stein, Z. (2009). *Eras in epidemiology: The evolution of ideas*. New York: Oxford University Press.

Webb, P., & Bain, C. (2011). *Essential epidemiology: An introduction for students and health professionals*. Cambridge: Cambridge University Press.

Webber, R. (2009). *Communicable disease epidemiology and control: A global perspective*. Wallingford, UK and Cambridge, MA: Cabi.

Websites

<www.who.int/csr/disease/en>

The World Health Organization (WHO) monitors epidemics and potential epidemic outbreaks. This information is available from Epidemic and Pandemic Alert and Response.

<www.cdc.gov/mmwr>

The Centers for Disease Control and Prevention (CDC) in the USA publishes a weekly update on figures for reportable disease called the *Morbidity and Mortality Weekly Report* (MMWR).

<www.abs.gov.au>

Information on population health can be found in the census. Whole population censuses are conducted every ten years by the Australian Bureau of Statistics.

<http://justice.vic.gov.au/wps/wcm/connect/DOH+Internet/Home/Births%2C=Deaths+and+Marriages>

Vital statistics (births, deaths, marriages) are often useful in epidemiology as they provide an ongoing record of information on health and mortality. In Australia, the states and territories collect vital statistics.

<www.health.gov.au/cda/Source/CDA-index.cfm>

Morbidity data, concerning incidence and prevalence of disease, is part of compulsory surveillance and reporting collected by the National Notifiable Diseases Surveillance System.

4 Human genetics and inheritance: Biological, social, cultural, and environmental perspectives

Sandra Taylor

TOPICS COVERED

This chapter covers the following topics:
- genes, chromosomes, and heredity
- the Human Genome Project
- genetic mutations, conditions, and risks
- genetic DNA testing
- public health genomics
- geneticisation
- subjective experiences of genetic risk
- gender and genetics
- genetic discrimination

KEY TERMS

Chromosomes
Genes
Genetic condition
Genetic determinism
Genetic discrimination
Genetic mutation
Genetic risk
Geneticisation
Genome

Genotype
Human Genome Project
Multi-factorial disorders
Phenotype
Predictive genetic test
Pre-symptomatic genetic test
Public health genomics
Single-gene disorders

Introduction

Genetic makeup is an important foundational factor that interrelates with a wide range of social, cultural, and environmental influences to determine people's health and well-being over the course of their lives. A person's genetic makeup does not operate in a vacuum or in isolation but rather in a complex web of interaction with many other factors in a person's internal and external environments. A person's individual and psychological makeup (age, life stage, and genetic makeup) is in constant interaction with multiple other factors ranging from very broad social, cultural, and socio-economic circumstances that determine so many of the contexts within which people operate right down to their own individual behaviour and unique biomedical characteristics like blood pressure or body weight. It is a complex and dynamic picture that changes over the course of a person's life.

See the broad coverage of determinants of health in Chapter 1.

Having a clear and accurate understanding of what determines and influences people's health and illness is fundamental for people who aim to work in the contemporary healthcare field. How we understand health and illness will inform the beliefs and attitudes we bring to our professional practice with people, the skills that we use to engage with them, and ultimately our capacity to maximise their health whether this be at an individual level or in communities and broader populations.

This chapter focuses on genes and genetic makeup, in interaction with a wide range of other factors, as determinants of health. The first part of the chapter introduces and reviews some basic genetic concepts within the contemporary context of human genetic science including the Human Genome Project. The roles played by genes and genetic mutations in the development of genetic conditions and disorders are outlined and genetic DNA testing is described. The second part of the chapter examines how people's genetic makeup interacts with a wide range of other factors in their psychological and social environments. Special attention is given to looking at how people's decisions and responses to their genetic makeup are moderated by factors like culture, socio-economic status, age, gender, and beliefs, to ultimately determine their health outcomes. The importance for health practitioners to acknowledge the complex picture of health determinants, only *one* of which is genetic makeup, and to understand people's subjective beliefs and experiences, is highlighted. Finally, a discussion of genetic discrimination shows how broad societal and political factors also operate as determinants of health and well-being.

See the discussion of the Human Genome Project in Chapter 5.

Human genetics and inheritance: Biological determinants of health

The importance of genetic makeup as a determinant of health and well-being has been acknowledged for a long time. In modern society, however, human genetics is a new and exciting scientific frontier, offering new frameworks for understanding human growth and development, health, and disease. James Watson and Francis Crick's 1953 discovery of the double helix structure of the DNA molecule made it possible for scientists to finally understand the mechanism of heredity in all organisms. Since then, there has been an exponential increase in genetic discoveries and developments including the cloning of the first human gene (insulin) in 1978 and of Dolly the sheep in 1997, the development in 1985 of 'DNA fingerprinting' for use in criminal investigations, and the isolation of specific genes that influence the development of many health conditions and genetic disorders (CGE 2007a, Fact Sheet 24).

In 2003, scientists in the USA, working collaboratively with others in many countries, announced that they had successfully achieved the primary goals of the **Human Genome Project** (HGP), namely to map all chromosomes in human cells and sequence all genes along those chromosomes. This extraordinary scientific achievement had, in effect, provided the complete genetic specification of a human being. Such a momentous scientific achievement was variously described as decoding the 'book of life', establishing the 'holy grail', and laying down the 'blueprint for life' (Alper et al. 2002). James Watson, Nobel Laureate, exclaimed, 'Now we know, in large measure, our fate is in our genes' (Alper et al. 2002, p. 1).

While not wanting to deny the significance of the HGP achievement, it is worth drawing attention to the assumptions and associated implications that underpin beliefs like that quoted above, which suggest that genes are essentially the determinants of people's health and behaviour. Such a perspective reflects **genetic determinism**, which assumes that people are the sum of their genes and that their health and behaviour are essentially predetermined by their genetic makeup, with social and other factors having minimal influence (ALRC/AHEC 2003).

A genetic determinist approach for understanding health and well-being is the opposite of the broader determinants approach that is argued in this book. A social determinants perspective asserts that people's health and well-being throughout the course of their lives are determined by the complex interplay between many factors, only one of which is genetic makeup.

Human Genome Project An international project begun in 1990 and completed in 2003 which aimed to map all chromosomes and sequence all genes in the human being.

Genetic determinism The belief that a person's health and behaviour are predetermined by their genetic makeup.

See Chapter 1 for an overview of other factors.

Stop and Think

» To what degree do you think your genes have determined your health as it is today? As it will be in the future?

» How might having a genetic determinist view impact on the practices of health professionals?

There are several concerns about adopting a genetic determinist approach. First, if we believe health and health problems are primarily determined by people's genetic makeup, any responses we make or 'solutions' we look for, by way of research, policy, practice, or interventions, are likely also to have a genetics focus. At its most extreme, such a view underpins a eugenics approach which aims to improve the human population through the controlled breeding of desirable characteristics. Eugenic practices were brutally imposed by the Nazi regime during the Second World War; they also underpin many contemporary conflicts that are characterised by ethnic cleansing of populations or minority groups. Where this is applied, a person's whole identity is subsumed by their genetic characteristics; if such characteristics are also socially or politically undesirable, as in, for example, a person's ethnicity or degree of disability, stigmatisation and discrimination can follow. Within the healthcare context, genetic determinist beliefs can result in people feeling fatalistic

Case Study 4.1   Belinda

Belinda is a single, 23-year-old mother of two small children aged 5 and 3 years. She suffers from severe asthma, which is exacerbated by the dampness of the caravan park she lives in. Belinda left school when she was 15 and has no formal qualifications although she would like to work in childcare; she can see little chance of this happening soon however. Belinda's family is interstate but she has recently been told that her father has been diagnosed as having high cholesterol and that this has been related to a relatively rare genetic disorder known as familial hypercholesterolaemia (FH); this means that Belinda could also have inherited an increased risk for developing coronary artery disease earlier in life, especially if her diet and lifestyle are not healthy. Belinda finds herself now worrying about this constantly and about how she can maximise her and her children's chances of being healthy in the future. She also fears that if she has inherited the faulty gene from her father, making her more prone to developing coronary artery disease, she might have unknowingly passed this gene on to her own children.

» *What are the key factors that are influencing Belinda's current health status as well as her future health prospects?*

» *How important is Belinda's genetic risk for FH in this picture?*

about their disease or illness, fearing that adopting a healthy lifestyle will bring them little benefit and that little can be done to actually affect their health outcomes. Evidence is clear, however, that even when a person's illness is primarily caused by genetic factors, adopting healthy practices and lifestyles can still significantly improve quality of life and health prospects (CGE 2007b, Fact Sheet 11).

See Chapter 15 for a discussion of stigmatisation of deviant characteristics.

Genes and chromosomes: The mechanisms of heredity

Genes Basic units in the body's cells which contain the genetic material that codes for heredity as well as health, growth, and development.

Chromosomes Long strands of a chemical substance known as DNA (deoxyribonucleic acid), along which genes are located.

Genes are the basic units of health and heredity in the body (CGE 2007c, Fact Sheet #1). They are located along **chromosomes**, which are tightly coiled strands of a chemical substance called DNA (deoxyribonucleic acid). Chromosomes are present in the nucleus of each cell in the human body and their structure is the well-known double helix discovered by Watson and Crick in 1953 and which enables heredity to occur.

Every cell in the body contains 46 chromosomes and these comprise 23 pairs: one pair has been inherited from the mother through her egg and one from the father through his sperm. Two of these chromosomes, known as X and Y, determine the person's biological sex; a man's and woman's chromosomes are described as '46,XY' and '46,XX' respectively. The 44 non-sex chromosomes (in 22 pairs) are numbered 1 to 22, representing the smallest to the largest in size; these are called autosomes. A *karyotype* is a chart or picture of all of an individual's chromosomes which have been photographed through a microscope and organised in a standard way according to their group and size. A karyotype can be used to indicate an individual's sex.

Genes are situated at particular locations along the chromosomes. Individuals inherit a gene from each parent for each locus of the chromosome and these can vary from each other according to the sequencing of their DNA. These alternative forms of genes are called *alleles* and they can produce different *traits* or inherited features in people; at the locus for eye colour, for example, the allele might result in the person having either blue or brown eyes. A person's physical and biochemical characteristics, as determined by their genetic makeup and/or their environment, is called their **phenotype**; their genetic makeup or constitution is called their **genotype**. The term '**genome**' refers to all of the genetic material contained in the cells of a person or a living organism.

It is now estimated that the 46 human chromosomes contain a total of between 20,000 and 25,000 active genes, a much smaller number than anticipated when the Human Genome Project first got under way (US Department of Energy 2010). These genes contain specific pieces of information that are in the form of a chemical code. This genetic code guides the production of protein in the body which in turn influences the formation of different types of cells, tissues, and organs. Having healthy tissues and organs clearly plays a very significant and fundamental role in determining a person's health and well-being as they grow, develop, and live life during their life course.

Genes that were mapped and sequenced in the HGP represent only about 25% of the known material on the human chromosomes, however. The remaining 75% of the genetic material constitutes what scientists call 'non-coding' or 'junk' DNA (CGE 2007a, Fact Sheet 24). It is now also known that certain genes are expressed only at different times in the life course and that the expression of such genes is strongly influenced by environmental conditions (CGE 2007b, Fact Sheet 11; Lin et al. 2007); understanding the nature of these interactions between genes and environment represents a key focus of ongoing genetic research (CGE 2007a, Fact Sheet 24; CGE 2007b, Fact Sheet 11). Another challenge for scientists lies in understanding exactly how genes function and interact within the body and how they contribute to human growth and development as well as health disorders and diseases (CGE 2007a, Fact Sheet 24; CGE 2007b, Fact Sheet 11; Metcalfe et al. 2009).

> **Phenotype** A person's physical appearance.
>
> **Genotype** A person's genetic constitution.
>
> **Genome** All the genetic material in the cells of a living organism.

Genetic mutations and conditions

Sometimes permanent changes occur in chromosomes or in genes that cause cells to be unable to accurately read the genetic codes within them; this is called a **genetic mutation** and the gene can be described as 'faulty'. Genetic mutations can occur spontaneously during or after conception; they can also accumulate naturally over a person's lifetime as they age and/or are exposed to external factors like radiation, viruses, or environmental chemicals. It is estimated that everyone has several faulty genes in their genetic makeup but that these do not cause any particular health-related problems. Some faulty genes are even associated with bringing health benefits to people, as in the case where being a gene carrier for the genetic condition *thalassaemia minor* is thought to be associated with having greater protection against malaria (CGE 2007d, Fact Sheet 4).

If a genetic mutation causes problems with how body systems develop or function, a **genetic condition** can occur (CGE 2007d, Fact Sheet 4). Genetic conditions can run in families when specific genetic mutations are passed from parents to children. There are three main patterns of inheritance relating to genetic conditions

> **Genetic mutation**
> A permanent change in a gene that prevents the cell from accurately reading the genetic code. Genetic mutations can occur naturally or they can result from exposure to chemical or physical agents; they can also sometimes be inherited.
>
> **Genetic condition**
> A condition or disorder caused by a genetic mutation that affects how body systems develop or function.

in families: dominant, recessive, and sex-linked (CGE 2007e, Fact Sheet 10). Because dominant and recessive inheritance patterns involve genetic mutations on the non-sex chromosomes or autosomes, they are referred to as autosomal; conditions that follow this inheritance pattern will affect men and women similarly. In autosomal *dominant* inheritance, a mutation occurs in one gene and this overrides or 'dominates' the other working copy of the gene; this is usually sufficient to cause a person to be affected by, or to be predisposed to develop, the genetic condition (CGE 2007f, Fact Sheet 9). Examples of autosomal dominant conditions are Huntington's disease (HD) and inherited predispositions to familial breast, ovarian, and bowel cancers.

See also Chapter 5 on the Human Genome Project.

In autosomal *recessive* inheritance, while a mutation may occur in one copy of the gene, the proper working of the other gene copy is sufficient to ensure normal functioning and the person will be unaffected by the condition; they are described as being a 'carrier' of the faulty gene (CGE 2007g, Fact Sheet 8). The faulty gene can be passed on to offspring, and children too can be carriers. Where both parents are carriers of the same faulty gene, there is a 25% or 1 in 4 chance in every pregnancy that a child will inherit both copies of the faulty gene; if this occurs, the child will be affected by the condition. Examples of conditions that follow an autosomal recessive inheritance include cystic fibrosis and thalassaemia.

Finally, *sex-linked* patterns of inheritance occur when genetic mutations occur on the X or Y sex chromosomes (CGE 2007e, Fact Sheet 10). Conditions associated with mutations on the X chromosome are more likely to occur, however, as the X chromosome contains more genes than the Y chromosome. The impact of genetic mutations on the sex chromosomes will differ for men and women. Sex-linked inheritance can also be dominant or recessive; Rett syndrome is an example of the former while haemophilia is an example of an X-linked recessive condition.

Genetic risk The probability that a trait, condition, or disorder will occur or recur in an individual or family more frequently than it occurs by chance.

Constructing a family history or genogram can provide an important picture of the pattern of inheritance of a genetic condition in a family (CGE 2007h, Fact Sheet 3). When an inherited condition in a family is objectively established, people are said to have a **genetic risk** or to be 'at risk' (Weil 2000). While being at risk for developing a genetic condition can be challenging for individuals and families, it can also be the basis for uniquely shared bonds and experiences (Taylor 2004, 2008b).

Single-gene disorders Genetic disorders caused by the inheritance of a mutation in a single gene; an example is Huntington's disease.

Some genetic conditions occur more frequently in particular populations or ethnic groups, reflecting ongoing adaptation of these groups to their environments but also group differences in susceptibility to disease (Lin et al. 2007). Higher occurrences of Tay-Sachs disease and cystic fibrosis occur in Ashkenazi Jewish families in central and northern Europe, for example; similarly β–Thalassaemia occurs more frequently among Middle Eastern, central and South-East Asian, and African communities (CGE 2007i, Fact Sheet 2). In Australia, the future health of immigrants who have originated from such areas, while relatively very small in number, is an important issue for health policymakers and genetic service providers to work with (Metcalfe et al. 2009).

Multi-factorial disorders Genetic disorders that are caused by a combination of factors including genetic mutations and environmental factors; examples are familial breast, ovarian, and bowel cancers.

Another important aspect of understanding genetic conditions is whether they are caused by mutations in one or more genes. Mutations that occur in a single gene can result in **single-gene disorders** and approximately 6000 such conditions have been identified; examples are cystic fibrosis and Huntington's disease (US Department of Energy 2008). Genetic conditions can also occur because of a combination of multiple factors, genetic and environmental, interacting to cause the disorder; these are called **multi-factorial disorders** (US Department of Energy 2008).

Many common conditions like heart disease, cancer, and diabetes are multi-factorial disorders. So too are rare inherited conditions like familial breast, ovarian, and bowel cancers where *one* of the causal factors can be a known genetic mutation. Inherited breast and ovarian cancers constitute only about 5–10% of these cancers overall; 90–95% are therefore associated with other factors that could include internal physiological processes like ageing as well as the person's diet or lifestyle plus exposure to other environmental factors like radiation, viruses, or chemicals. Exposure to the sun is also an environmental factor that is known to damage DNA (CGE 2007j, Fact Sheet 47). Understanding why some people develop health conditions when exposed to particular environmental factors while others do not is an area of great interest to genetic researchers (US Department of Energy 2009) as it promises advancement in more accurate risk assessment and potential intervention strategies.

Genetic DNA testing and screening

One of the major genetic technologies to emerge from the Human Genome Project has been the development of DNA genetic tests, of which more than 1000 are now available (US Department of Energy 2010). Gene or DNA-based tests involve a direct examination of the DNA molecule itself (US Department of Energy 2010) and are based on a clear understanding of genetic mutations that may have occurred. Other genetic tests are based on the examination of chromosomes and the biochemical products of genes (CGE 2007k, Fact Sheet 21). Most DNA genetic tests require tissues from the human body including blood, skin, saliva, or hair follicles; for a prenatal genetic test, a sample of tissue from the embryo, placenta, or amniotic fluid is required (CGE 2007k, Fact Sheet 21; US Department of Energy 2010).

Genetic DNA testing and screening are widely used in many medical, health, and forensic domains. They can be used to diagnose disorders in pregnancies as well as to screen the health and normal development of newborn babies and even embryos in certain circumstances (Metcalfe et al. 2009). Genetic DNA tests can also be undertaken where there is a family history of an inherited condition or to confirm the diagnosis of a person who has symptoms of a specific genetic condition. Genetic tests are used also to confirm the identity of people like refugees who are likely to arrive in countries without formal identification, or of deceased people (ALRC/AHEC 2003).

In addition, genetic tests are available for people with known inherited conditions in their family, to *predict* the future possible development of the condition themselves. Two types of such tests are available and each one yields different information. A test that relates to a multi-factorial condition like familial cancer is called a **predictive genetic test**. In the case of inherited breast and ovarian cancer, for example, a predictive test can establish if the person has inherited changes in specific genes known as BRCA1 and BRCA2, which are associated with developing these cancers. Where the person has inherited the mutations, they will have an increased *risk* of developing the condition in the future, relative to the risk of the general population (CGE 2007j, Fact Sheet 47). Khoury et al. (2000) propose that predictive tests will have strong potential in future public health because many common disorders like diabetes, obesity, hypertension, coronary artery disease, and inflammatory bowel disease are multi-factorial.

Predictive genetic test A DNA test to establish the statistical probability that a person has inherited an increased risk of developing a multi-factorial condition.

A second type of genetic test relates to single-gene disorders like Huntington's disease. Here, the test can establish with certainty whether the person will develop the condition in the future or not, based on whether they have the relevant faulty gene.

Pre-symptomatic genetic test A DNA test to establish if a person has or has not inherited a faulty gene associated with developing a single-gene disorder.

The genetic test for single-gene disorders is called a **pre-symptomatic test** as it can establish if the faulty gene has been inherited or not; where the faulty gene *has* been inherited, the person will eventually develop symptoms of the disease as long as they live to the age of onset. Pre-symptomatic testing can provide more certain genetic information to people than predictive testing, which can give risk-based or statistical probability information only.

Predictive and pre-symptomatic testing present ethical challenges because no genetic conditions can as yet be cured (CGE 2007k, Fact Sheet 21). This means that testing can give people *knowledge* about future risks or disorders but as yet no effective treatments are available. Nonetheless, many people with family histories of inherited illnesses have already undertaken predictive or pre-symptomatic testing. Reasons for testing include wanting to remove the uncertainty about whether the genetic condition is going to develop in the future or not, future planning including career and reproductive decisions, and helping others like offspring clarify their risks (Evers-Kiebooms et al. 2000; Taylor 2004). Where people carry the mutations for familial cancers, there are also possible health benefits associated with having regular health monitoring for the early detection of disease.

Stop and Think

» The field of ethics is broadly associated with questions about what is morally right or wrong. Why might predictive or pre-symptomatic genetic testing be considered an issue for ethical or moral consideration?

Most predictive and pre-symptomatic tests are accessible only through specialist clinical genetics services in Australia (Human Genetics Society of Australasia 2010). Genetic counselling is a requirement before a predictive or pre-symptomatic test result is given; this is because it is considered necessary for people to be fully informed about ethical, legal, and social issues associated with such

Case Study 4.2   Brian

Brian is 20 years old and acutely aware that cancer runs in his family. His grandmother and other relatives died of cancer in the past and Brian's mother died of breast cancer when she was in her late thirties. At that time, Brian was only a young boy and losing his mother was very traumatic for him as well as for his siblings and the whole family. Since then, one of his mother's sisters has died of breast cancer and a second sister has been diagnosed with it. It has recently been established that the BRCA2 gene is the mutation that has been associated with breast and ovarian cancer in Brian's family; this now makes it possible for Brian to have a predictive genetic test to see if he has inherited the BRCA2 gene. If he has, Brian will have increased risks of developing male breast cancer, as well as prostate and pancreatic cancer, in the future.

» *What are some of the issues that Brian might be considering as he decides whether to be tested or not?*

Adapted from CGE 2007l, Fact Sheet 48.

testing. Gaining important genetic knowledge about oneself is a big decision; not only will such information be clearly relevant to the tested person themselves but, because genetics is inherently about relationships between family members, one person's genetic test result may contain implicit information about other family members like siblings and children. Genetic test information is also irreversible: once a person's 'knows' about their future risk of developing a genetic condition, they can no longer 'not know'; further, this is knowledge that they will potentially have to carry with them for many years. Other third parties such as life insurance companies or employers may also be interested in a person's genetic test result; when applying for life insurance in Australia, for example, people are legally required to disclose any genetic test information they have acquired (ALRC/AHEC 2003; Taylor et al. 2008b).

Predictive testing and public health genetics

Predictive genetic testing also has the potential to bring benefits to broader populations. **Public health genomics** aims to improve the health of populations and to prevent disease by using predictive testing on a broad scale (Khoury et al. 2000; Metcalfe et al. 2009); this is called *predictive genomic testing*. Here it is proposed that predictive testing would be used, first, to screen healthy individuals to detect their susceptibility to common multi-factorial diseases like heart disease, obesity, or cancers. Once high-risk people are identified, interventions could be offered that aim to prevent these conditions from developing in the future or lessen their impact; such interventions could include surveillance of identified at-risk people for early detection, advice and education regarding positive health behaviours and lifestyle options, and individually targeted medicines aimed at reducing their chances of developing illnesses in the future. Molster and colleagues (2009) describe this as being a scenario where 'the focus of genetic research and technology will shift from single gene disorders to multi-factorial conditions and from "illness and disease" to "health and risk"'.

> **Public health genomics** An emerging scientific field that aims to understand genetics in the contexts of populations and public health.

Stop and Think

» What are the potential benefits for a healthy person in having a genetic DNA test to predict their future risks of developing conditions like heart disease or diabetes?

» Is *knowing* about health risks enough to guarantee people's health? Where people do have knowledge about health risks, what other factors might prevent them from maximising their health in the future?

There are, however, many challenges if predictive genomic testing is to become a viable population health option. These include the potential cost-effectiveness of DNA-testing on large populations, plus numerous ethical, social, and legal concerns. Hall and colleagues (2004, p. S23) argue that 'our knowledge about most disease genes and their roles is far from sufficient to make reliable predictions about a patient's risk of actually developing a disease. In addition, genomic medicine will create new political, social, ethical and economic challenges that will have to be addressed in the near future'. While Australians appear generally to accept that genes play an important role in determining health, the accuracy of people's understanding of genetics, that is, their genetic literacy, would need to be ensured if predictive genomic testing is to be offered effectively and ethically on a broad scale (Molster et al. 2009; Taylor 2012). A related ethical concern in promoting the potential benefits of predictive testing in large populations is the fact that powerful private commercial imperatives are now driving many of the biotechnologies associated with genetic science. These are multi-billion dollar enterprises that are operating within the global context; as Willis (2005, p. 162) argues, the 'economic and commercial imperative...often masquerades as a technological imperative'.

Willis (2005) gives an interesting analysis of several case studies involving the potential use of predictive testing in public health and raises questions about some of the associated legal and ethical challenges. In one example, he examines melanoma, a gene for which was identified and patented in 1997 by the biotechnology company Myriad Genetics. Holding the patent for the MTS1 (Multiple Tumour Suppressor 1) gene theoretically allows Myriad Genetics to develop a genetic test to identify people in the general population who have inherited an increased susceptibility to developing melanoma; once identified, melanoma-prone people and groups can be advised and guided about appropriate health behaviours they should undertake in order to prevent melanoma from developing. Willis then superimposes this example onto a population like that in the southern Chilean city of Punta Arenas which, in 2000, experienced significant exposure to very high levels of ultraviolet, melanoma-causing radiation, caused by a significantly large hole in the ozone layer. In such a case, is it the responsibility of individuals alone to undertake predictive testing and what happens if people are unable, or refuse, to do so? What is the responsibility of government and public health authorities to ensure the maximum health of their citizens in such a circumstance? Also, whose responsibility is it to meet the costs of this testing as it will be expensive, largely because the company that has patented the melanoma gene and developed the relevant test has commercial imperatives to make a profit? At an even more fundamental level, what are the ethical and legal issues associated with gene patenting? These questions reflect some of the complex and challenging questions to be explored and addressed in regard to predictive genetic testing and their implications for the health outcomes of people in the public health domain: in particular, how to balance the rights and responsibilities of not only individuals but also governments and the broader community as a whole (ALRC 2004; Bunton & Petersen 2005; Willis 2005).

Stop and Think

A patent is a right of protection that is granted to the inventor of a product, method, or process in a field of technology. Holders of patents can maximise the commercial potential of their invention for the patent's duration.

» Compare an invention and the discovery of a natural phenomenon. Are genes inventions or do they represent a naturally occurring phenomenon?

» What might be some of the key arguments for and against the patenting of a gene?

Genetic factors in interaction with cultural, psychological, social, and political factors
Genes, genetic science, and culture

According to Falk (1985), the history of the body is the history of culture. This statement can be extended to argue that the field of human genetic science as we know it today is also a product of culture and history. Science, including biomedical science, has not always occupied the prominent position in society that it does today. Rather, the rise of science in Western society had its origins in the unique historical and cultural conditions of 18th-century Europe where state and religion were disentangled and religion was replaced by science as the primary paradigm for explaining health and illness (Samson 1999). During this time, the belief that good health reflected people's *moral* virtues and their positive alignment with broader cosmic forces was replaced by growing esteem for, and confidence in, scientific reason, rational thinking, and scientific methods. In sociological terms, this is referred to as the emergence of the age of reason or the era of modernity (Grbich 1999; Samson 1999). While we have since moved beyond this period, high esteem for science remains a fundamental characteristic of contemporary Anglo-Western culture and society. This has provided a fertile context for developments in many specialist areas in science including human genetics. It is worth remembering from an historical perspective, however, that biomedical science as a dominant framework for understanding health and illness in Western cultures is less than 200 years old and is therefore relatively young; further, other cultures do not necessarily position biomedical science in the same way (Hardey 1998; Samson 1999).

Human genetic science, it can be argued therefore, occupies a privileged place in contemporary Western culture, as evidenced for example by the allocation of billions of dollars to support the Human Genome Project. Some argue that, as a result, Western culture has become 'geneticised' (Nelkin & Lindee 1995). Samson (1999, pp. 18–19) describes the HGP, for example, as being 'a logical extension of [our] medical obsession with the body as a machine'. Nelkin and Lindee (1995, p. 164) claim that 'genetic explanations appear to locate social problems within the individual rather than in society...They are thus a convenient way of addressing troubling social issues'.

It is argued that, as a result of **geneticisation**, attention and resources are focused on identifying genes and their roles in human health and well-being, at the expense of research and resources being allocated to addressing the many other factors that are known to influence health, well-being, and quality of life (Samson 1999; Petersen & Bunton 2002; Willis 2005). Using breast cancer as an example, Willis (2005, p. 163) argues that the 'emphasis on the 5–10% of cancers which are heritable has the potential to divert attention (and possibly research funding) from research on the 90–95% which are not and for which ongoing research on the environmental and other non-medical determinants remains crucial'.

However, it is important to state that this discussion by no means denies the real and actual burden of genetic disease that affects those individuals and families who have known family histories of genetic illnesses. Such individuals and families require appropriate and accessible genetic and

See Chapter 5 for discussion of the expectations and impact of the Human Genome Project on chronic disease management.

Geneticisation
Explanations of social, cultural, or health phenomena with reference to genetic frameworks.

other specialist health services to address their needs and maximise their health; it is acknowledged also that their hopes for cures and treatments of the conditions in their families lie squarely within the realm of genetic science.

Genes, ethnicity, and beliefs

Sociologists Richards and Ponder (1996) point out that people's lay beliefs about genetics, inheritance, and concepts like genetic risk can vary significantly from scientific explanations and are likely to be influenced by factors like cultural, ethnic, and family beliefs about kinship and inheritance. Understanding the health-related *beliefs* of clients or patients can help health practitioners understand health-related *behaviours*. In the genetics context, the importance for contemporary health practitioners, policymakers, and genetic health services to understand and work respectfully with the different cultural beliefs of people they serve is being increasingly advocated (Pour-Jafari & Pourjafari 2009).

See the discussion in Chapter 1 on beliefs about the nature of health and illness.

In a recent Australian study, Eisenbruch and colleagues (2004) investigated the beliefs and understanding of Chinese-Australian people who had known family histories of hereditary breast, ovarian, and colorectal cancers; this research was partly aimed at identifying potential barriers this group might be experiencing to using genetic counselling services. These researchers found that even where Chinese-Australians were highly acculturated within Australian society and accepted scientific and biomedical explanations for the hereditary cancers in their families, such beliefs coexisted with their traditional Chinese cultural beliefs about genes, inheritance, and genetics. Here, the paternal line was believed to shape the transmission of genes and natural and supernatural forces were believed to be in operation when hereditary cancers developed; the inheritance of cancer was also associated with having offended ancestors or with retribution for ancestors' misdeeds. The researchers concluded that barriers to the use of scientifically based genetic counselling services emanated from an incompatibility between Western and traditional Chinese belief systems. The researchers urged health professionals to take full account of differences in people's cultural and family beliefs regarding concepts like inheritance and genetics, not to be judgmental or stereotyping in their views, and to develop 'culturally competent' approaches to genetic counselling and education when working with Australian-Chinese patients.

A second interesting example of how genetic factors interact with social and cultural factors to determine health outcomes is provided by Lin and her colleagues (2007). In the late 20th century, Native Hawaiian people were recording higher than national average rates for a wide range of health problems including diabetes, obesity, heart disease, cancer, and infectious diseases. Their declining health status was attributed to a combination of cultural factors, dietary changes, and genetic factors. Because of their genetic makeup, Native Hawaiian people (as with other indigenous people) lack a particular enzyme that is required to metabolise fat. With colonisation, however, traditional lands and farming practices were lost and a diet that was built upon the staple food taro, which does not contain any fat or cholesterol, was progressively replaced by other foods. Since the late 1970s, initiatives to address the poor health status of Native Hawaiians have been successfully introduced. These initiatives have largely focused on a revival of traditional Hawaiian values and customs, which in turn have led to measures like the renewed cultivation of taro and the development of the 'Hawaiian Diet' which address the specific requirements of the Hawaiian people because of their genetic makeup.

Genetic makeup and health decisions: Subjective experiences and social locations

Interactions between people's genetic makeup and their health outcomes are not only moderated by particular cultural or ethnic beliefs and backgrounds. Health decisions and outcomes can also be significantly influenced by complex interactions between people's subjective knowledge and understanding of genetics, their age and family-based beliefs and experiences, their gender, the degree of education they have attained, their current personal and family circumstances, the income they have at their disposal, and the resources they can mobilise in order to be proactive about their health (Blaxter 2004). For people who are poor, who have insecure housing, limited income, or opportunity to plan and work for a secure future, proactively seeking information about genetic risks for illnesses that may or may not develop in the future may be a long way down their list of immediate priorities and concerns. Thus, regardless of genetic makeup or family history in these instances, other social factors are likely to dominate to determine people's health decisions and well-being. It is a significant concern that people from lower socio-economic classes or different racial or ethnic backgrounds, and who have less education, may have less access in the future to genetic technologies in the healthcare system (Ponce et al. 2007).

Recently, Molster and colleagues (2009, p. 89) reported findings from a Western Australian study about public knowledge of genetics and health. They found that people who achieved high scores in genetic knowledge were more likely to be younger, to be from a higher socio-economic status, to be women, and to be people who were proactive about seeking information in the health area. They concluded that 'lay knowledge of genetics [was] personal, social, biographical and shared...Evidence shows that people develop *situated* [emphasis added] understandings of genetics through experience [and that this] can impact upon genetic-related decisions and actions'.

Stop and Think

» How might genetic literacy be affected by a person's age? Their socio-economic status? Their gender?

A person's understanding of identified genetic risks they might carry because of their family history can also differ considerably from the scientific or 'objective' assessment of their risks. Even ideas about what constitutes high risk or low risk can vary from one individual to another: the same scientifically established risk of 50% for developing an illness in the future can seem very high to one person but not high at all to someone else. Whether we think a health risk is high or low will usually determine what we do about it! It is essential that health practitioners acknowledge and understand people's lay knowledge and 'subjective' experiences of health risks in order to relate meaningfully to them and to provide health services that meet their needs (Sullivan 2003). In the genetics context, understanding how people *subjectively* experience their genetic risks can be a key to helping practitioners make sense of what might seem like people's apparent failure to take up 'logical' genetic service options, like genetic counselling, screening, and predictive or pre-symptomatic genetic testing (Leggett 2009).

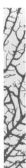

Mythbuster

1   What societal values and assumptions underpin the following two statements:

Undertaking a predictive genetic test to identify risks for developing future disorders is a logical *course of action to take to ensure one's health.*

Undertaking a predictive test is a course of action that people should *do if they are acting responsibly.*

2   To date, only about 5–20% of at-risk people have voluntarily undertaken pre-symptomatic testing for the serious genetic condition Huntington's disease in the 18 years that such testing has been available (Evers-Kiebooms et al. 2000). For other conditions also, such as inherited cancers, uptake appears variable (de Snoo et al. 2008).

»   Why do you think the uptake of predictive genetic testing by people with family histories of inherited conditions might not be as high as anticipated?

At face value, lower-than-expected usage of genetic tests might seem difficult to understand because there are many 'logical' reasons why an at-risk person could, and even *should*, be tested for serious conditions that they might develop in the future (Bunton & Petersen 2005). However, a scientifically established genetic risk is only one important part of the knowledge that at-risk people are working with at any particular time; many other aspects of people's lived experiences come into play and are interacting to guide and determine health decisions and behaviours. For example, in research about the beliefs of people at risk for developing the serious genetic condition Huntington's disease, Cox and McKellin (1999, p. 641) concluded that 'while Mendelian genetics may provide a coherent framework for calculating the odds of inheriting a disorder...they do not recognise the liveable framework...for understanding risk as it emerges within everyday life'. Taylor (2004) showed that even when people had a 50% risk of developing Huntington's disease, they considered a wide range of issues when deciding whether or not to have a pre-symptomatic test. They considered, for example, how much they felt they needed the test information, or could cope with it, at any particular time (bearing in mind there is no current treatment for HD following a positive test result) and how much they felt others in their family could benefit from, or cope with, them being tested. People's past and ongoing experiences of HD in the family also influenced their thinking about whether or not to be tested, even when they felt they had social or moral obligations to do so. Other researchers have shown that people who have undertaken testing can have very resilient personalities and very well-developed coping strategies (see Evers-Kiebooms et al. 2000). All of this demonstrates how factors like genetic makeup, psychological factors, and family experiences can work together to influence people's health decisions about genetics, and ultimately, their health outcomes.

Case Study 4.3   Kylie

Kylie is at 50% risk of developing Huntington's disease. She is 18 years old and her mother Jenny, who is 40 years old, is in a nursing home because with HD she can no longer live at home. Jenny's quality of life is now very limited and it is likely that she will live only for several more years as the disease is progressing rapidly. Kylie still lives with her father Doug and younger sister Anna, who is aged 15. Kylie and Anna's upbringing was difficult because no one knew for a long time what was wrong with their mother; there was no history of HD in the family because Jenny had been adopted as a baby and it took a long time to unravel the family history. Once Jenny's HD diagnosis became clear, however, Kylie and Anna's 50% risk for developing HD also became clear. Now that Kylie has turned 18, two of her aunts are urging her to take the pre-symptomatic test for HD; they say she has a responsibility to find out if she has the faulty HD gene or not, so that she can plan her life responsibly, be fully honest with any possible future partners, and also know whether or not to have any children. In her heart of hearts though, Kylie is afraid of being tested. Going through testing and knowing there is no available treatment if the result is positive seems too hard to cope with emotionally and its value in her life seems unclear. Kylie also secretly worries that, because her physical appearance is very like her mother's, she is going to get a positive test result; she often tries to remind herself though that the clinical geneticist the family saw in the past specifically said that whether a person develops HD had nothing to do with how much they might look like their parent who had HD. Kylie also thinks of the impact that a positive test result could have on Anna and feels she just couldn't put her sister through this. As the older sister, Kylie has tried hard to make sure Anna's life has been as normal as possible, even though they have both experienced the heartache of watching both their mother and father trying to deal with HD over the years. Kylie would like to go to university soon and hopes to enjoy at least a period of her life when HD is not pressing in on her all the time; if she has inherited the faulty HD gene, she knows that symptoms of HD could start within the next ten years. Kylie also wants to visit her mother as much as she can but knows the road ahead will be difficult as her mother continues to deteriorate; Kylie knows she and Anna will be losing their mother in the not too distant future.

» *From a scientific perspective, Kylie's genetic risk for developing Huntington's disease is a clear 50%. Compare this with her subjective or lived experience of having a 50% risk. Discuss how the genetic risk that is part of Kylie's genetic makeup is being influenced and mediated by her psychological makeup and family experiences to determine her actions in regard to being tested.*

Genetic makeup and health behaviour

Simply having health-related information does not necessarily guarantee a change in someone's health behaviour or health outcomes. This is clear in relation to current issues like alcohol or drug overuse, unsafe sex, cigarette smoking, or drink-driving where a lot of health promotion and education occurs that is aimed at increasing people's knowledge and awareness about these issues. Most people when asked *know* that these practices are potentially bad for their health, but knowledge alone does not necessarily change their risky behaviours (Keleher & Murphy 2004). Similarly, people might know they have genetic risks or are susceptible to developing inherited disorders in the future but this does not necessarily result in a decision to have a predictive genetic test or even to engage in health behaviours like regular breast or bowel screening. Such decisions and behaviours can also change over time; people's views often change, for example when they have children. Health beliefs, decisions, and behaviours are dynamic: they change over time and with changes in circumstances. Best professional health practice is built on understanding that health is determined by complex and dynamic interactions of many factors and by adopting a *person-in-context* approach to understanding and working with people who use health services (Taylor et al. 2008a).

Genes and gender

A person's gender can interact with their genetic makeup and other factors to determine health decisions and outcomes at any given point in time (Newman et al. 2002; Charles & Walters 2008; Taylor 2008b). From a sociological perspective, a person's 'gender' is socially and culturally constructed and relates to the social notions of 'being feminine' and 'being masculine' and the social roles, behaviours, and expectations that are associated with these categories (Connell 2002; Broom 2009). 'Sex' on the other hand is about a person's biological characteristics and is determined by having an XX or an XY chromosome which then codes for differences in the hormonal and physiological features of males and females (Keleher & Murphy 2004).

See also the discussion of the social construction of health in Chapters 1 & 12.

In the genetics context, gender can influence how people understand, experience, and respond to the idea of inheritance, to having identified genetic risks, or to making a decision about genetic testing. Richards (1995) describes how men and women in Western cultures adopt different roles in families in relation to family histories of illness. Women in particular appear to automatically assume responsibility for keeping information on family history. Thus, women generally take up roles as 'genetic housekeepers' and 'kinkeepers' in families, actively seeking information about issues of inheritance that might be relevant and documenting family history; this seems to apply even where a genetic condition might affect male family members only (Richards 1995). Women also often act as orchestrators for family members in the healthcare context, proactively organising healthcare appointments for family members and negotiating the 'interface' between individuals, families, and healthcare service providers (Stacey 1995). This is consistent with the broader picture of 'gendered health' in Australia where women are generally more proactive than their male counterparts in seeking health information and in using healthcare services (Broom 2009).

Women appear also to have predictive genetic testing more frequently than men, including where genetic conditions are inherited equally by men and women (Hayden 2003; Gaff et al. 2006; Taylor 2008a). This could be attributed to differences in how men and women perceive and respond to risk and threat in general terms, as well as to genetic risk in particular (Shiloh 1996; Sarafino 2006). Women may also undertake genetic testing more often because they are said to have greater psychological capacity to cope with the emotional challenges of testing (Marteau & Croyle 1998; Hayden 2003) and because they are more closely involved with reproductive issues and possible risks to offspring (Sarafino 2006; Charles & Walters 2008; Taylor 2008b). But there are no biological explanations for such differences; rather the explanation lies in the broader social and cultural context of how men and women in Western society are socialised (Connell 2002). However, thinking about the differences in men and women's health behaviour as if they represent a simple constant dichotomy or binary is not necessarily useful either, because not all men nor all women behave in exactly the same way with regard to any health issue, including the decision to undertake a genetic test. Once again, a health determinants approach is based on understanding that a person's health decisions and outcomes at any one time emanate from interactions between their unique genetic characteristics, their gender, and other factors like cultural beliefs, age, class, income, and occupation (Taylor et al. 2008a).

Genes and the socio-political context

On the broadest scale, a person's genetic makeup can also be seen to interact with societal and political factors to significantly influence health-related decisions, behaviour, and ultimately, health outcomes. The fear of being discriminated against by insurance companies or employers on the basis of genetic makeup, for example, is consistently documented as a concern and disincentive for people to undertake predictive or pre-symptomatic genetic testing (Taylor et al. 2008b; Taylor 2012). **Genetic discrimination** is defined as the unfair treatment of an otherwise healthy person on the basis of their genetic characteristics (Taylor et al. 2008a). Concerns about genetic discrimination in Australia and elsewhere have been shown to be realistic because multiple accounts of such discrimination have already been documented. People have been discriminated against or treated unfairly in Australia by life insurers and employers, within family relationships, and in access to health services (Taylor et al. 2008b). Before undertaking predictive or pre-symptomatic genetic testing, individuals and families now receive direct advice from genetic professionals about the possibility of discrimination, especially regarding life insurance (Human Genetics Society of Australasia 2008), and such information is also readily available on genetic education and support group websites (CGE 2007m, Fact Sheet 23a).

> **Genetic discrimination**
> The unfair treatment of an asymptomatic person on the basis of their genetic characteristics or makeup.

Under the *Disability Discrimination Act 1992* in Australia, it is illegal to discriminate against people on the basis of any future disorders they might develop including those associated with genetic factors (Human Rights Commission 2011). It is not illegal in Australia, however, for life insurers to discriminate against people on the basis of genetic test information, although many people regard this as unfair because people cannot be held responsible for the genes they have inherited (ALRC/AHEC 2003). Decisions relating to socio-legal issues like this are made at the highest level of society and its institutions and are therefore political in nature. While Australia currently takes this approach, not every country does. In the UK, for example, the Association of British Insurers established a moratorium in 2001 against the use of predictive genetic test results for purposes of getting life, critical illness, and income protection insurance, provided the policies do not exceed capped amounts of money; this moratorium has now been extended to 2014 (Montia 2008). A person with a positive genetic test result for Huntington's disease in the UK could therefore successfully apply for life or other insurances at capped levels, thus ensuring a sense of financial and emotional security for the person and their family; in Australia this is not currently possible. The USA recently responded to concerns about genetic discrimination by introducing a special piece of legislation called the *Genetic Information Non-discrimination Act (GINA) of 2008* which aims to provide baseline protection for citizens against genetic discrimination, although people remain unprotected from discrimination in various other domains (Department of Health and Human Services 2009). These are examples of how institutions within society have the power to establish what will be legal and acceptable, or illegal and thus not acceptable, for people who live in that society. It demonstrates how people's health-related decisions and behaviours regarding their genetic makeup and genetic risks can interact with very broad societal and political factors over which they have no control, to determine and influence their health and well-being.

Summary

Genetic makeup is an important determinant of people's health, growth, and development; it operates at biological and molecular levels within the human body and has unfolding influence throughout the life course. It is important to remember that genetic factors do not in themselves determine health or operate in isolation: a person's genetic makeup is constantly mediated and moderated through interaction with environmental, cultural, social, and psychological factors to affect health decisions, behaviours, and outcomes. The Human Genome Project and subsequent discoveries have significantly increased scientific knowledge and understanding about how genes, chromosomes, and genetic mutations operate to influence heredity, health, and illness. Genetic tests are also being increasingly used in healthcare to diagnose conditions and establish people's genetic risks. To undertake a genetic test can be a complex decision: it is potentially influenced by factors like gender, family, or cultural beliefs and subjective experience, as well as broader commercial and political factors that can determine whether tests are available and accessible. The potential for people with family histories of genetic illness or genetic test results to experience genetic discrimination also reflects how broad social, legal, and political factors may interact with people's knowledge about their genetic makeup to influence their health decisions and outcomes. For healthcare to be effective, relevant, and meaningful to the people it services, contemporary health practitioners should understand and acknowledge that people are more than the sum of their genes; genetic makeup is one health determinant only, operating in conjunction with multiple other factors. Assessing and responding to people in their multiple contexts underpins best professional practice.

Tutorial exercises

1   Watch the 1997 science fiction film *Gattaca*. What are the implications for people and society more broadly of adopting genetic determinism as a guiding principle?

2   Bring some media pieces about genes and recent developments in human genetic science to your tutorial. Analyse and discuss with your tutorial members the language and messages contained in the media pieces and the underlying assumptions about genes as health determinants.

3   Discuss in small groups what the 'lived experience' of being 'at risk' of developing a genetic disorder might be like. How might a person's age or level of income influence their lived experiences of being at risk?

Further reading

Australian Law Reform Commission and Australian Health Ethics Committee (2003). *Essentially yours: The protection of human genetic privacy in Australia.* <www.alrc.gov.au/publications/report-96>.

Blaxter, M. (2004). *Health*. Cambridge: Polity Press.

Bunton, R., & Petersen, A. (eds) (2005). Genetics and governance: An introduction. In *Genetic governance: Health, risk and ethics in the biotech era*. London: Routledge Press, 155–70.

Marteau, T., & Richards, M. (eds) (1995). *The troubled helix: Social and psychological implications of the new human genetics*. Cambridge: Cambridge University Press.

Nelkin, D., & Lindee, M.S. (1995). *The DNA mystique: The gene as a cultural icon*. New York: W.H. Freeman & Company.

Petersen, A., & Bunton, R. (2002). *The new genetics and the public's health*. London: Routledge Press.

Richards, M. (1995). Families, kinship and genes. In T. Marteau & M. Richards (eds), *The troubled helix: Social and psychological implications of the new human genetics*. Cambridge: Cambridge University Press, 249–73.

Sullivan, M. (2003). The new subjective medicine: Taking the patient's point of view on healthcare and health. *Social Science and Medicine*, 56, 1595–604.

Websites

http://aihw.gov.au/publications/aus/ah10/11374-c01.pdf

This government website for the Australian Institute of Health and Welfare (AIHW) provides a comprehensive overview of health and current health issues in the Australian population. *Australia's Health 2010* is the most recent report available.

<www.genetics.com.au>

The NSW Health Centre for Genetics Education website provides reliable and up-to-date Australian-based information for students, health professionals and members of the general community regarding human genetics, genetic conditions, and genetic testing.

<www.hgsa.org.au>

The Human Genetics Society of Australasia (HGSA) provides a forum for human genetics-related professional disciplines in Australia. Their website gives a range of information relevant to human genetics and the provision of services in Australia.

<www.ornl.gov/sci/techresources/Human_Genome/home.shtml>

This website is one of the US Department of Energy (DOE) genomic websites and provides up-to-date scientific information and reports regarding the ongoing Human Genome Project.

<www.councilforresponsiblegenetics.org/Help/About.aspx>

The Council for Responsible Genetics website is an interesting and comprehensive website which aims to provide accurate and up-to-date information for the broader community regarding key social, ethical, and environmental implications of genetic technologies.

5 | Chronic illness and the genome

Chris L. Peterson and
Evan Willis

TOPICS COVERED

This chapter covers the following topics:
- definitions of chronic illness
- explanations of biological, social, behavioural, and environmental determinants of chronic disease
- explanations of the Human Genome Project
- discussions on the extent to which the Genome has offered cures for chronic disease

KEY TERMS

Behavioural factors
Biological basis
Chronic disease
Disease genetics
Environmental determinants
Gene mutations

Gene therapy
Genetic reductionism
Human Genome Project
Ideology
Social determinants
Stress

Introduction

The average age of the population is increasing, particularly in the developed world. The extent of chronic disease has also been increasing as the population gets older. It has been argued that 'deteriorating health leads to a greater likelihood of economic inactivity late in a person's working life' (Peterson & Murphy 2010, p. 623). Further, Peterson and Murphy argue that in countries such as Australia, the USA, and the UK chronic illness is a major factor in retirement from the workforce, and as a consequence a high cost the community has to bear. The Intergenerational Report (2010) argues that there will be extensive population growth over the next generation or more and there will be substantial increases in costs such as increased healthcare.

Generally, chronic conditions are characterised by having complex causal factors. These result from a number of risk factors: they have an extended period in latency, the illness runs over a long time, and there may be some impairment of function and/or resulting disability. Most chronic conditions are not completely cured. Some chronic diseases, cardiovascular disease for example, can be life-threatening, and others may need intensive management, for example diabetes (AIHW 2010a). In other cases, disease persists through a person's life (e.g. arthritis) but may not be a cause of death.

Dimensions of chronic disease

Chronic disease refers to an illness that is persistent, lasts a long time, and may result in death (Chronic Illness Alliance 2010). Charmaz (1991) refers to several types of chronic illness experience, from mild, which has only small effects on lifestyle, to the type of illness that rips a person's world apart, where a person is severely compromised, their ability to support themselves diminished or not possible, and their family and friendship circle severely inhibited.

> **Chronic disease**
> A long-term illness that has complex causes and multiple risk factors, and in most cases has no immediate or long-term cure.

Less than 100 years ago, people with chronic conditions were labelled 'incurables' or 'chronics'. According to Walker and colleagues (2003, p. 2), 'they sought treatment from medical practitioners, apothecaries or others until they were no longer able to work and their money ran out'. If their families were not able to take care of them and hospitals would not, they could be sent against their will to public institutions. More recently, however, Walker and colleagues (2003, p. 2) suggest that 'people with chronic illnesses have found themselves both the preserve of highly specialized physician care and a group vilified in politics as contributing to increased health budgets'.

Some chronic conditions have been known about for centuries, such as diabetes and arthritis. However, medicine has been dominated by acute care for a very long time and while chronic disease has been rapidly increasing, there has been less focus on it than for acute conditions. Overall, the total number of people dying from chronic diseases worldwide is twice that compared to those who die from infectious diseases (WHO 2011c). The World Health Organization cites globalisation, urbanisation, and the ageing of populations as major contributing factors.

This chapter will look at major chronic diseases occurring over time. It will examine biological determinants, the influence of social factors on prevalence, and behavioural and environmental factors found to be conducive to the development and growth of chronic diseases. The impact of the

Human Genome Project on chronic diseases will be also examined. It has ushered in new medical ways to develop potential cures for a number of diseases; yet for how many chronic conditions have these met expectations of success?

What are chronic diseases?

Most recently, chronic disease has focused on 12 conditions that had previously been identified by the National Public Health Partnership: ischaemic heart disease (known also as coronary heart disease); stroke; depression; lung cancer and colorectal cancer; arthritis; type 2 diabetes; asthma; chronic obstructive pulmonary disease; osteoporosis; oral disease; and chronic kidney disease (AIHW 2010b).

In Australia, cancer is the leading cause of death (about 19%), closely followed by cardiovascular disease (16%) and mental disorders (13%). Diabetes is expected to become the leading cause of disease burden in little more than a decade. For 25–64-year-olds, coronary heart disease for men and breast cancer for women are leading causes of death. For older Australians, heart disease followed by stroke and cancer are the leading causes. Consequently, for Australians over 24 years of age, chronic illnesses are by far the largest causes of death as well as the bases of the disease burden (AIHW 2010a). Tamlyn (2003) has reported in a study of rural and regional Victoria (Australia) on the cost of having a chronic illness. For those with low incomes even the cost of medications and some treatments such as by allied health providers is a significant burden for some individuals and families with a member with a chronic illness.

The paper *Preventing chronic disease: A strategic framework* (National Public Health Partnership 2001, p. 1) argues that 'the health priority areas and associated conditions are responsible for approximately three quarters of the total burden of disease in Australia'. There are many common risk factors, and much of the burden of disease could be prevented, or the effects modified, through early detection or prevention, therefore reducing the reliance and overuse of healthcare services. In Australia the National Chronic Disease Strategy of 2005 (National Health Priority Action Council 2006) focused on approaches for prevention, treatment, and community integration. The Australian Institute of Health and Welfare (2008a) recommends that prevention, early identification and treatment, continuity of prevention and care, and self-management be carried out. Over the past decade, there has been a growth in self-management and related education programs for people with a number of chronic diseases (Cooper et al. 2008; Hoey et al. 2008).

Determinants of chronic illness

There are many factors contributing to health and well-being: 'they result from complex interplay between societal, environmental, socioeconomic, biological and lifestyle factors, nearly all of which can be modified to some extent by healthcare and other interventions' (AIHW 2010a, p. 63). Biological factors include genetics and ageing. Socio-economic factors include education, type of employment, income, wealth, and housing. Health behaviours include smoking, drinking alcohol, physical activity, and diet. In addition, environmental factors include air quality, the spread of pesticides and other chemicals, and related factors. All of these may exacerbate attempts at prevention and treatment of chronic disease.

Biological factors

Biological factors are those that affect health through genetics and as a result of ageing. In terms of genetics, an individual has traits passed on from parents which can lead to risk of serious chronic disease or death (AIHW 2010c). The later part of this chapter has a detailed discussion of biological factors, in particular the role of genetics in chronic disease.

> See Chapter 4 for a discussion of the role of genetics in illness.

Ben-Shlomo and Kuh (2002) present biological factors in relation to childhood asthma, and how they may interact with social and epidemiological factors. Chang and colleagues (2008) also report that a relationship has been found between biological markers and chronic diseases such as hypertension, type 2 diabetes, and heart disease. The incidence of chronic disease increases with ageing. Stoppard (2010) contends that more must be done by government about the increasing health issues of the growing ageing population. Geithner and McKenney (2010) argue that physical exercise is one of the key ingredients to reducing the risk of chronic disease.

A Canadian study (Griffith et al. 2010) found that foot problems, cognitive impairment, heart disease, arthritis, and vision had the biggest effect on functional ability for older people. In addition, Brownie (2006) also reports that reduced nutrition intake for older people can exacerbate the the onset of chronic illness and affect the management of some chronic conditions. Adams and colleagues (2009) report that older people with chronic illnesses tend to rely more on the use of complementary and alternative forms of medicine.

Social factors

There is increasing agreement in the research community that the **social determinants** of chronic disease are influenced by experiences such as chronic *stress* due to economic hardship, racism, a lack of physical activity, and poor nutrition (Taylor & Bury 2007; Blas & Karup 2010). Based on the WHO Commission's Final Report on the social determinants of health (WHO CSDH 2008), Hawe (2009) argues that social determinants and their effects on chronic disease onset can too easily be dismissed as ideology. The public may acknowledge structural factors such as poverty as important but consider personal health to be more closely related to health behaviours.

> **Social determinants** Socio-economic factors such as income, education, and location that affect the incidence of chronic illness.

Most other determinants such as behavioural and environmental are closely related to social determinants (such as social class) and the inequities manifest there. Denton and colleagues (2004) use the vehicle of gender to examine the interaction between different determinants of chronic disease (see also Vlassoff 2007). Groake and colleagues (2005) also examined the relationships between several variables and disease outcomes for women with rheumatoid arthritis. Other studies have identified the importance of social and structural factors such as poverty in a person being susceptible to mental health problems (Kazi et al. 2006).

The social determinants of health and therefore of chronic disease is not a new idea. Metzler (2007, p. 2) contends: 'It is actually an idea that has been part of the public health story when concerned practitioners noted the need to improve poverty, sanitation, and other living conditions to improve health.' The rapid increase of chronic diseases such as obesity in the early 21st century has heralded the need to reduce risk factors as public health strategies. The advent of evidence-based

See Chapters 1 and 12
for discussion of the
social construction of
health.

medicine also addressed social factors contributing to disparities in health, including gaps in mortality, for factors such as socio-economic position, race, and indigenous status. Harvey (2006) has argued for adopting public health approaches to chronic illness. Much can be learnt about chronic illness from the history of public health (Leeder 2007); reduction in inequality and poverty are required.

Currently not on the public health agenda is reform in education, transport, and housing to improve health. Metzler (2007) refers to the need to collect public health data on social conditions, and argues that there needs to be more understanding of the concept of empowerment to deal with chronic disease. Metzler (2007, p. 2) puts it that 'developing reciprocal, trusting and equitable relationships with communities is a more effective strategy'.

Wilkinson and Marmot (2003, p. 7) argue that 'even in the most affluent countries, people who are less well off have substantially less life expectancies and more illnesses than the rich'. This social injustice and these differences have drawn scientific attention to some of the most important determinants of health. According to the AIHW (2010a), disentangling the effects of social and other determinants and health outcomes is complex, largely because it can be difficult to argue the causal direction. In Australia, living standards are generally increasing each year, but the gap between those who are wealthy and those below the poverty line is widening. Australia is an advanced neoliberal economy, as are many other developed economies such as the USA, Europe, and the UK. In each of these economies the gap between the wealth of rich and poor is getting wider, and has led to wider differences in health with increased disadvantage for the poor (Coburn 2000; Navarro 2007). This also includes a greater propensity for those at the poorer end to have a higher incidence of chronic illnesses.

Glover and colleagues (2004) undertook an Australian study of the socio-economic gradient of chronic illness. They found that diabetes and circulatory diseases for the 25–64-year-old group occurred mostly among poorer groups. For older people (over 64 years), the greatest inequalities were found for behavioural and mental health problems, diabetes, and diseases of the circulatory system. They also found that risk factors match inequalities, particularly for smoking and lack of exercise.

Risks for chronic disease based on social disadvantage, socio-economic status, or ethnicity are avoidable. Metzler (2007, p. 2) argues that poverty, for example, is responsible for 'multiple disparate health outcomes through a variety of pathways, including reduced social standing and limited access to healthy food and safe neighborhoods'. Unwin and colleagues (2010) argue that out of 285 million people worldwide with diabetes, 209 million (or 73%) live either in low- or middle-income countries. And in countries with high incomes, the prevalence of type 2 diabetes is most common among the poorest people. While the incidence of diabetes is relatively high in some wealthy countries, people's ability to manage it is far greater than in poorer countries (see Buckner-Brown et al. 2011).

In their study of the precursors for cardiovascular disease in the British civil service, Marmot and colleagues (1991) found that there was an increase in cardiovascular disease among those lower down the occupational hierarchy. In their ground-breaking study in the UK, they found a strong association between social class (as determined by level of employment) and health/illness (note Caan 2010). The lower the grade of employment, the higher the risk. In particular, ischaemia, angina, chronic bronchitis symptoms, and related disorders were more prevalent in the lower classes. Marmot and colleagues found that a lower level of employment was characterised by routine work and a lack of support, both of which were conducive to stress. This in turn led to a risk of conditions such as ischaemic heart disease and other chronic cardiovascular conditions. The relationship between lower classes and the propensity to develop chronic diseases has been demonstrated in a number of other studies: for example between socio-economic status and exercising control at work; stress also affects the onset of chronic illnesses (see Karasek et al. 1981; Marmot et al. 1991; Peterson 1999).

Karasek and colleagues (1981) demonstrated that cardiovascular disease was more pronounced in men who worked at lower-level occupations who had restrictions on job latitude and opportunities for control. Peterson (1999) argues that those working at lower occupational levels exercise less control and when under pressure this results in increased cortisol levels. This can lead to more depression, reduced ability of the immune system to function effectively, and a resulting susceptibility to chronic illness (see also Wahlqvist 2002). Wilkinson (1997b) also argues that those least well off have physiological disadvantages based on poorer housing, inadequate heating, poorer diets, and pollution. There is also the indirect effect of stress, including smoking, poor eating, and drinking, all of which lead to chronic physical and emotional stress.

Chronic stress 'wears us down and wears us out' (Wilkinson & Pickett 2009, p. 86). It can depress immune systems, growth in children, ovulation in women, erectile function in men, and contribute to digestive disorders in all.

Behavioural factors

Health behaviours are important to developing chronic diseases: these arise from individual makeup, cultural and family factors, and socio-economic status and opportunities. These largely lifestyle factors include quality of diet and nutritional intake, level of physical inactivity, misuse of alcohol, smoking, high blood pressure, high blood cholesterol, and excessive weight or obesity.

The extent of these risky **behavioural factors** can be seen in that 17% of people over 14 years of age in Australia smoke tobacco and 10% consume alcohol at a risky level; at least half the 25-year-old and older population have high blood cholesterol, 30% have high blood pressure, and 60% carry excessive weight (AIHW 2010c).

Behavioural factors
Risk factors such as diet, exercise, smoking, and alcohol consumption and their effects on the incidence of chronic illness.

According to the AIHW, smoking is the single most important factor associated with death and ill health in Australia, with lung cancer being a major preventable health condition. In 2004–05, the total cost of smoking to the community was $31.5 billion. Alcohol consumption is a major risk factor for a range of chronic conditions, namely some cancers, stroke, and coronary heart disease, and has been strongly associated with depression and other mental health states. The total cost of alcohol consumption in 2004–05 in Australia was $15.3 billion (AIHW 2010a). Physical inactivity is associated with a number of chronic conditions, for example coronary heart disease. Exercise is seen to be protective against arthritis and type 2 diabetes; it can also moderate the effects of coronary disease. Type of work performed can moderate some chronic diseases, with sedentary jobs posing the greatest threat to health. Illicit drug abuse is problematic in Australia and is increasing in frequency and effect. It has strong associations with depression and other mental health states. Dietary intake is associated with some chronic diseases also. The recommended intake is from five food groups (vegetables and legumes, fruit, cereals, dairy, and meat (or alternatives)). Incorrect fat and nutrient intake can exacerbate certain chronic conditions such as type 2 diabetes. Unprotected sex can lead to conditions such as certain kinds of cancers (anal and cervical). In addition, a lack of sun protection can lead to skin cancers, with

Australia having a very high incidence of melanoma (AIHW 2010a, b). Many of these behaviours are linked to social and structural location. For example, young people with chronic mental health problems can be taught how to engage in health-enhancing behaviours (Gorski et al. 2004), which may include adopting behaviours associated with lifestyles of higher socio-economic status.

Stop and Think

» To what degree do you think your behaviours (especially risk factors) are associated with your social location (class or socio-economic status)?

» How might changing socio-economic status/location change pressure on people to display certain types of health risk behaviours?

» How may this be done?

Environmental factors

Environmental determinants Effects of factors in both the physical and social environment. These include air quality related to pollution, chemicals, water quality, and outcomes of climate change and global warming.

See Chapters 1, 9 & 10 for environmental factors affecting health.

According to the AIHW (2010b), the environment includes not only physical surrounds but social surrounds, referred to as social capital. Baum (2008) examines the relationship between public health and social capital—it is often the lack of community and social relationships that make dealing with chronic diseases so difficult. Other **environmental determinants** include the quality of food, water, and air, the health and safety of the built environment, and the quality of social relations and relationships, including in the local community (Auffrey 2008).

One of the major causes of health disadvantage for cardiovascular disease and respiratory conditions results from air pollutants and chemical exposure in the workplace. In some cases, chemical contaminants can have an effect on chronic illness and can exacerbate conditions such as chronic respiratory disorders. Both natural and artificial air pollutants can have an effect, particularly on conditions such as asthma. In Australia, people with asthma are known to suffer greatly from air pollution caused by bushfires, and metropolitan air pollution levels (from industry, cars, and so on). The air pollutants of most concern are particulates and ozone, both of which are related to high temperatures (AIHW 2010a). There is also an important impact on childhood asthma from the bacterial community in household dust (Maier et al. 2010). Coal miners are particularly vulnerable. Breathing excessive coal dust often leads to symptoms of 'black lung disease' (Human Diseases and Conditions 2010). Water quality also has an impact.

Climate change and global warming are two important issues for health. Human activities contribute through greenhouse gases, aerosols, and clouds. There are both direct and indirect effects on health. Direct are the number of extreme weather events such as bushfires and floods, exacerbating current illnesses and making some people more vulnerable, particularly older people. Indirect effects are increased exposure to air pollution and food and water that is contaminated. Finally, in Australia the living environment is primarily urban and this leads to reduced physical activity, a risk factor for type 2 diabetes and cardiovascular disease. It also promotes greater air pollution, increasing the risk of asthma and related symptoms.

See also Chapters 1, 9 & 10 for environmental determinants of health.

Stress and the onset and development of chronic disease

There are complex associations between stress and the ability of the immune system to protect the individual from illness or disease. Schneiderman and colleagues (2005) argue the importance of the stress response, triggered by events in personal/or work life that are negative or cause strain. If these negative events are constant and persist they can damage health (see Selye 1956). The relationship between stressors and disease is influenced by the nature and strength of the stressors and by the biological vulnerability (i.e. constitutional and genetic factors) and coping resources people have (also based on their socio-economic status and availability of personal and social resources) (Mechanic 1974; Peterson 1999).

Schneiderman and colleagues (2005) argue that the ability to influence and mitigate the effects of stress-related disorders can affect the development, course, and impact of chronic diseases. Riso and colleagues (2002) also refer to the strength of the stress reaction, particularly through adolescence, in affecting the onset of chronic mental health disorders, especially depression. Brooks (2008) maintains that stress for those with chronic diseases can be reduced by what is called health-related hardiness and this can affect the outcomes of illnesses.

What has been learnt about the precursors to chronic illness is that a complex range of factors is responsible for the increase in chronic disease in the population. Lifestyle factors and stress associated with these contribute, as well as biological and environmental factors. However, as a backdrop, social factors such as class or socio-economic status, and the income people earn, form very important conditions that can affect the influence of other determinants.

Case Study 5.1   Ischaemic heart disease

Shisana (2010) argues that a relatively few main risk factors contribute to most mortality and disability for major lifestyle chronic illnesses such as cardiovascular disease, some types of cancer, and type 2 diabetes. Main contributing factors were elevated fat levels including serum cholesterol levels, high blood pressure, physical inactivity, being overweight or obese, a poor diet, and using tobacco.

Ischaemic heart disease is one of the major chronic conditions in Australia. It has been associated with age, a sedentary lifestyle, socio-economic status (type of job performed and level of job in the status hierarchy), and poor diet. The US Department of Health and Human Services National Institute of Health (2011) argue that cardiovascular disease is the main cause of disability and death in the USA. A number of environmental factors have not been clearly identified as contributing, but those that have include air pollution, some pesticides, and heavy metals. They maintain that studies are needed to assess the continuing impact of these environmental factors in early childhood and adolescence on the development of heart disease in adulthood.

More research is needed to identify the mechanisms contributing to heart disease: the effects of passive smoking on blood vessel cells of children and the extent to which obesity expands this effect. Furthermore, the extent to which cholesterol metabolism is influenced by pesticide exposure needs investigation. And finally, there is a need to examine the impact of arsenic exposure on vascular function.

Case Study 5.2   Type 2 diabetes

The risk of getting type 2 diabetes is much higher for those living a Western lifestyle (e.g. having a diet high in fats and low in carbohydrates). In the USA, for example, ethnic groups adopting Western diets are much more at risk of getting type 2 diabetes (American Diabetes Association 2011).

More than a decade ago Glasgow and colleagues (1999) proposed that diabetes needed to be treated as a public health problem, due to the enormous social and personal costs of uncontrolled diabetes, including complications, its effects on patient quality of life, and also its utilisation of healthcare resources. For a long time, diabetes was treated with acute episode resources in the healthcare system that were not suited to the disease and were also very costly. A population-based provision of resources is proposed which many developed healthcare systems either have or are adopting. This means that the individual with diabetes, their family, healthcare team, and community are linked in the development and delivery of preventive and treatment services. Epidemiology and population health, public health, and related disciplines are now working together more. The fairly recent development of self-management programs and the use of expert patients for chronic conditions such as diabetes is an example of the development of this more integrated approach (see Taylor & Bury 2007; Hoey et al. 2008).

Genetic factors

The debate about the extent to which aspects of what might broadly be called human existence are more the result of nature or nurture is a debate that has raged for decades if not centuries. Is how a child turns out more the result of the card they draw in the genetic lottery of life or the influence of environmental factors? Many trees have been felled to provide the paper to debate these issues!

Human Genome Project A research program in molecular biology to map the genes on the 23 different chromosomes.

See Chapter 4 on genetic factors influencing health.

Advances in the genetic understanding of disease have been associated with the **Human Genome Project**. The 'Genomic Age' was ushered in by the announcement in 2003 that the project of mapping the human genome had been completed. It occurred almost 50 years to the day after Watson and Crick announced that they had identified the double helix structure of DNA (see Lorentz et al. 2002). These rapid developments in molecular genetics, which have collectively become known as the Human Genome Project, have resulted in the completion of the task of mapping the human genetic code. The HGP is an international research program in molecular biology, based in the USA, to identify and map the 30,000–35,000 genes on the 23 different human chromosomes, and sequence the approximately 3 billion nucleotide bases from which these genes are composed. Funded initially through the US Department of Energy, some US$3 billion is involved, making it the largest scientific project since the Moonshot.

Beginning in 1988, rapid progress was made with a first draft announced with much fanfare at the White House in late June 2000. At the launch, President Clinton argued that the HGP was a revolution aimed at the prevention, diagnosis, and treatment of most, and perhaps all, diseases (Wade 2010). Since 2003 the focus has turned to applying the discoveries and knowledge gained not only to human genetic disease generally but also to a search for monetary profits from patenting those discoveries. Although some of the genetic discoveries predated the formal establishment of the project, two directions of research have arisen out of this basic mapping expedition. The first direction is what could broadly be called '**disease genetics**'. This is the search for specific **gene mutations** thought to cause particular ill health conditions: on the one hand, single gene disorders such as Huntington's disease, and on the other, a predisposition to common diseases such as certain types of breast and ovarian cancer. The second and much more controversial direction has been in the area of 'behavioural genetics'. This has involved a search for genes that are thought to be likely to affect behaviours that some define as socially undesirable and therefore potentially amenable to 'alteration', such as depression, alcoholism, homosexuality, obesity, and—the 'holy grail'—intelligence.

So, how has this greater understanding of the genetic basis of disease flowed through so far into the treatment of chronic illness? The genetic makeup of a person may impact on chronic illness in several ways depending on how penetrant the genetic abnormality or mutation is that has health implications. By 'penetrant' is meant the likelihood that the genetic makeup of a person will result in ill health. The extreme case is Huntington's disease; having the mutation is 100% penetrant and therefore totally determinant of the onset of the disease. If genetic testing reveals a person has that particular mutation, they will get the disease. Others are much less penetrant. With cystic fibrosis (CF), for example, the most common genetic disease among Caucasians, if both parents carry a mutation of the relevant gene, then the chances of their offspring having the mutation and therefore experiencing CF is much lower (see Horsley et al. 2009). So, in this category of direct causation of ill health, a distinction is drawn between single-gene disorders (e.g. sickle cell anaemia) and chromosomal abnormality (e.g. Down's syndrome).

Of more interest here as it relates to chronic illness are multi-factorial or polygenic genetic disorders. Here, a number of genes appear to interact with environmental as well as lifestyle factors. For these conditions, penetrance is low; they may 'run in families' but do not have the clear inheritance pattern of single-gene disorders and chromosomal abnormalities. Most chronic diseases appear to fall within this category. These include diabetes, asthma, inflammatory bowel disease, obesity, heart disease, hypertension, and autoimmune diseases such as multiple sclerosis.

Another way to conceptualise this is to think of illnesses along a continuum. At one pole (left side) are those that have clear genetic causation (such as Huntington's disease). At the other pole (right side) are those where there is a multi-factorial interaction between genetics and lifestyle, or where interaction between inheritance and environment is more pronounced, complex, and as yet unclear. Most chronic illnesses on this measure are towards the right side of this continuum.

So, what impact have the advances in genetic understanding associated with the HGP had on these common chronic illnesses? The argument to be made here is very little. While there is much hope and some promise, there is very little impact as yet. A decade after the completion of the first draft, the promised benefits to medical treatment remain largely unfulfilled.

Genetic diseases generally are very difficult to treat. Most treatment technologies involve screening; the only way to avoid a serious genetic illness is not to be born with it in the first place! The classic example is Huntington's disease. Effective screening technology is available that can say whether a person will or will not contract the disease. This screening can be performed on unborn foetuses as well, and, if the value system of the parents allows it, can result in termination. But at present, nothing can be done for a person for whom screening shows that they have

Disease genetics
The search for gene mutations thought to cause ill health conditions.

Gene mutations
Thought to cause particular ill health conditions.

See Chapter 4 on genetic influences on health.

the genetic mutation. There is no cure or effective treatment—all of which raises the question of 'would you want to know'?

Biological basis The genetic basis of chronic illness, and also refers to the effects of ageing.

What we call the **biological basis** of chronic disease is accompanied by a pervasive discourse of hope and promise, but so far there is very little to show of actual success in reducing the burden of genetically caused chronic illness. The assumption (which is what is called a 'modernist' one) is that the advance of medical science and technology will eventually develop forms of treatment, known as genetic biotechnologies, based on an improved understanding of the genetic basis of illness. The literature is full of references to 'not yet' and 'soon'. In the context where discoveries of the location on particular genes on human chromosomes have been allowed to be patented, such 'genohype' has to be understood in the politico-economic context of venture capitalism where the share prices for impending discoveries were talked up to the point where they constituted a 'Genobubble' of speculation that has long since popped (see Pollack 2010). Indeed, it has become clear that the HGP has been much more about increments in biological science than it has been about advances in medical treatment. As Harold Varmus, the director of the National Cancer Institute has argued: Genomics is a way of doing science, not of doing medicine (Wade 2010).

What then are the technological advances held up as being of 'promise'? There are a number of biotechnologies that have been mooted as arising out of the HGP. Gene therapies, long anticipated as a technological innovation, are still largely at the potential, 'cautious optimism' stage of development, and according to the HGP information website run by the US Department of Energy,

Gene therapy The insertion of DNA into cells to correct genetic defects. This involves supplementing or replacing a gene where its abnormality or absence leads to a disease.

have not proved very successful in clinical trials. Little progress has been made since the first **gene therapy** clinical trial began in 1990. It has remained at the experimental stage, beset with many difficulties, not the least of which is its short-lived nature. As they affect the chronic diseases that are the focus here, the difficulties stem from the multi-factorial nature of any genetic link—they result from the interaction of many genes. Indeed, in 1999 the FDA placed a halt on all gene therapy trials in relation to liver disease, one of the main areas being investigated, after the death of a patient receiving gene therapy.

Likewise, genetic screening can be used as the basis for predicting illness events. An example is a study that investigated genetic predictions for heart disease. To investigate this multi-factorial health condition, a US medical team in Boston collected 101 genetic variants that had been statistically linked to heart disease. But the variants turned out to have no value in forecasting disease among 19,000 women who had been followed for 12 years. The authors

Stop and Think

» To what extent do you think genetic makeup has contributed to the chronic illnesses among your family, friends, or other people you know?

» How might taking a genetic approach provide a different explanation to a risk factor/behavioural explanation for having developed a chronic condition?

» How can both approaches be used?

Case Study 5.3   Cystic fibrosis

An example of a genetically induced chronic disease is cystic fibrosis (see Willis et al. 2001). The discovery of the genetic mutation that caused this disease actually predated the genomic era, having been discovered in 1989. While there have been significant advances in life expectancy over the decades, gene therapy has long been held out as the great promise for combating this disease, and a realistic treatment option. However, as Anson and colleagues (2006) demonstrate, a practical and effective gene therapy has not eventuated in the time since. They argue that there are a number of reasons for this, including the lack of a suitable technology for delivering the gene. Gene therapy may be available in the future, and anyone who has ever had any association with this debilitating disease fervently hopes that this or some other treatment technology will reduce the burden of this genetically based disease. The point is that it remains at the stage of hope at this time.

concluded that the traditional (and for some old-fashioned) method of taking a family history was a better indicator of an individual's likelihood of having heart disease (Paynter et al. 2010).

Likewise, with the possibility of pharmocogenomics, the possibility of tailoring drug treatments to meet the individual illness needs of patients can be achieved but a development is still 'on the horizon'. The same can be said of treatments flowing from a better understanding of the biological basis of chronic disease, including the genetic basis. In the meantime, the discourse of hope continues, not only that the genetic roots of chronic diseases can be found, but that actual effective treatments follow.

The social context of genetic biotechnologies

Health sociologists are not only interested in what happens to individuals and their chronic illnesses but also in the social context in which the illnesses occur in regard to their biological and genetic basis (see Willis 1998). The determinants of health, in both individuals and populations, are a combination of medical and nonmedical. Developments in the genetic understanding of ill health have meant a vastly increased understanding of the genetic determinants of ill health alongside bacteriological and virological determinants. But the understanding of the non-medical determinants has also increased vastly.

See also Chapter 12 on the social construction of health.

The discipline of public health indeed was founded on the understanding that there is more to health than medical services and that the most basic non-medical determinants are class and gender. Chadwick argued back in 1840 that the Englishman's life expectancy depended on his social class. Many studies have come to a similar conclusion about the class gradient of disease from the Black report on (Black 1980). Indeed, it may well be that, in a population sense, the best predictor of longevity is how much an individual earns (see Macklin 1992).

See Chapter 7 on health promotion and the Ottawa Charter.

Genetic reductionism
Attempts to understand and present complex sets of relationships/precursors to disease by genetic explanations only. By focusing on these, important social and related factors which can contribute to illness are ignored.

Ideology A collection of beliefs or ideas particular to a group or discipline.

The point is that the need remains great to consider ill health not narrowly as an individual, biological, and, by a process of reductionism, a genetic phenomenon but more broadly as a social and political phenomenon. The World Health Organization has played an important part in crystallising such an awareness and has been responsible for a considerable focus around activities such as the Alma Ata Declaration, the Healthy Cities program, and the Ottawa Charter for Health Promotion. The problem is that the new public health is being overtaken by outside social, political, and economic forces so that the basic messages of public health are in danger of being lost. The developing emphasis on an individualist rather than a collectivist paradigm of health has been strengthened by a reductionist focus. Indeed, **genetic reductionism** operates as an **ideology** to legitimise these broad changes in the political economy of the global order. By focusing on the individual (a sort of 'Genes R us' approach), it diminishes the effects of social environments. If people are the way they are, it is because of their genes rather than the social environment in which they find themselves. One example is mature onset diabetes where modest upstream interventions such as improved diet and exercise may well be considerably more cost-effective than genetic medicine. Likewise, with breast cancer, emphasis on the 5–10% of cancers that are heritable has the potential to divert attention (and possibly research funding) from research on the 90–95% which are not and for which ongoing research on the environmental and other non-medical determinants remains crucial.

So, the social context of the new genetics provides a rationale and a justification for inequality. If people with chronic illnesses are the way they are because of their genes rather than the sort of society in which they live, government programs are not likely to make any impact.

There is a Swedish saying to the effect that 'when you're holding a hammer, everything looks like a nail'. For those holding the new genetic biotechnological hammer, what ill health conditions are genetic 'nails' and what are more like public health 'screws' is being actively negotiated. Advances in the understanding of molecular genetics *will* reduce the burden of suffering from genetically caused illnesses. But the social and societal context of the new genetics must be carefully considered. The social relations of genetic biotechnologies are complex and the debate intense over the social and political meaning of having particular genes. The temptation is to use the new improved design hammer on screws rather than the traditional screwdriver!

Genetic determinants of health in general and chronic disease in particular are important, and as we have seen, multi-factorial. But so are non-medical determinants, as well as the relationship between the two. In terms of health policy, the important questions are ones of priorities in attempting to address the major health issues, especially those resulting in premature morbidity and mortality. Genetic illness is undoubtedly one of these, but in the rush to embrace and promote the benefits of the 'new genetic medicine', in the clamour of demands for a shrinking research funding pie, more traditional public health concerns are in danger of being marginalised. The danger is that the ideology of genetic reductionism is legitimating the abandonment of collectivist responses to social problems and focusing instead on individual solutions. The 'new genetics' thus has the potential to strengthen the narrow, reductionist biomedical paradigm of ill health as an individual and biological phenomenon rather than the broader paradigm that the 'new public health' has advocated of being more of a social and political phenomenon.

Mythbuster

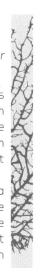

» *Consider whether you see the following as questionable. What does this tell you about your own values?*

- Your government is introducing new measures to deal with the upsurge of chronic illness in the population. They are investing in providing more access to medical services (such as increases in the number of 24-hour clinics), and in increasing the number of available medical staff and the number of hospital beds available for treatment. This is using much of the healthcare budget and some groups in the community are very critical, arguing that there are other approaches to reducing chronic disease that should be tried.
- The government has used this policy in the past and claims it is effective. However, a growing group of health experts and consumer advocates maintain that prevention is the key to reducing the incidence of chronic disease and that this starts with addressing the determinants of health, particularly inequity in the population. The government claims that outcomes from addressing these issues take too long and may be hard to link to prevention strategies. Which group is right and how might the differences in approach be resolved?

Summary

Chronic illness is increasing. Internationally as well as in Australia, more than two-thirds of the burden of disease is due to chronic diseases. There are several determinants of chronic disease, and these include biological (which can be largely explained through an examination of genetic factors), social, behavioural, and environmental, and also the role that stress plays in the onset and management of chronic conditions. Both biological and social factors (e.g. poverty) underpin the other determinants of chronic illness, and each should be seen as not only interacting with the other factors, but as having an important effect on the influence of these other factors. The social location of a person (e.g. social class and associated wealth and lifestyle) interacts with both behavioural risk factors and the environmental conditions they are exposed to. Government policymakers need to be aware that treating chronic conditions with the traditional acute healthcare model is both costly and inefficient.

Through the Human Genome Project (regarding the key biological determinant) important precursors to a number of chronic diseases have been identified. In fact, there have been extensive advances in identifying genetic structures and therapies. With chronic conditions such as the genetically induced cystic fibrosis we should be close to finding cures for these chronic conditions. Yet, given the advances, we are really just at the 'hoping for a cure' stage. Taking a genetics approach does not mean we should ignore other determinants, in particular the social factors that are associated with increased chronic disease uptake. A multi-factorial approach is required.

Tutorial exercises

1   Form a group of five with your peers in the class. Each of you needs to write down what you think chronic disease means and how it can affect people's lives. Then compare your answers with your peers in the group. Are there similarities? Are there differences? Discuss the similarities and differences that you have noted in the group and how they have come about.

2 After finishing this chapter, make a list of what you consider are the most important determinants of chronic diseases. Can you list the most important determinants for five chronic diseases?

3 Who are the most vulnerable to developing chronic diseases? What can the government do to reduce these risks?

4 As a group discuss how an understanding of genetics can inform about chronic disease risk and offer potential cures. Do you see this as the way in the future for chronic diseases or does it need to be tempered by an understanding of other (e.g. social) determinants?

Further reading

Anson, D., Smith, G., & Parsons, D. (2006). Gene therapy for cystic fibrosis airway disease: Is clinical success imminent? *Current Gene Therapies*, 6(2), 161–79.

Australian Institute of Health and Welfare (2010a). *Australia's health 2010*. Canberra: AIHW. <www.aihw.gov.au>.

Baum, F. (2008). *The new public health: An Australian perspective*, 2nd edn. Melbourne: Oxford University Press.

Ben-Shlomo, Y., & Kuh, D. (2002). A life course approach to chronic disease epidemiology: Conceptual models, empirical challenges, and interdisciplinary perspectives. *International Journal of Epidemiology*, 31, 285–93.

Charmaz, K. (1991). *Good days, bad days: The self in chronic illness and time*. New Brunswick, NJ: Rutgers University Press.

Leeder, S. (2007). The scope, mission and method of contemporary public health. *Australian and New Zealand Journal of Public Health*, 31(6), 505–8.

Peterson, C.L. (2003). *Work stress: Studies of the context, content and outcomes of stress: A book of readings*. Amityville, NY: Baywood Publishers.

Walker, C., Peterson, C.L., Millen, N., & Martin, C. (2003). *Chronic illness: New perspectives and new directions*. Croydon: Tertiary Press.

Willis, E. (2009). The human genome project: A sociology of medical technology. In J. Germov (ed.) (2009), *Second opinion: An introduction to health sociology*, 4th edn. Melbourne: Oxford University Press, 328–46.

Websites

<www.aihw.gov.au/publications/phe/ifcdtd08/ifcdtd08-c01.pdf>
This website provides useful information about AIHW indicators of chronic diseases and their determinants.

<www.aihw.gov.au/cdarf/index.cfm>
This site has very useful summary data on the range of chronic illnesses.

<www.aihw.gov.au/cdarf/data_pages/prevalence_risk_factors/index.cfm>
Presentations are provided on the role and impact of a number of risk factors for chronic disease.

<www.diabetes.org/diabetes-basics/genetics-of-diabetes.html>
This gives a useful comparison to the Australian AIHW sites.

<www.chronicillness.org.au>
Details on chronic illnesses and member organisations in Australia.

<www.humanillnesses.com/Behavioral-Health-Br-Fe/Chronic-Illness.html>
Information on a range of chronic diseases.

<www.health.gov.au/internet/main/publishing.nsf/content/7E7E9140A3D3A3BCCA257140007A
B32B/$File/stratal3.pdf>
An outline of the approach the Australian Government adopted in controlling the prevalence of
chronic diseases.

6

Ageing and health: Biological, social, and environmental perspectives

Colette Browning and
Chyrisse Heine

TOPICS COVERED

This chapter covers the following topics:

- population ageing
- models of ageing
- determinants of ageing and health
- stereotypes and successful ageing
- population ageing and policy development

KEY TERMS

Active ageing
Baby boomers
Biomedical model of ageing
Functional health
Healthy ageing
Individual ageing
Life expectancy
Longevity
Older adults

Old-old population
Population ageing
Positive ageing
Productive ageing
Psychosocial models of ageing
Quality of life
Stereotypes
Successful ageing

Introduction

Ageing is a significant global issue that impacts on society both socially and economically. While many have characterised **population ageing** as a 'burden', we argue that population ageing is in many ways a triumph for society, where today many people live healthy and productive lives well into later life. This perspective does not deny the heterogeneity of the ageing process. Age-related chronic illness and frailty have negative impacts on our experience of ageing. However, the factors that contribute to ill health in old age, such as sedentary lifestyle, poor diet, and poor social networks, are potentially modifiable. Health and welfare professionals need to take an active role in their community and clinical work in addressing these modifiable risk factors.

Population ageing The increase in proportion of older people in a population caused by mortality, fertility, and migration.

Population characteristics differ worldwide, for example between industrialised and non-industrialised countries and rural and urban contexts. Therefore, **life expectancy** (mortality rate) in different regions has been influenced by different population ageing patterns in relation to change, pace, determinants, and consequences (Satariano 2006). In particular, a wide variety of biological, social, behavioural, and environmental factors have been associated with health status and survival. Satariano (2006) lists a number of factors associated with survival: gender (women live longer), race and ethnicity (social minorities have decreased survival rates), socio-economic status (the lower socio-economic groups have decreased survival rates), the physical environment, social capital, living arrangements, health behaviours, having a sense of control, self-efficacy, having fewer diseases and co-morbidities, experiencing fewer falls and injuries, and retaining good physical and cognitive functioning. This chapter emphasises that understanding ageing requires readers to examine the topic from different perspectives and in doing so this may challenge your views of ageing and older people.

Life expectancy The average life span at birth for a given society.

See Chapters 1, 11 & 12 for further discussion on the social determinants of health.

Older adults (those aged 65 years and over) constitute the largest growing sector of the population. Currently, many older people are living well into older age. At the individual level, new technologies to sustain life, medical innovations in the management of chronic illness, and the promotion of healthy lifestyles have contributed to this phenomenon. Lower rates of fertility, migration, and mortality have driven population ageing. According to the Australian Bureau of Statistics (ABS 2005), in 2004 those aged 65 years and over constituted 13% of the population, and in 2021 it is predicted that this proportion will rise to 26–28% of the population. On a global level, by 2050, 16.5% of the world's population will be aged 65 years and over (Wilson 2005). While the median age of the Australian population has risen from 20.1 years in 1881 and 30.7 years in 1947 to 36.4 years in 2004 (ABS 2005; Borowski & Encel 2007), so has the average age of the older adult population. According to ABS data (ABS 2008), the male life expectancy at birth has increased from 55.2 years in 1901–10 to 78.5 years in 2003–05, while female life expectancy at birth increased by 24.5 years from 58.8 years in 1901–10 to 83.3 years in 2003–05. In accordance with this increase in the age of the older adult population, there has been a rapid expansion in the number of those people aged 85 years and older (the **old-old population**).

Older adults Refers to that segment of the population that is aged 65 years and above.

Old-old population Refers to that segment of the population aged 85 years and above.

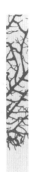

Mythbuster

Over 30 years ago Erdman Palmore published the 'Facts on Ageing Quiz' that was designed to assess people's knowledge of ageing. He and others have demonstrated that many of us endorse a number of myths about ageing (see e.g. Palmore 1977; Luszcz et al. 1985).

»   *Go to the website <www.webster.edu/~woolflm/myth.html> and complete the quiz but do not score it.*

»   *After reading this chapter do the quiz again and score your first and second attempts. How did you score? Do you think that our views about ageing have changed over the last 30 years?*

By 2051, it is predicted that 1.6 million people (6–8% of the total population) will constitute the old-old population (ABS 2005, 2006).

This chapter addresses a number of issues important to our understanding of individual and population ageing. First, what approaches/models influence our understanding of the experience of ageing and life expectancy? Biomedical theories of ageing propose that ageing and life expectancy are largely dependent on cellular and physiological changes and exacerbated by the onset of chronic and degenerative diseases such as heart disease (Bengston et al. 2009). This approach focuses on the inevitability of decline and does not consider the role of potentially modifiable behavioural, psychological, social, and environmental determinants of ageing. Advances in the prevention, treatment, and management of chronic illnesses and disability and the role of the environment in health have contributed to our understanding that ageing is more than biology. Our understanding of the role of psychological factors such as resilience and adaptation and social factors such as socio-economic disadvantage, social networks, social support, and attitudes to ageing has also shifted the view that ageing equates with inevitable decline. Current conceptualisations of ageing are focused on 'successful ageing' and 'healthy ageing'. As noted by Lupien and Wan (2004, p. 1423):

> To strive towards a more optimal view of the ageing process, research on successful ageing needs to focus not only on models of biological and cellular ageing that consider the gradual deterioration of the organism, but also on psychological and sociologically related factors that are related to improvements or maintenance of function.

This shift from a biomedical approach to ageing to a broader social model requires the adoption of new innovative health and well-being programs which recognise that many factors that influence ageing are potentially modifiable. Our roles as educators, researchers, and professionals will need to accommodate this different approach.

In this chapter, the authors also consider the role of stereotyping in the health and well-being of older people and the shift on the part of researchers and policymakers to examine more positive views of ageing and of older individuals through the use of concepts such as successful, healthy, active, productive, and positive ageing. In regard to stereotyping, do we have a typical view about older people? Does old imply grey hair, wrinkled, and ill? Can we move away from this stereotype to acknowledge individuality and that many older adults are living longer, more active, and happier lives? As professionals involved in promoting health, it is important to understand these positive approaches to ageing as they have informed current ageing and aged care policy development and will no doubt influence our approaches to individual and population ageing as the **baby boomers** enter old age. Finally, this chapter describes the policy approaches in Australia and internationally that are designed to address population ageing.

Stop and Think

Edith is an 84-year-old woman, living in her own home. Her spouse of 60 years recently passed away. Edith has diabetes, controlled by insulin injections, and has mild high blood pressure controlled by medication. She is mildly visually impaired (wears glasses) and does not drive. She walks with the aid of a stick. She has home help once a week for two hours. She has three children and only one child lives in the same city as her. She occasionally participates in religious/community services and sees family and friends approximately three times a week. She speaks on the phone to family and friends daily although her mild to moderate hearing loss at times leads to frustration with her communication. Edith does not use or want a hearing aid.

» Is Edith a typical example of our ageing population?

» Do we have preconceived ideas of older people?

» Is there a typical ageing stereotype?

Baby boomers Those born during the post-Second World War baby boom. They are usually defined as those born between 1946 and 1964.

The biomedical approach to ageing and health

The biomedical approach to understanding ageing focuses on the ageing process at different levels of biologic organisation, including the molecular, cellular, and systemic levels. This model assumes that the likelihood of malfunction (on a biological level) will occur with increased time and with age (Satariano 2006; Bengston et al. 2009). Molecular theories of ageing focus on the extent to which molecular functioning and integrity (such as gene regulation and genetic expression) change with age. In contrast, cellular-level theories of ageing consider cellular functioning and the link between ageing and metabolism, while systemic theories are based on the regulation and coordination of organ systems over time (Satariano 2006; Hayflick 2007).

The underlying assumption of the **biomedical model of ageing** is that life expectancy and morbidity are determined by biological functioning and that decreased life expectancy is expected due to physical and mental deterioration and disability (Bowling & Dieppe 2005). For example, the free-radical theory (which occurs on a cellular level) links ageing with metabolism. In this theory, free or unstable oxygen molecules damage cells and contribute to the ageing process. At the chromosomal level, the shortening of telomeres (structures at the end of chromosomes) impedes cell division and contributes to biological ageing (Hayflick 2007). **Successful ageing** according to the biomedical model is thus determined by the intactness and efficiency

See also Chapters 1 & 5 on biological and genetic determinants of health.

Biomedical model of ageing Emphasises the role of age-related biological changes and chronic illness (morbidity) on the ageing process.

Successful ageing Ageing is said to be successful when an individual stays free of illness and disability into old age, and is likely to function well physically, mentally, and socially (Rowe & Kahn 1997).

of these levels of the body systems. Biomedical ageing research therefore focuses on the biological and medical contributors that interfere with body functioning and life expectancy.

Longevity The length of one's life, often used to describe the state of someone who has lived beyond their natural life expectancy.

A consequence of the biomedical model of ageing is the concern that increasing **longevity** would lead to increases in the burden of illness and disability in later life, for example dementia, cardiovascular disease, cancer, stroke, among other diseases, and dependence in terms of everyday activities of daily living (ADLs). Fries (1980, 1989, 2002) proposes the Compression of Morbidity hypothesis to explain this concept. In this hypothesis, the burden of illness could be reduced if the timing of the illness could be moved closer to the point of death. Under this hypothesis, successful ageing is aimed at early intervention to ensure that people live longer free from illness or disease. There is evidence that as many as one-fifth of centenarians survive 'without the diagnosis of the 10 most age-associated diseases' (Evert et al. 2003, p. 234) and that early intervention in reducing risk factors for disease is effective (Fries 2002).

Rowe and Kahn's (1997, p. 433) model of successful ageing is influenced by the biomedical approach. They defined successful ageing (within the 'normal', non-disabled older population) according to three components that are hierarchically organised: 'low probability of disease and disease-related disability, high cognitive and physical functional capacity and active engagement with life.' If an individual can stay free of illness and disability, then they are more likely to function well both physically and mentally, which in turn are preconditions for active engagement.

However, many have argued that successful ageing should not be judged simply as increased longevity but in terms of quality of life in old age that is in turn influenced by psychological, social, and environmental factors. The literature on defining and measuring quality of life is vast and complex and beyond the scope of this chapter. For the purpose of the current discussion quality of life in old age refers to individual and general well-being (Browning & Kendig 2003; Glass 2003; Kendig & Browning 2010).

Psychological, social, and environmental approaches to ageing and health

Psychosocial models of ageing Acknowledge the importance of psychological resilience and adaptation, mental health, life satisfaction, and social environments including social support and social networks.

See the broad coverage of health and illness in Chapter 1.

Functional health Is seen as well-being, not merely as the avoidance of disease and disability,

Although biological ageing and chronic illness are important factors in older adults' longevity and well-being, **psychosocial models of ageing** acknowledge the importance of psychological resilience and adaptation, mental health, life satisfaction, and social environments including social support and social networks as important influences on the experience of ageing and on longevity. *Environmental models of ageing* incorporate the role of the physical environment in health and well-being.

Recognising the importance of psychosocial and environmental factors in ageing and health parallels the World Health Organization's definition of health which is 'a state of complex physical, mental and social well being and not merely the absence of disease or infirmity' (WHO 1952, p. 100). In relation to ageing, it is not merely physical health that needs to be considered. More specifically, Hall and colleagues (1989) describe health as a multidimensional construct that includes **functional health**, emotional health, physiologic health, social activity, and cognitive functioning. Applying this approach to ageing requires a shift from conceptualising ageing as merely the avoidance of disease and disability to thinking of it in positive terms such as healthy ageing.

Ageing models should not therefore encompass only survival and physical health criteria, but should be extended more broadly to acknowledge the importance of psychological and social factors. Lamb and colleagues (1988) maintain that positive health is dependent on factors such as the ability to cope with physical disability and stressful situations, the maintenance of strong social support systems, integration in the community, high morale, life satisfaction, and psychological well-being. More recently, Bowling (1997, p. 4) defines functional status as 'the degree to which an individual is able to perform socially allocated roles free of physically (or mentally in the case of mental illness) related limitations'. Positive health thus implies efficient functioning of the mind and body, which in turn leads to adequate social functioning. As health is central to older people's well-being, recognising the multiple determinants of health leads us to a more optimistic view about the extent to which the experience of ageing is modifiable.

Psychological models recognise that not all older adults will age in the same way. Baltes and colleagues (1984) make important contributions to the way we understand **individual ageing**. They describe cognitive ageing as a process of adaptation that includes three components:

Individual ageing The biological, psychological, and social changes in an individual over time.

- *Selection:* Growing older may lead to restrictions in functional capacities.
- *Optimisation:* Older people have the capacity to improve their level of functioning.
- *Compensation:* Older people learn to adapt when capacities are reduced or lost.

Baltes and Baltes (1990) further develop this psychological model based on the premise that successful individual development (including ageing) is a process involving the three components mentioned above, namely selection, optimisation, and compensation. This model has come to be known as the SOC model of ageing. In this model, successful ageing means reaching the goals that the person has selected as important. Furthermore, those who age successfully make more use of the three psychological processes. Those who are rich in sensorimotor, cognitive, personality, and social resources are more likely to use these psychological processes as well.

There is now a plethora of research on the role of social environments on health. Seeman and Crimmins (2001) reviewed research on the effects of the social environment on health and ageing. A number of conclusions were drawn about the role of social integration measured by ties with spouse, friends, and community participation. They concluded that 'decreasing levels of social integration...are associated with increasing mortality' (p. 90) and that social integration protects against morbidity and the severity of disease, particularly in heart disease and stroke. They also concluded that social networks are protective of health when they promote 'the individual's self-esteem, sense of belonging, and efficacy or mastery through positive, supportive actions' (p. 94). More recently, researchers have examined the role of physical environments and neighbourhood socio-economic disadvantage in the health and well-being of older people. Clarke and Nieuwenhuijsen (2009) reviewed the evidence linking the environment and healthy ageing. They reported that car-dependent neighbourhoods and neighbourhoods with streets in poor condition have been linked to dependence in daily activities in older adults, especially in those with disabilities or those who are socially disadvantaged. Neighbourhood disadvantage is also associated with poorer self-rated health and more chronic illness in older adults. Thus, encouraging age-friendly social and physical environments has the potential to improve the quality of life of older people.

Stereotyping and successful ageing

Extending the notion of the role of social factors in ageing, stereotyping and attitudes to ageing can also impact on the experience of ageing and on an individual's well-being. According to Levy (2009), stereotyping can affect physical and cognitive outcomes for older people. Stereotyping older adults is common. That is, we associate particular features, symptoms, behaviour, and diseases with old age. For example, it is unusual to see a 40-year-old with grey hair since we associate grey hair with old age. When we admit to forgetting something and refer to it as a 'senior's moment', we imply that 'forgetting' is a behaviour of older people. Although both positive and negative **stereotypes** exist, it is the negative stereotype that predominates and marginalises older people. For example, older people may be categorised as a group that has regressed to childhood (Levy 2000). This categorisation is illustrated when younger people address an older person using patronising speech. Older adults can also be characterised as debilitated, frail, or unproductive (Levy 2000). An older person may be the last to be hired and the first to be retrenched.

It is, however, not only younger people who apply these stereotypes; older adults may accept these stereotypes themselves. According to Levy (2003, p. 203), ageing self-stereotypes exist and characteristically 'originate in the form of ageing stereotypes as early as childhood and are reinforced in adulthood; [they] can operate below awareness; and…in old age, the ageing stereotypes become ageing self-stereotypes'.

Interestingly, there is also debate in the literature about the use of the term 'successful ageing'. Successful ageing, and related terms such as healthy ageing, **positive ageing**, and **productive ageing** are concepts that were in part coined to counter the negative stereotypes of ageing. However, it has been argued that the concept of successful ageing does not take into account the varied context of the ageing experience and the broader psychosocial determinants of successful ageing (Holstein & Minkler 2003). For example, Holstein and Minkler applied critical gerontology and a feminist perspective to examine the concept of successful ageing. They examined the contradictions and assumptions underlying successful ageing and the roles that gender, class, and race have to play. In particular, they argued that successful ageing as conceptualised by Rowe and Kahn (1997) implies an individual responsibility for health with little emphasis on the roles of economic, social, cultural, and physical environments, and healthcare systems in healthy choices and health outcomes.

Criticisms of the concept of successful ageing include its implication that ageing with an illness or disability is 'unsuccessful' ageing or even 'a transgression against cultural rules' (Holstein & Minkler 2003, p. 792), thus further stigmatising the older person (Minkler & Fadem 2002). Similarly, Angus and Reeve (2006) argue that the term reinforces negative stereotypes of ageing and marginalises older people. Yet, as Minkler and Fadem argue, providing supportive environments for people ageing with a disability can affect their perceptions of their functional abilities and their ability to sustain good quality of life. An overemphasis on an individual responsibility or individual capacity approach to successful ageing ignores the role of factors beyond the individual's control.

Stereotyping older people is outdated, particularly since there is heterogeneity among older people and no consensus regarding what constitutes 'old' or a typical profile of ageing that can be

Stereotype
A conventional, formulaic, and oversimplified conception, opinion, or image; one that is regarded as embodying or conforming to a set image or type.

Positive ageing Refers to numerous concepts such as one's ability to live to an old age with little or no disability prior to death as well as attitudes towards ageing, e.g. having a positive attitude towards older people.

Productive ageing
Refers to an individual's or population's ability to maintain productivity and participate actively in the social and economic advancement of the nation.

applied to all older people. According to Bowling (2005), the acceptance of any categorisation by age obscures the diversity of older people. Ageing is a natural phenomenon and a natural transition that occurs with time. Since there is individual variation in ageing (determined by, for example, social and environmental influences), ageing needs to be viewed more broadly than just as a biomedical phenomenon. There has been a move away from 'negative models of ageing' to the positive view of ageing as a 'natural component of the lifespan' (Bowling 2005). As health professionals, we need to consider heterogeneity, individuality, and the social and environmental influences on ageing that are open to intervention.

Stop and Think

When we think of an older person, we think about a person who looks 'old' (wrinkled, shorter stature, grey hair), has one or more diseases (e.g. cardiovascular disease, stroke, high blood pressure, diabetes), has one or more sensory disabilities (e.g. hearing loss, vision loss), is ill (perhaps needs frequent hospitalisation for falls, or requires surgery, e.g. cardiac surgery), is dependent on others (e.g. requires home help for completion of ADLs, cannot complete many Instrumental ADLs independently), is inactive (physically and socially), and needs adjusted living conditions (e.g. needs to live with a child or be placed in a nursing home).

» In 2011, is this really the typical older adult? Do we know what contributes to successful ageing and do we have a specific successful ageing stereotype in mind? Does ageing solely depend on health or are there other factors that lead to longevity? Do you view older people you know differently from older people in general?

Case Study 6.1   Women living in different social and cultural environments

Rose is an 82-year-old woman living in a low-care residential facility in a suburban area of a bustling city. She is a widower—her husband passed away 25 years ago. She has two children who visit her on alternate days for approximately one hour per visit. In the residential facility, she mainly watches television in the communal lounge, and plays cards with other residents about three times a week. On Sundays, she joins in with the entertainment offered at the facility. Rose has suffered numerous falls recently and has osteoporosis (for which she takes daily calcium and vitamin D). Rose also has high blood pressure (currently medicated) and type 2 diabetes (currently medicated by tablets).

Maria is an 82-year-old woman living with her son, daughter-in-law, and three grandchildren. The family is from an Italian background and lives in a close-knit community in a three-bedroom house in a suburban area of a large city. She is a widow—her husband passed away two years ago, and her son insisted that she live with his family. Maria accompanies the family to religious services and joins in all activities offered by the local religious centre, where she has many friends. She is in good health and only takes tablets daily for Vitamin D and stroke prevention (aspirin).

Li is a 67-year-old woman who lives with her husband in a three-bedroom government-subsidised apartment in a bustling city. She has two sons, both married and with children. One of Li's sons lives on the other side of the city, two hours away by car; her other son lives in another country. Li and her husband are retired. Li was a factory worker and her husband was a government official. They frequently participate in social activities with their neighbours since their neighbours come from a similar background. Li is spiritual (but not religious), participates in regular exercise, and does not take any medication.

Josephine is a 73-year-old widow living in rural South Africa (in a kraal). She lives in a small tin house among other members of the community. Her house is home to three of her five grandchildren, and her two great-grandchildren. Her seven children and their spouses work in the city and visit only occasionally during the year and for Christmas. Josephine sings in the church choir and participates in social activities at her local church. She has not had any major illnesses and does not take any medication. When she is sick, she consults the local healer (witchdoctor/sangoma), who usually prescribes some herbs or potions.

» *Are these women ageing in the same way?*

» *What is the influence of their social and physical environments on ageing?*

Determinants of ageing well

We have discussed how ageing is influenced by a range of biopsychosocial factors. The best evidence for these influences comes from longitudinal studies that have followed older people as they age. Browning and Thomas (2007) conducted a major review of longitudinal studies that have examined the predictors of ageing well. They were particularly concerned with identifying factors that were potentially modifiable. They found that most studies focused on predicting the negative aspects of ageing, such as functional decline, morbidity, and mortality while others focused on predicting positive aspects of ageing such as happiness and good physical and mental functioning. Table 6.1 summarises the study results in terms of how the outcomes were measured or defined and the significant predictors of the outcomes. The predictors that are potentially modifiable can be categorised as risk factors for poor outcomes or protective factors for good outcomes. The modifiable risk factors for poor outcomes are high blood pressure, high cholesterol levels, and being overweight or underweight. The modifiable protective factors for good outcomes are engaging in social and productive activities, moderate alcohol intake, not smoking, and moderate levels of physical activity. Many of these modifiable risk and protective factors are linked to the probability of developing disease such as diabetes and cardiovascular disease, which in turn have been shown to be associated with poor outcomes in old age. In addition, social and physical activities are often associated with the quality of the physical environment and access to age-friendly facilities. Depp and Jeste (2006) also note that there are a number of potential predictors of successful ageing that have received little attention in the research literature. These include genetic markers, allostatic load, access to health services, nutrition, and psychological variables including spirituality and resilience.

Table 6.1   Summary of the predictor variables for poor or good outcomes in old age

Outcome Measure/Definition	Predictor Variables
Alive, not living in nursing home, ADL independent and mentally competent (Roos & Havens 1991)	Spouse alive and not in nursing home, better self-rated health, not retiring because of poor health, high mental status score, free of cancer and diabetes
Happiness, high physical and mental functioning, mortality (Menec 2003)	Social and productive activities
Mortality and maintenance of high levels of physical functioning (top 20%) as measured by composite ADL and physical activity score (Guralnik & Kaplan 1989)	Absence of high blood pressure and arthritis, past or non-smoker, moderate body weight and alcohol intake
Minimal interruption of usual function, although minimal signs and symptoms of chronic disease may be present (Strawbridge et al. 1996)	Absence of diabetes, not often depressed, often walking for exercise, five or more social contacts, moderate alcohol, not smoking
Functional decline (Balfour & Kaplan 2002)	Neighbourhood noise, inadequate lighting, heavy traffic
Reaching old age without experiencing serious chronic illness and having maintained high levels of physical and cognitive functioning: Fewer years of successful ageing post-baseline (Newman et al. 2003)	Cardiovascular disease, diabetes, smoking, low levels of physical activity
Alive, stability in self-rated health or remaining functionally independent (Havemen-Nies et al. 2003)	Good diet, physical activity, not smoking
Sustained (2 years) living in the community with no assistance in ADLs (Ford et al. 2000)	Younger age, being male, higher capacity in performing activities, fewer medical conditions, not smoking
'Happy-Well': high level of well-being in a number of domains of health, life satisfaction, and social supports (Vaillant & Mukamal 2001)	Some regular physical exercise, no depressive symptoms, low levels of smoking, stable marriage
Surviving to late life free of major life-threatening illnesses and maintaining the ability to function physically and mentally (Reed et al. 1998)	Not smoking, not obese, low blood pressure, and low blood glucose levels
Living to old age with little or no disability prior to death (Leveille et al. 1999)	High levels of physical activity
No disability (Ferucci et al. 1999)	Physical activity, not smoking
Low disability or recovery from disability (Mendes de Leon et al. 1999)	Social networks
Decline in physical performance in high-functioning group from MacArthur Studies (Seeman et al. 1994)	Older age, lower income, higher education, higher weight and blood pressure, lower peak expiratory flow, diabetes, hospitalisation

(continues)

Colette Browning and Chyrisse Heine

Table 6.1 Summary of the predictor variables for poor or good outcomes in old age (continued)

Outcome Measure/Definition	Predictor Variables
Improvement in physical performance in high-functioning group from MacArthur Studies (Seeman et al. 1995)	Moderate or strenuous physical activity, greater frequency of emotional support
Less decline in physical performance in high-functioning group from MacArthur Studies (Unger et al. 1999)	More social ties
Satisfaction with ageing, lack of agitation, and absence of emotional and social loneliness (Freund & Baltes 1998)	Life management strategies
Successful mental health ageing: MMSE greater than 24 and GDS-15 was 5 or lower (Almeida et al. 2006)	High school or university education and physical activity (unsuccessful mental health ageing associated with consuming full cream milk and coming from non-English-speaking background)

Case Study 6.2 Health and successful ageing

Dennis is 83 years of age, a widower who until recently lived alone in his own home without any need to access any services. He has two children; one son is married and lives interstate while his other son is divorced and lives near him. Dennis has recently moved into an aged care centre (low-care facility) following a period of hospitalisation due to a fall. Dennis has a mild hearing loss (age-related) and recently discovered that he has macular degeneration. Dennis also has mild arthritis that affects his dexterity. He also takes medication for high blood pressure and osteoporosis and takes Vitamin D. Dennis has very few friends and can no longer drive or socialise independently. He has also had to give up his regular bowls and bridge games.

» *What biological, behavioural, social, and environmental factors may be influencing Dennis' experience of ageing?*

» *Is Dennis ageing well? What is 'successful' ageing for Dennis?*

Policies for ageing populations

Since the older adult population is now a large segment of the overall population, governments and society now face many public policy issues. The health and vitality of older people is of serious concern as the ability to minimise disability and maintain their well-being and quality of life become major goals for health professionals and policymakers (Browning & Kendig 2003, 2004; Satariano 2006). These questions are being asked: Will the increase in the proportion of older people lead to an increase in the prevalence of chronic disease and disability? How are services going to be provided when there is increased demand? What policies have been put into place to accommodate population ageing? How can we promote healthy ageing?

Much government policy is concerned with older people who need significant support to live at home or in residential care. In response to the recognition that aged care is an important component of Australia's health system and that significant reform is required, the Australian Productivity Commission (2011) developed a draft report entitled *Caring for older Australians*. In this report, a number of challenges were identified including, first, increased demand for services with ageing of the population and second, significant shifts in the type of care required (e.g. increased preference for independent living and choice in aged care services; greater level and disparity of affluence among older people; changing patterns of disease and associated costs to manage these diseases; reduced access to carers and family support; diverse geographical spread; and the increased need for psychogeriatric care and palliative care). The third challenge identified was to secure expansion of the aged care workforce. The Commission recommended increased government funding of services and regulation of their delivery. Reforms should target both aged care providers (e.g. there is a need for providers to provide a minimum quota of supported residents) and older Australians and their carers (e.g. care and support needs should be assessed via a gateway agency).

The recognition that ageing is not associated with inevitable decline has also led to policies related to healthy and **active ageing**. Health Canada has promoted healthy ageing concepts since the early 1970s and further developed policy frameworks and programs during the 1990s <www.hc-sc.gc.ca/seniors-aines>. **Healthy ageing** is defined by them as 'a lifelong process of optimising opportunities for improving and preserving health and physical, social and mental wellness, independence, quality of life and enhancing successful life-course transitions' (Health-Canada 2001, p. 2).

In Australia, in the International Year of Older Persons, the Commonwealth Government developed the National Strategy for an Ageing Australia (NSAA) (Bishop 1999b), which included four themes: independence and self-provision; world-class care; healthy ageing; and attitudes, lifestyle, and community support. The healthy ageing theme was concerned with health promotion, chronic disease management and the management of disability, and focused on maintaining health in old age by promoting physical activity, healthy eating, and the management of chronic diseases and disabilities such as diabetes, heart disease, urinary incontinence, and sensory loss. Bishop (1999a, p. 3) defined healthy ageing as an approach to ageing that aims 'to maintain and improve the physical, emotional and mental well being of older people'. The other themes of the NSAA linked with the healthy ageing theme. For example, the attitudes, lifestyle, and community support theme recognised the influence of community attitudes and the physical and social environment of older people on their health. Attitudes to ageing are a central component of the concept of positive ageing discussed below. Andrews (2002, p. 52), in updating the NSAA, expanded the definition to include 'disease prevention and optimal well being' and 'maximizing capacities to participate and contribute' to society.

The World Health Organization has contributed significantly to the importance of promoting health and well-being in old age. The active ageing policy framework (WHO 2002) challenged stereotyped views of older people as ill and dependent. Active ageing is defined as 'the process of optimizing opportunities for health, participation and security in order to enhance quality of life as people age' (WHO 2002, p. 12). This approach has been prominent in ageing policy frameworks, particularly in the UK and Europe.

The framework recognises that optimising well-being in old age is not just about personal health actions such as engaging in physical activity or accessing good nutrition. The WHO (2002)

Active ageing Optimising health, participation, and security to enhance quality of life.

Healthy ageing The process of achieving optimal health and well-being through active adaptation to ageing processes.

active ageing policy framework listed five determinants of active ageing, with culture and gender as cross-cutting influences: personal; behavioural; economic and social; the physical environment; and health and social services. This approach recognises that access to transport, housing, and safe neighbourhoods impacts on health actions such as physical activity, as well as on access to appropriate services. Similarly, Heikkinen (1999) lists hereditary factors, socio-economic circumstances, gender, behavioural factors, and attitudes to ageing as the primary determinants of healthy ageing.

Walker (2002) argues that the WHO active ageing concept is not just concerned with making people work longer but focuses on health, independence, and quality of life as we age and as such combines productive ageing with promoting well-being. He outlines seven key principles of active ageing (Walker 2002, p. 124):

- Activities should include meaningful pursuits and not just paid work.
- All older people should be included, not just the more healthy 'young-old'.
- Prevention should be emphasised across the life span.
- Intergenerational fairness and intergenerational activities should be emphasised.
- Rights and obligations should embody active ageing.
- Strategies for active ageing should be empowering and encourage participation.
- Cultural diversity should be respected.

See also Chapter 13 on health throughout the life course.

Walker (2002) also argues for a life course perspective on active ageing. He discusses strategies to promote active ageing for key points in the life course. For young people ('first age'), he suggests raising awareness about the benefits of healthy lifestyles and lifelong learning and addressing ageist attitudes and promoting intergenerational interaction. As people move through adulthood ('second age'), they need to manage their own ageing with support from government and employers, particularly in the areas of employment choices, retirement, and healthy lifestyles. Approaching retirement and beyond ('third age'), older people need choice in activities and encouragement to participate in society. Later in life ('fourth age'), older people and their carers need to be empowered to engage in self-reliance and self-determination in collaboration with the health and social care systems.

Summary

Ageing is a significant global issue and today many people live healthy and productive lives well into later life. Population characteristics differ worldwide and therefore life expectancy in different regions has been influenced by local social, economic, and environmental factors as well as biological factors. Biomedical theories of ageing explain the ageing process as largely dependent on biological factors and the onset of chronic and degenerative diseases. Advances in the prevention, treatment, and management of chronic illnesses and disability, and the roles of psychological and social factors and the environment in health, have contributed to our understanding that ageing is more than biology. Current conceptualisations of ageing are thus focused on 'successful ageing' and 'healthy ageing' and many of the risk and protective factors for outcomes in old age are modifiable. The modifiable risk factors for poor ageing outcomes are high blood pressure, high cholesterol levels, and being overweight or underweight. The modifiable protective factors for good ageing outcomes are engaging in social and productive activities, moderate alcohol intake, not smoking, and moderate levels of physical activity. In addition, social and physical activities are often associated with the quality of the physical environment and access to age-friendly facilities. Our challenge is to avoid stereotyping older adults as 'unwell' and incapable of change and create environments and programs for older people that encourage optimal well-being while supporting vulnerable older citizens.

🔏 Tutorial exercises

1   Watch the film *About Schmidt* starring Jack Nicholson, which portrays the life of a 66-year-old man whose wife has died. The film follows his journey to make sense of a life without a partner. What does this film tell us about the role of relationships in ageing well? Is Schmidt ageing successfully?

2   Newspapers often portray older people as either high achievers ('Look at Granny parachuting out of an aeroplane') or as dependent ('Nursing home crisis'). Look at the pictures and stories about older people in your city newspaper. What stereotypes are being portrayed?

3   Watch the episode of *The Human Body* titled 'Immortal'. <www.sbs.com.au/shows/secretsofthe humanbody/tab-listings/page/i/3/h/Immortal>.

   Discuss: Do you think that we should strive to extend life indefinitely? What would a society look like where older people significantly outnumber younger people?

4   'Population ageing and climate change are the two most important challenges facing society.' Do you agree? What impact might climate change have on ageing? See <www.epa.gov/aging/resources/climatechange>.

Further reading

Bengston, V.L., Gans, D., Putney, N.M., & Silverstein, M. (2009). *Handbook of theories of ageing.* New York: Springer.

Buettner, D. (2010). *The Blue Zones: Lessons for living longer from the people who've lived the longest.* Washington, DC: National Geographic Mass Market paperback.

Marmot, M., & Wilkinson, R.G. (eds) (1999). *Social determinants of health.* Oxford: Oxford University Press.

Phillipson, C., & Dannefer, D. (2010). *The Sage handbook of social gerontology.* Los Angeles: Sage Publications.

Snowdon, D. (2002). *Aging with Grace: What the Nun Study teaches us about leading longer, healthier, and more meaningful lives.* New York: Bantam Books.

Websites

<www.activeageingnetwork.org.au/Pages/default.aspx>
This website contains information about Active Ageing Network.

<www.ageingwell.edu.au>
In this website, readers can see information regarding the Ageing Well Research Network.

<www.un.org/ageing>
This is the website about the United Nations Programme on Ageing.

<www.who.int/ageing/en>

Readers can find information about ageing and life course of the WHO on this website.

<www.cdc.gov/aging>

It provides information about US Centers for Disease Control and Prevention.

<www.halcyon.ac.uk>

This website contains information about HALCyon Healthy Ageing across the Life Course.

<www.eastwestcenter.org/fileadmin/stored/misc/FuturePop08Aging.pdf>

Readers can find information about ageing in Asia on this website.

7 | Introduction to health promotion

Alana Hulme Chambers and
Rae Walker

TOPICS COVERED

This chapter covers the following topics:
- defining health promotion
- the determinants of health
- a conceptual framework for health promotion
- evidence-based health promotion
- improving equity
- community enablement
- working collaboratively

KEY TERMS

Best practice
Climate change
Collaboration
Communicable disease
Determinants of health
Equity

Evidence-based
Food security
Health promotion
Non-communicable disease
Population health

Introduction

Health promotion
A discipline that takes a holistic approach to positively maintaining and improving the health and well-being of individuals, communities, and whole populations.

Health promotion is a discipline that takes a holistic approach to positively maintaining and improving the health and well-being of individuals, communities, and whole populations. The aim of health promotion is to enable people to improve their health (WHO 1986; Raphael 2000). As both a distinct discipline with its own knowledge (Green & Tones 2010) and its own standing alongside other health disciplines, health promotion has an important and necessary role in addressing contemporary health issues for which responses are complex and contested. Therefore, it is timely to explore or, for some, revisit the concept of health promotion. It seems inevitable that, for any student of health sciences, knowledge of this discipline will be essential.

This chapter is an introduction to health promotion. It begins with a definition of health promotion. It then draws on a framework for planning and delivering health promotion programs (Victorian Government Department of Human Services 2003) to help readers explore the elements that comprise best practice approaches to health promotion. Sections in the chapter outline these elements and respond to key questions faced by any health professional when undertaking health promotion. These key questions are:

- *The determinants of health*: What are these and why are we concerned with them?
- *A conceptual framework for health promotion*: What is the Ottawa Charter for Health Promotion and how do we utilise it?

Once we have an understanding of the determinants of health and the Ottawa Charter as our foundation for understanding health promotion, we turn to the other elements that are common in

Best practice
Theoretically based activities and/ or practices that have a rigorous and systematic evidence base to support their recognition as effective and appropriate means for delivering programs or services.

best practice approaches to health promotion:

- *Evidence-based health promotion*: What is 'evidence' and why is it needed?
- *Improving equity*: How do we create conditions that ensure everyone has a fair opportunity to thrive?
- *Community enablement*: Why is it important and what are the benefits?
- *Working collaboratively*: How do we work with others to create sustainable change that improves health and well-being?

Three case studies are presented to help readers understand health promotion in practice.

Defining health promotion

There are a number of definitions of health promotion, with subtle differences between them (e.g. Tannahill 2008a; Jirojwong & Liamputtong 2009; Green & Tones 2010). Among these, and within the health sector, the Ottawa Charter remains a reference point when it comes to defining health promotion. The Ottawa Charter was developed in 1986 at the First International Conference on Health Promotion, which took place in Ottawa, Canada. The definition used in the Ottawa Charter is given below, with a longer discussion of the Charter continuing later in the chapter.

> Health promotion is the process of enabling people to increase control over, and
> to improve, their health. To reach a state of complete physical, mental and social
> well-being, an individual or group must be able to identify and to realize aspirations,

to satisfy needs, and to change or cope with the environment. Health is, therefore, seen as a resource for everyday life, not the objective of living. Health is a positive concept emphasizing social and personal resources, as well as physical capacities. Therefore, health promotion is not just the responsibility of the health sector, but goes beyond healthy life-styles to well-being. (WHO 1986, p. 1)

Prior to the Ottawa Charter, health promotion focused on disease and physical ill health (Antonovsky 1996; Breslow 1999; Baum 2008). Individual behaviour change was common in many early definitions of health promotion (Baum 2008), as was taking a linear approach to altering behaviour (Crosby & Noar 2010). Behaviour change and health education were hallmarks of health promotion in its infancy. However, the Ottawa Charter moved health promotion away from these approaches and, instead, clearly articulated the need to recognise and respond to the **determinants of health**, to look beyond narrowly focused, individually based issues and involve groups and communities, and to consider health from a well-being perspective.

> **Determinants of health** A range of individual, social, economic, environmental, and cultural conditions that have the potential to contribute to or detract from the health of individuals, communities, or whole populations.

The Ottawa Charter was successful in reshaping health promotion into what we see today. Indeed, the Charter remains a key conceptual framework utilised by health promotion practitioners. Because of its significance, the Ottawa Charter will be discussed in more detail later in this chapter. Before this, we need to delve further into understanding some of the elements of best practice in health promotion. The first of these are the determinants of health.

The determinants of health

Health promotion is informed by and draws from a range of disciplines including medicine, sociology, political science, psychology, and ecology. This is why health promotion is concerned with more than just medically based issues. It considers the whole picture surrounding an individual, group, or population, taking into account the economic, environmental, political, and social forces that have a role in influencing health.

These forces, which are known in the health sector as the 'determinants of health' (and also referred to as the social determinants of health) have the potential to either contribute to or detract from the health and well-being of both individuals and populations (WHO CSDH 2005). Figure 7.1 displays the main determinants of health.

> See also Chapters 1 & 11 on the determinants of health.

At the centre of the diagram are determinants over which we have very little control as they are largely what we are born with. However, the circles outside these are the ones that are of interest to health promotion. Note that, as the diagram moves outward, the way in which health promotion can be applied also broadens. The inner circles demand a health promotion response that is individually focused, but as you move out further in the diagram, the issues become broader. In turn, the response changes from being concerned with the individual and individually focused lifestyle factors to social, political, and economic arrangements that underpin, or determine, those lifestyle factors.

Many of the factors in the diagram, at first glance, may seem to have little to do with health. Why is health concerned with agriculture and food production, or education, or employment? The determinants of health approach encourages health promotion practitioners to look further afield at other sectors, and to gather and make sense of evidence that may come from any discipline in order to understand and address what is influencing health and well-being (Keleher & MacDougall 2009).

Figure 7.1   Determinants of health

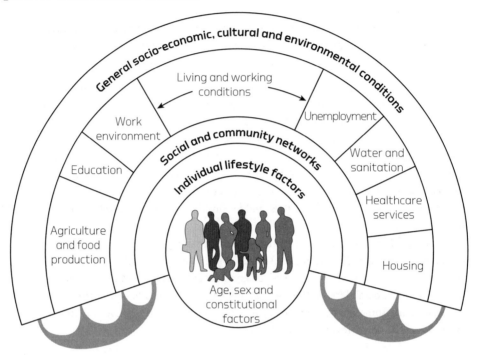

Source: Dahlgren & Whitehead 1991

This holistic approach has the benefit of also raising the question why certain forces may have a particularly potent effect on health and well-being.

Addressing the determinants of health, rather than just focusing on the factors immediately surrounding the silhouettes in the diagram above, is a way of getting at the roots of the cause. The Stop and Think box below provides an example of this.

Stop and Think

Antony presents at your community health service to see a drug and alcohol counsellor because he feels he is drinking too much alcohol. Heather, his counsellor, asks some questions in the first consultation: where he is living, his family situation, his employment, and his social networks. She discovers that Antony's drinking is linked to the breakdown of his marriage, his subsequent move from the family home into a caravan, and no access to his children. Antony's despair at his situation has led him to not turn up at work, and he has been fired, in the process losing his network of work colleagues with whom he used to socialise. While concerned about the amount of alcohol he is consuming, one of Heather's first responses is to arrange for Antony to see a housing provider and a relationships counsellor.

» As a drug and alcohol counsellor, why is Heather helping Antony with housing and relationships? What has this got to do with alcohol?

The determinants of health approach in health promotion works effectively when we collaborate with other sectors such as education, local government, agriculture, or transport. **Collaboration** between health promotion and these other sectors (which will be discussed later in the chapter) is necessary to make any significant progress in working on the determinants of health (Sparks 2010). Health promotion or, indeed, the health sector cannot 'go it alone' in improving conditions that promote health and well-being. As readers can see in Figure 7.1, this is because most of the determinants that influence health are outside the control of the health sector.

As readers can appreciate, addressing the determinants of health is not simple or straightforward. It requires substantial commitment and effort in a number of sectors. It also requires considering people in relation not just to their age, gender, and lifestyle habits, but also where they live, the type of education they have, their employment status and type of employment, and their connections to their cultural and social networks. Such considerations mean that the actions we take to address health issues need to be multiple and target a range of determinants.

Collaboration
A process involving different parties who are committed to working interdependently to achieve a common goal or address a common issue.

Determinants of health: Population health

In the health sciences, **population health** is a common term that you will encounter, and is often discussed in relation to the determinants of health. Population health

Population health
An approach to improving the health of populations by introducing interventions that have the potential to affect everyone.

Stop and Think

Below is a diagram of a tree. It can be used to help you understand the determinants of health. Imagine the canopy of the tree as representing a health issue to be addressed and the roots of the tree as being the connections to the determinants of health that underlie the health issue. Using the tree to note your observations, consider the following health issues by discussing what determinants of health might have contributed to the health issue:
- rising rates of obesity among children in the UK
- rising rates of obesity among adults in China
- cholera outbreaks in Haiti
- harmful alcohol use by young people in Australia.

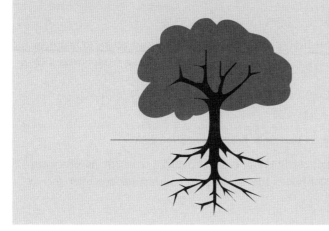

focuses on improving the health of whole populations by intervening in risk factors that affect everyone (Baum 2008). An example of this is legislation requiring all passengers in a car to use a seatbelt. This is an intervention that has the potential to have a significant effect on the health of a whole population.

A population health approach is concerned with reducing inequity, and requires collaboration between different sectors and participation by the community to be effective (Victorian Healthcare Association 2010). The population health approach is complementary to the determinants of health approach. Population health is concerned with the forces and factors underlying the more visible issues that can result from the determinants of health.

Taking a population health approach is useful for issues that require a whole population to be targeted in order for a positive change in health and well-being to be observed (Green & Tones 2010).

A conceptual framework for health promotion: The Ottawa Charter

As mentioned previously, the Ottawa Charter (WHO 1986) is perhaps the best-known health promotion document. Since its adoption in 1986, the Charter remains a key conceptual framework for planning, implementing, and evaluating health promotion programs.

Characteristics of the Ottawa Charter

Besides offering a comprehensive definition of health promotion, the Ottawa Charter has a number of characteristics that distinguish it as a comprehensive framework for planning, implementing, and evaluating health promotion.

The Ottawa Charter recognises factors that are required for good health

The Charter nominates a number of prerequisites for health (many of which are now often referred to as determinants of health, as discussed earlier in this chapter). These are seen as necessary to any improvements in population health and include peace, shelter, education, food, income, a stable eco-system, sustainable resources, social justice, and equity.

The Ottawa Charter focuses on wellness

The Charter encourages a focus on the health-enhancing factors that assist people to maintain and improve their health rather than simply addressing factors that cause disease (Antonovsky 1996).

The Ottawa Charter provides principles for guiding health promotion activity

There are three principles in the Charter that guide health promotion action:

- *Advocate*: to recommend or support conditions or factors conducive to health. Advocacy can take many forms. Chapman (2004b) notes that advocacy in health promotion often focuses on factors that are usually contested, meaning there is often no common agreement about them; and that advocacy takes advantage of opportunistic and responsive situations, such as having access to a decision-maker or being in a circumstance where there is an opportunity to motivate or convince.

- *Mediate*: to intervene between parties in order to bring about an agreement on health (WHO 1998). Health promotion is concerned with improving people's health, and this can be an emotive, even passionate issue. As a result, conflict can occur about how to improve health. Mediation skills are useful here for providing a process by which all stakeholders and their interests can be considered within a context that is conducive to promoting health. Methods used in mediation may include facilitated community meetings or public debates where stakeholders can hear and consider each other's opinions.
- *Enable*: to create conditions or provide resources to help people achieve improvements in health at an individual or community level. The key here is that health professionals work in partnerships, rather than in isolation, with the people or community that are experiencing the health problem (WHO 1998). This enables people to determine what they need, and ensures that the community owns the outcome.

The Ottawa Charter provides actions for undertaking health promotion

The Charter articulates five action areas that give health professionals domains to target in planning and implementing interventions. Implementing interventions based on a number of these action areas is common practice in health promotion. Rarely do we only use one or two since the most effective improvements in health often arise from interventions associated with using several action areas.

- *Build healthy public policy*: This action area involves engaging policymakers in health and other sectors on how policy can impact directly and indirectly on people's health.
- *Create supportive environments*: This refers to social, natural, economic, and built environments. It is concerned with creating the contexts in which it is possible for people to live healthy lives.
- *Strengthen community actions*: This means involving, enabling, and ultimately empowering the community to determine, lead, and implement actions relating to their health and well-being.
- *Develop personal skills*: This action area is concerned with increasing people's ability and capacity to achieve better health throughout life by supporting personal and social skill development within a variety of settings including school, work, and home.
- *Reorient health services*: This encourages health services to embrace health promotion as a philosophy and a practice by which to plan and deliver services, and educate and train health professionals. This gives credence to, and a means for, promoting the wellness approach to health, particularly in settings where there is a strong clinical focus to health.

These action areas reflect opportunities to undertake health promotion using different interventions, working across many settings and within different contexts, so enabling a comprehensive approach for acting on health issues.

The Ottawa Charter can be used on different scales

Finally, the Charter encourages health professionals to plan and implement health promotion interventions on different scales. It does this through the action areas. Some of these areas, such as 'build healthy public policy', are suited to implementation on a broad scale because they affect people at the community or population level, while others, such as 'develop personal skills', occur on a smaller scale because they are focused on individuals and small groups. The key to effective health promotion is to utilise action areas on different scales in order to have a wide-reaching impact on people's health.

Climate change
A variation in climate that is either attributable to natural environmental changes or stemming from human action.

Food security Having access to sufficient food that is nutritionally and culturally appropriate.

Case Study 7.1   A health promotion approach to climate change

It is now accepted that **climate change** is not only occurring, but at faster rates than anticipated (Baum 2008). The effects on human health globally range from direct, such as extreme weather events which can result in threats to physical health, to indirect, such as a reduction in **food security** and an increase in communicable disease.

Recognising the need to respond to climate change at a local level, the Southern Grampians and Glenelg Primary Care Partnership (PCP) developed *Climate change adaptation: A framework for local action* to assist their catchment population in addressing the health and social impacts of climate change (Rowe & Thomas 2008).

The Framework aims to identify local issues related to climate change, guide planning and action, and encourage intersectoral planning and partnerships to respond to the issues identified. The Framework uses the Ottawa Charter to provide strategies for action on the indirect effects of climate change. Some of these indirect effects include increasing prices and reduced availability of household energy, water, and affordable food supply; the increasing price of fuel; and decreasing community strength and resilience. Below is an example of how the Ottawa Charter has been used in the Framework in relation to affordable food supply. Refer to the explanations of the Charter action areas and then read below to understand how these have been put into practice:

Build healthy public policy: Advocacy for increased competition in the fresh food retail market may help to stabilise fresh food prices. This would make fresh food available to more people.

Create supportive environments: Planting of edible foods, such as fruit, in streetscapes can provide a cheap, local supply of fresh food, meaning more people can have access to nutritious food.

Strengthen community action: Partnering with local community organisations that have an interest in gardening and food production in community gardens can assist communities to have some control and self-determination over food availability.

Develop personal skills: Developing food preparation and storage skills in those groups identified at high risk. This can assist those most vulnerable to food security to consume fresh and healthier food.

Reorient health services: Building capacity of the health workforce on the issues of food security (Rowe & Thomas 2008, p. 20) can help health services to identify situations and clients where food security is an issue, and provide proactive responses.

These examples demonstrate how health promotion can be applied to an issue that at first glance may seem more connected to environmental matters than a health issue. It also exemplifies the holistic nature of health promotion.

In health promotion there are a number of elements we need to consider and utilise to ensure that what we are doing is going to be appropriate, accepted by the community, sustainable, and effective. The remainder of this chapter will focus on exploring these elements in greater detail: **evidence-based** health promotion, improving equity, enabling communities, and working collaboratively.

Evidence-based
Using good-quality information to develop a policy, position, strategy, or action.

Evidence-based health promotion

Using evidence in health promotion is crucial for a number of reasons. First, we can use evidence to help us identify health issues; when considering a health issue, we can use evidence to determine its magnitude. Second, evidence informs us about the determinants of health related to the issue; that is, what are its causes. Third, we can use evidence to guide us in how to address the issue, helping to ensure we are using best practice interventions. Finally, evidence assists us in evaluating whether the ways in which we addressed the issue were effective (Raphael 2000).

Tannahill (2008b) provides an excellent summary of what might count as 'evidence' in health promotion. In simple terms, evidence can be seen as good-quality information that is useful in and relevant to being able to make an informed decision, judgment, or conclusion.

While, traditionally, only scientific, quantitative knowledge was considered to be good-quality evidence, there is now a growing argument that other forms of knowledge, such as qualitative information and systematically prepared reports, should also be considered as evidence (Hill et al. 2010) because of the value of this in informing practice. Qualitative knowledge, for example, can give insight into people's feelings about, and experiences of, particular issues (Liamputtong 2009b). Unpublished information, such as progress reports or evaluations of a health promotion intervention, can offer alternative insights into how we understand health issues. Both of these forms of knowledge can contribute greatly to how we might perceive and take action on a health issue (see Liamputtong 2010b).

Regardless of the type of evidence, any information that forms the basis for an evidence-based approach needs to be critically appraised, before being used, for considerations such as age, source, replicability, adaptability, and relevance to the issue at hand (Tannahill 2008b; Hill et al. 2010). We need to ensure that any evidence we utilise is appropriate and credible.

In relation to sourcing evidence, the Cochrane Collaboration is an international organisation that makes available systematic reviews of the effectiveness of healthcare interventions (Doyle 2004).

It has a number of fields that focus on different areas of health. The health promotion and public health field aims to provide best available evidence to guide health promotion policy and practice.

To summarise, evidence-based health promotion is an approach that prioritises information that has met a number of prerequisites. This information helps to ensure that best practice and the most sustainable and effective outcomes are achieved when addressing a health issue.

Improving equity

Equity Creating conditions and eliminating structural barriers to ensure that everyone has a fair opportunity to thrive.

See also Chapter 17 for a discussion of social justice.

Equity is about creating just and fair opportunities for everyone to grow and thrive regardless of race, class, gender, income, level of education, sexuality, religion, political beliefs, or geographic location (Sparks 2010). Inequity occurs then when there are no opportunities or when opportunities are unjust or unfairly distributed.

Inequity is the cause of many of the differences in health experienced within and between communities and populations. Consider these sobering statistics: if you happen to be born in a country like Sweden or Japan, you can expect to live to at least 80 years of age. However, if you happen to be born in an African country, your life expectancy may not even reach 50 (WHO CSDH 2008). Currently, in Australia you can expect to live to at least 75 years of age unless you are Indigenous; then your life expectancy is going to be at least 16–17 years less than the overall Australian population (AIHW n.d.). These examples reflect how inequity exists not only between countries, but also between population groups within a country.

Stop and Think

>> What are some of the causes of the gap in life expectancy between Indigenous and non-Indigenous Australians? How do these causes relate to equity?

Inequity in health is avoidable. This is why improving equity is a key concern for health promotion; because it is avoidable we have an opportunity to prevent it and, in turn, improve health. So, what are the ways in which health promotion can improve equity? The following section takes a practical approach to exploring how to improve equity relating to the social determinants of health.

Social determinants of health and equity

The Commission on Social Determinants of Health (CSDH) was set up by the World Health Organization in 2005 to gather evidence on ways to promote health equity and foster a global movement to achieve it (WHO CSDH 2008). The report from the CSDH made three overarching recommendations on reducing health inequalities globally. These are described below, along with examples from the CSDH report that indicate practical ways to improve equity.

See also Chapter 11 for a discussion of social inequality and health as a global concern.

Improve daily living conditions

This recommendation from the CSDH report reinforces our need to collaborate if health promotion is to make any difference in people's daily lives. For this to happen, change is required to the determinants that lie outside the health sector such as education and employment. This reflects one of the key challenges for health promotion professionals: gaining the involvement of governments and global institutions whose first priority may not be health.

What does equity look like in this context?

Focusing on where people live, as a determinant of health, will help to reduce inequities arising from poor living conditions. A policy that could help to improve where people live might include changing urban planning policies to reflect healthier environments, such as providing easy access to retail environments with healthy food choices.

Tackle the inequitable distribution of power, money, and resources

Unless there is more equal access across society to decision-making opportunities, the ability to have more control of one's life, to gain a decent financial income, and have access to economic, social, and environmental resources, populations will continue to experience the health differences that result from inequity.

What does equity look like in this context?

How a government leads a nation is key to that nation's prosperity. Governments need to be reminded of their responsibility to ensure that all constituents have equal access to the nation's resources whether they are natural, built, financial, or social resources. Health promotion can do this by advocating just resource allocation for the most vulnerable groups in society.

Measure and understand the problem and assess the impact of action

While those working in health promotion may understand the fundamental importance of addressing the determinants of health, this understanding is not always shared by those with the power and ability to create change. As such, this recommendation calls for improving knowledge around health equity and determinants of health among policymakers, other health professionals, and the public.

What does equity look like in this context?

Training health workers about the determinants of health would help in building capacity to identify and act upon determinants as seen in various health contexts.

In summary, improving equity in health is about ensuring everyone has a fair opportunity to thrive by eliminating various structural barriers and oppressive conditions. Improving equity around the determinants of health has the potential to have significant and far-reaching effects for the health of all peoples.

Non-communicable disease A term applied to a diverse group of diseases. These diseases do not involve infectious agents, so cannot be passed from person to person, but tend to be ongoing and to have persistent symptoms. The term 'chronic disease' is often used interchangeably with non-communicable disease.

Case Study 7.2   Minimising the impact of non-communicable diseases on populations

Non-communicable disease (NCD) is a growing problem worldwide. The risk factors that are common to most NCDs are a lack of nutritious diet, physical inactivity, and tobacco use (WHO 2005a). These risk factors are linked to socio-economic, cultural, and environmental determinants of health including urbanisation, income, housing, employment status, and access to healthcare services. The following figure shows this link:

Figure 7.2   Links between the determinants of health and the risk factors for NCD

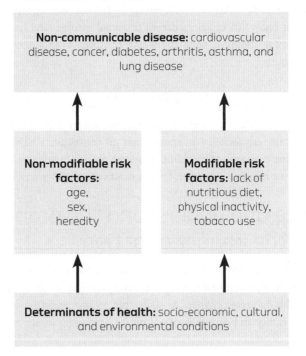

Health promotion can be used to minimise the impact of NCDs. Health promotion interventions can improve the determinants of health, prevent or minimise the modifiable risk factors of obesity, physical inactivity, and tobacco use, or assist those with NCD to manage their condition. This case study focuses on assisting populations with NCD to manage their condition.

NCDs have persistent physical and ongoing implications for the health and well-being of populations. This can mean that the mental and social well-being of populations are also affected. Any form of self-management for NCDs needs to take a holistic approach to ensure that physical, mental, and social well-being are all addressed.

Health promotion can play a key role in helping populations to develop personal skills to manage their NCDs. Skills that are common to and helpful for managing all NCDs include pain management, managing emotions, ensuring good nutrition, taking regular exercise, using breathing techniques to help with relaxation, and managing fatigue (Lorig et al. 2006).

The following table outlines the types of health promotion interventions that can be used to help those with NCDs to manage their condition.

Table 7.1 Health promotion interventions and methods for managing NCDs

Health promotion interventions

Individual focus ←————————————————→ Population focus

Methods for Managing NCDs	Screening Individual Risk Assessment	Health Education & Skill Development	Social Marketing Health Information	Community Action	Settings & Supportive Environments
Pain management	✕	✕	✕		✕
Managing emotions	✕	✕	✕		✕
Nutrition	✕	✕	✕	✕	✕
Exercise	✕	✕	✕	✕	✕
Breathing techniques	✕	✕	✕		✕
Fatigue management	✕	✕	✕		✕

Source: Adapted from Lorig et al. 2006 and Victorian Government Department of Human Services 2003

The table shows that the management methods for NCDs can be used by individuals or whole populations. For example, exercise could be improved at an individual level by assessing how much a person is exercising and then helping them to increase the amount of exercise. Health promotion could also be useful in creating supportive environments so that those who use exercise to manage their NCD have greater opportunity and a helpful and encouraging environment in which to do so.

This table can be used where management of the NCD is being approached from a health promotion perspective. It shows the various individual to population-level interventions that could be used to implement methods for managing NCDs. The result can be that those with NCDs are exposed to the management method in different ways, which can help in understanding, uptake, and continued use of the method to maintain well-being.

Community enablement

When we talk about enabling the community and having members actively participate in health promotion, what we are doing is making sure there are genuine and meaningful opportunities for people to work together in identifying key health issues for their community, discussing various solutions to these issues, and developing interventions to implement these (Jacobs 2011). Enablement and a focus on the determinants of health have been acknowledged as the key defining features of health promotion (Kickbusch 2007).

Community enablement is advantageous in health promotion for a number of reasons. Enabling communities to lead the work in improving their health can help to engage hard-to-reach populations; it can mean that the health promotion intervention is more relevant because it has been designed and carried out by those whose health is in question, and it can lead to more sustainable outcomes because local ownership over the issue and the intervention is generated (Merzel & D'Afflitti 2003).

As health professionals we need to understand that, although we may have expert knowledge of a health problem, communities experiencing the problem have personal knowledge and understanding that is equally important. For community to be truly enabled, our role as health professionals needs to be guided by the lived experience of the population we are working with.

As simple as this message may seem, in reality it can be quite difficult for professionals to let go of their expert role and allow the community to lead the analysis of a health issue, plan how to address it, and then implement interventions. This has been noted in several studies which have found that, as health professionals, we can feel a need for control, we can find it hard to understand our role, and we can struggle with accountability over outcomes when at the same time we are also encouraged to allow communities to guide the direction of an intervention (Jacobs 2011).

There are other obstacles to enabling communities: differences between the priority of a funding body and the priority identified by the community; lack of time to develop a trust-based relationship with the community; communities having competing priorities that require their time; and confusion about roles and responsibilities of community and that of health professionals (Merzel & D'Afflitti 2003).

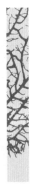

Mythbuster

» Consider the following statements. Which ones reflect community enablement and why? Why couldn't the remainder be considered community enablement?

Communities should only have a say in issues about which they have expert knowledge.

Keeping the community informed about how the issue is being addressed can be considered community enablement.

When health professionals and the community are equal partners in identifying and addressing a health issue, then community enablement occurs.

What this means for us as health professionals is that we need to be clear about both our role and that of the community before embarking on a community-led health promotion intervention. We need to ensure that communities have adequate support, skills, and resources to be able to take on the tasks that community enablement suggests. Where necessary, we need to advocate to our funding bodies the need to change policies where these inhibit community enablement. Finally, we need to realise that community enablement is an ongoing process of learning for both communities and health professionals. Reflecting on this learning and how we work together can provide a way of ensuring that community enablement is sustained.

Working collaboratively

Collaboration is a process or activity involving different parties who are committed to working interdependently to achieve a common goal or address a common issue (Hulme 1998). Collaboration has long been recognised in health promotion as a process for working effectively with other individuals, agencies, or organisations (i.e. stakeholders) in order to achieve health outcomes, particularly those where sectors outside health need to be involved.

There are many benefits of collaboration. Involving others in addressing health issues can result in greater efficacy (Kickbusch & O'Byrne 1995). Collaboration can result in the better use of health resources, reduce duplication of services and ensure quality of care, share the load in finding solutions to complex issues, and provide a way of developing sustainable solutions (Harris et al. 1995).

However, some of the difficulties associated with collaboration include potential stakeholders not seeing collaboration as necessary, not having the time, resources, or available staff to be able to collaborate, a lack of trust between stakeholders in relation to working together, and difficulties in achieving a shared vision of what the collaborative process can achieve (Hulme 1998).

What this indicates is that we need to be very clear on our motives for wanting to use a collaborative approach in health promotion. We need to be able to articulate clearly the role we would like our stakeholders to take on in the collaborative process. Finally, we need to ensure that we enable all stakeholders to have an equal voice in determining the aim and outcomes of the collaborative process.

Case Study 7.3   A health promotion approach to communicable disease

Influenza is a **communicable disease** that poses a real and continuing threat to health globally. With new strains of the influenza virus appearing regularly, the role of health promotion is vital in minimising the spread of this highly contagious disease. This case study will help you to understand how health promotion can be used to prevent communicable diseases like influenza.

Influenza is spread from person to person. The virus can be spread through respiratory droplets (e.g. infected people coughing on or near non-infected people) or contact spread (e.g. non-infected people introducing the virus into

Communicable disease
The transmission of an infectious agent from one person to another.

their body by touching something with the live virus on it (e.g. recently used tissues) and then touching their mouth, eyes, or nose (Department of Health and Ageing 2009).

One of the most effective ways to stop the spread of communicable disease is to prevent the disease from even occurring. Vaccination is a way of doing this. If we vaccinate against communicable disease, we are not only gaining protection for ourselves, but if enough people in the population are vaccinated against a particular disease we can build up what is known as 'herd immunity'. This occurs when enough people are resistant to a disease and so the less likely is the chance of a susceptible person coming into contact with an infected person.

One of the reasons why influenza spreads so rapidly is because not enough people get an annual influenza vaccination. So, how can health promotion improve vaccination rates?

Using the guiding principles in this chapter, let's look at how health promotion can be used to improve vaccination rates.

First, we might decide to use a *population health* approach, providing free influenza vaccinations for whole populations, such as people over 65 years, pregnant women, and those who care for small children and babies, because we know that these populations are particularly susceptible to influenza.

We might achieve this by using the *Ottawa Charter* strategy of *advocacy* to lobby government to provide free influenza vaccinations because they are an important way of preventing the spread of this disease, particularly for those who have less access to the influenza vaccine such as Indigenous peoples in remote areas and people on low incomes. This would help to *improve equity* in access.

We might look at *developing personal skills* by educating people about the benefits of getting an influenza vaccination. At the same time, we could also use social marketing strategies, such as posters and information sheets, to educate people on hygiene measures to prevent the spread of influenza.

Finally, we may *reorient health services* by training health professionals in various health settings to talk about the benefits of vaccination if working with population groups susceptible to influenza.

As readers can see, health promotion can play a varied role in relation to communicable disease.

Summary

Health promotion as a discipline addresses complex issues in the contemporary approach to health. Concerned with more than just medical matters, health promotion takes a holistic approach to positively maintaining and improving the health and well-being of individuals, communities and whole populations. The goal of health promotion for whole populations can necessitate intervening at local, national and international scales.

The Ottawa Charter of 1986 clearly articulates this approach to health promotion. As a framework it encourages the consideration of health from a well-being perspective and nominates some prerequisites for health. Central to health promotion is an understanding of the social, political, economic, and environmental determinants of health; health promotion seeks to counteract the presence of adverse conditions of life that undermine health and well-being.

Four elements can be used to ensure that health promotion is appropriate, sustainable, and effective. *Evidence-based health promotion* can help by identifying the causes of illness, and determine the magnitude of an issue and the most effective ways to address it. *Improving equity* can counter the frequent inequitable access to health. *Community enablement* is a way to ensure genuine opportunities for people to work together in identifying key health issues and developing interventions. Finally, *collaboration* is essential if the various health bodies are to promote health in a realistic way.

Tutorial exercises

1 You are a member of a student health committee at your university. Students have recently been notified by the university campus health service that there has been an outbreak of the sexually transmissible infection Chlamydia among campus students. The university asks your health committee for ideas and approaches on how to combat the outbreak and prevent it from spreading further.

» What types of evidence might you need to consider before you come up with any ideas?
» How could you use the Ottawa Charter to explain to the university how they could approach the issue?

2 A member of your health committee suggests that every student on campus should be tested for Chlamydia, citing the population health approach as an effective way to stop the outbreak.

» What equity issues might you need to consider if you recommend taking a population health approach?
» How could you 'sell' this approach to a student population that might see getting tested as intrusive and unnecessary?

Further reading

Baum, F. (2008). *The new public health*, 3rd edn. Melbourne: Oxford University Press.

Green, J., & Tones, K. (2010). *Health promotion: Planning and strategies*, 2nd edn. London: Sage Publications.

Laverack, G. (2007). *Health promotion practice: Building empowered communities*. London: Open University Press.

Liamputtong, P. (2009b). *Qualitative research methods*, 3rd edn. Melbourne: Oxford University Press.

Liamputtong, P. (2010b). The science of words and the science of numbers: Research methods as foundations for evidence-based practice in health. In P. Liamputtong (ed.), *Research methods in health: Foundations for evidence-based practice*. Melbourne: Oxford University Press, 3–26.

Naidoo, J., & Wills, J. (2009). *Foundations for health promotion: Public health and health promotion practice*, 3rd edn. Edinburgh: Bailliere Tindall.

Websites

<www.who.int/social_determinants/en>

The World Health Organization website on social determinants of health provides links to publications, tools, and resources.

<www.vichealth.vic.gov.au/en/Publications.aspx>

This is a link to the many health promotion publications released by the Victorian Health Promotion Foundation.

<www.health.vic.gov.au/healthpromotion/evidence_res/index.htm>

This is a Victorian Government website that contains information on health promotion issues, approaches, and guidelines.

<www.aracy.org.au/index.cfm?pageName=adv_collaboration_publications>

This site, maintained by the Australian Research Alliance for Children and Youth, provides an excellent list of downloadable publications on collaboration.

8 Anthropogenic change and human health

Rebecca Fanany

TOPICS COVERED

This chapter covers the following topics:
- how human efforts to alter their living environment can impact on health
- examples of human activity that have the potential to affect health
- the potential impact of increasing population and population density on human health
- the ways in which changes effected by human beings may allow opportunities for new diseases to affect human populations

KEY TERMS

Anthropogenic change
Built environment
Emerging disease
Population density
Psychosocial factors

Social capital
Urbanisation
Vector-borne
Zoonosis

Introduction

Human beings have always tried to alter the environment around them to better meet their needs and provide the material items they required. This process continues today and encompasses the physical, social, and personal environment of individuals and populations. This chapter explains the meaning and nature of anthropogenic change in these three contexts and discusses the observed and potential impacts on human health. The effects of increasing population density and urbanisation are described, and a number of recent examples of anthropogenic change and its impact on specific health issues are given to show the way in which changes intended for a particular beneficial purpose may have unintended side effects on health and disease.

Anthropogenic change

Anthropogenic change
Caused by human activity.

Built environment
All the buildings, structures, infrastructure, etc. created by human beings in an effort to improve their living environment.

See also Chapter 10 on the impact of the living environment on health.

Zoonosis A disease that originated in an animal species but that has adapted such that it can affect human beings.

Since prehistoric times, people have attempted to change the environment around them to make it more beneficial to them. This change that results from human activity is called **anthropogenic change**. Increasing technology over the centuries has allowed people to dramatically alter their surroundings in ways that make it easy for them to survive. These include the development of modern agriculture, housing, infrastructure, the **built environment**, industry, and, more recently, the generation of electricity, management of water, use of motor vehicles, and many more.

Not surprisingly, changes people make to their environment have the potential to influence health, for better or worse. Most of the time, any effects on health have been unintentional; that is, people have attempted to change their environment for a different reason, such as to produce more food or live more comfortably, but a side effect of this has been some effect on health. Human beings are part of the natural interactions between organisms on earth, and changes that we make also affect other species. Sometimes, the effect on other species (especially microorganisms that cause disease and insects that act as vectors of disease) makes it easier for them to infect us.

An interesting example of this is measles, a common childhood disease now routinely vaccinated against. The earliest known historical records of a measles outbreak occurred in the 9th century, and there were later epidemics recorded in the 11th and 12th centuries (McNeil 1976; Griffin 2007). It is now known that a vulnerable population of about 250,000–500,000 is required to maintain measles transmission (Black 1966; McNeil 1976; Black 1997); this can be calculated through statistical analysis. Populations of this size existed in the Middle East by about 3000–2500 BC, but the historical record does not mention any disease whose symptoms are compatible with measles, although smallpox is clearly identifiable. The measles virus belongs to the genus *Morbillivirus* and is related to the viruses that cause canine distemper, rinderpest (a serious disease of cattle), and other animal viruses (Sheshbaraderan et al. 1986; Barrett 1999; McCarthy & Goodman 2010). It is hypothesised that measles emerged as a human disease as a result of human efforts to domesticate cattle beginning in the earliest human settlements (McNeil 1976). Over centuries, a common virus of cattle mutated in such as way as to be able to infect humans. A human disease with an animal origin is called a **zoonosis**, and many common human diseases have come about through contact with animals.

Changes to the physical environment

The changes that human beings make to the environment have an impact on health because they create new opportunities for disease to spread or because they allow people to change their lifestyle and habits in such a way that they become more vulnerable to disease. Often, the effect on health is unexpected and unintended and may not appear for some time. Nonetheless, looking back, it is often possible to connect some change in the living environment with a particular health effect.

The earliest changes people tried to make were to their physical environment. Settlement in permanent locations, agriculture, the building of roads, and management of water resources all required that changes be made to the physical location in which people lived, both through building and by altering the natural environment. We still make constant changes to our physical environment today and have much greater ability to control more aspects of the world in which we live.

See Chapter 10 on health and the living environment.

Agriculture is thought to have begun about 10,000 years ago as early human populations began to shift from a nomadic existence to living in permanent settlements (Bellwood 2005). The aim of agriculture was to secure the food supply, but farming and the handling of animals greatly changed the work and living environment and, with it, the health status of communities. On the one hand, the development of agriculture led to better and more consistent nutrition for human populations. Being able to predict with some certainty what food and how much would be available allowed for planning and storage and also the potential to support larger populations, although often storage of food over a long period reduced the nutritional value. Agriculture is dangerous work, however, and even today many injuries occur in this sector (Day 1996; McCurdy & Carroll 2000). Archaeological study of early human settlements suggests that a range of health changes followed the introduction and intensification of agriculture and includes evidence of traumatic injury, decline in adult stature, increase in dental caries, and the effects of a more sedentary lifestyle (Lovell 1997; Judd 2004; Roberts 2005). The practice of animal husbandry that brought people into close contact with animals also created situations in which new diseases could develop (as with measles), and approximately 61% of human disease is thought to have an animal origin. This includes anthrax, brucellosis (related to tuberculosis in humans), cholera, salmonellosis, listeriosis, dengue fever, bubonic plague, trichinosis, and many more (Berenson 1990).

Work is another human activity that has had a profound impact on health. At one time, work was largely informal, with each person doing the tasks needed for individual survival and to support family members. Daily activities were much less structured than today, and each person had a greater degree of control over their own occupation. Gradually, however, work became a societal institution with many of the restrictions we are familiar with today. Over time, the length of the working day became standard; tool and material use developed in individual professionals; and eventually technological development allowed for increasingly mechanised workplaces (Weindling 1985; Abrams 2001). It is perhaps not surprising then that work has always been associated with injuries and accidents. Occupational exposures to chemicals were also known to be associated with illness from an early date (the first writings on occupational medicine date from the 15th century), but it was not until the 20th century that governments began to be concerned about the toll on health from unsafe and unregulated workplaces. The first workers' compensation programs were established in the late 19th century in Europe (Fishback & Kantor 1998, 2006), and occupational safety and health authorities began to be set up in the second half of the 20th century (Lee 1973; Rosner & Markowitz 1987).

Over time, one of the most significant changes human beings have made to their physical environment relates to increasing population and **population density**. Not only are there more people in the world than at any time in the past, but more people are living in urban areas with larger populations occupying smaller physical areas. Australia, a country with a very low population in relation to its land area, had a population density of 1 person per square kilometre in 1950; today population density has reached 3 people per square kilometre. By contrast, India, a large nation with a very large population, had a population density of 113 people per square kilometre in 1950 which rose to 369 people per square kilometre in 2010 (United Nations 2009). In both cases, population density has tripled over the last 60 years, but the impact is likely to be very different because of the absolute levels of population in each country.

Population density
The number of people per square unit of land; often reported as some number of people per square mile or square kilometre.

Increasing population and population density often goes along with increasing urbanisation, where more people are living in cities. Urbanisation is characterised by higher population density but also by concentration of services. This means that infrastructure, services, and facilities tend to be located in population centres instead of spread out evenly across a country. People are drawn to areas where facilities are better, causing a growing net gain in population of cities and towns in many parts of the world. The World Health Organization (WHO 2010d) estimates that more than 50% of the world's population now lives in a city and projects that this will reach 70% by 2050.

Urbanisation and increasing population density have been associated with a number of health conditions. Early in the 20th century, many cities around the world, including those in developed countries, experienced epidemics of influenza, typhoid, cholera, and tuberculosis (Rosen 1993). Large numbers of people living in close proximity facilitated the spread of these diseases, and unsanitary living conditions were often the cause. By the 1970s, much of the disease associated with water and food hygiene had been eliminated in the developed world (although it remains a serious problem in developing countries), but it was observed that rates of infectious disease, chronic disease, and mental illness were rising among urban residents (Dohwenrend & Dohwenrend 1974; Webb 1984; Vlahov & Galea 2004). Urban residents also tend to be more seriously affected by social problems associated with high-density living, such as stress, domestic violence and violence related to crime, and drug abuse (Vlahov et al. 2007). Urban residents in developing countries face a range of infectious and vector-borne disease (malaria, dengue fever) but also the same chronic diseases that are rising in the developed world and a very high incidence of urban social problems that relate to health, such as traffic accidents and violent crime (Murray & Lopez 1997b; McMichael 2000).

Urbanisation
The increasing concentration of human population, activities, and services in towns and cities.

Rapid urbanisation and increasing population density has required changes in construction practices and the nature of the built environment. Building for high-density areas has been characterised by taller, more enclosed buildings, often on the model of the 'glass and steel' skyscraper frequently used for public buildings and offices in urban areas (see e.g. Ford 1992). These buildings, while fulfilling one set of needs for more space used more efficiently and providing more comfortable accommodation for workers, have created new health problems not previously experienced by human societies. One example of this is the condition often referred to as 'sick building syndrome'. Sick building syndrome is a constellation of non-specific symptoms experienced by workers in particular modern buildings. The illness, which can be severe enough to prevent people from working, disappears by itself when the affected person is away from the building that is felt to be the cause (Edvardsson et al. 2007). While no specific etiology for this condition has been developed, it has been hypothesised that the symptoms are related to the air-conditioning systems or to a combination of volatile organic chemicals in use in the building or used in its construction (Jaakkola et al. 2007). Interestingly, sick building syndrome is most common in buildings that are in full compliance with current design standards (Burge 2004). Although the exact nature and cause of sick building syndrome is not known, it is clear that it is related to changes in the work environment and work practices of urban residents.

Stop and Think

The changes we make to our physical environment are usually intended to improve people's experience and living conditions. We rarely anticipate the possibility that these changes will have an adverse impact on health. If we take sick building syndrome as an example, we see that best practice in design and construction is not a guarantee of a healthy environment.

» How can we use our knowledge and experience of health and disease to develop our physical environment in ways that are better for people's health?

» What aspects of the physical environment seem to be associated with better health for users?

» What aspects are associated with health problems?

Changes to the social environment

As people change the environment around them to meet their needs for food, shelter, work, entertainment, transport, and the whole range of human activity, the social environment changes as well. The social structure of any society is closely related to its culture but also to the physical nature of the environment in which it exists. That is, while social structures develop in line with cultural practices in various parts of the world, they evolve because of opportunities or limitations placed on people's behaviour by the physical environment. For example, in many parts of the world, small-town living where a majority of people lived in separate houses and had much in common with their neighbours has been replaced by high-density dwellings (apartments) where people are segregated largely by income and proximity to their workplaces (see e.g. Rudlin & Falk 2009). The complaint that nowadays many people do not know their neighbours is a perception of the social setting that many people feel relates directly to changes in the living environment (see e.g. Williamson 1981; Ginsburg & Churchman 1985; Gifford 2007).

The social environment, which includes how people relate to one another, the possibility of establishing and maintaining social networks, interactions between individuals of different races, religions, and cultures, the expression of extended family relationships, and many other aspects of human experience, can have a profound effect on mental and emotional health. Most people seem to need satisfying social relationships to fulfil their potential and have a good quality of life. Urbanisation, changes to the work environment, and changes to how people live have all been observed in many locations around the world to be associated with a range of **psychosocial factors** with the potential to affect health and well-being.

Psychosocial factors
Aspects of the living environment that have the potential to affect people's feelings, perceptions, and cognitive state.

One example of how the demands of the modern workplace have the potential to affect health is the relatively new phenomenon of workplace rage, sometimes referred to as 'going postal' because of a series of highly publicised incidents of workplace rage that took place in the USA from the early 1980s onward and involved US postal employees. One of the best-known of these events occurred in Edmond, Oklahoma in 1986 when a mailman shot and killed 14 of his co-workers, injured six others, and then committed suicide by shooting himself in the head. In fact, similar instances of rage have occurred in many different work settings as well as in other social contexts and are now well known, especially in the USA (see Ames 2005, for a detailed discussion of this social phenomenon). It is generally agreed that incidents of murderous rage, wherever they occur, arise from feelings of isolation and inability to control their own fate in a vulnerable individual who may feel trapped in a low-autonomy job (such as in the postal service) or large institution that does not value their individuality (such as a school or the military) (Newman & Baron 1998; Denenberg & Braverman 1999; LeBlanc & Kelloway 2003; Barling et al. 2009).

There is growing evidence of the importance of the social environment in contributing to the health of individuals and communities. At the individual level, meaningful social relationships, a sense of belonging and of being valued are important for good health and well-being. At the community level, higher levels of social capital are also associated with better health and better quality of life, a subjective measure based on the perception of the people in question.

Social capital The intangible factors that create networks and linkages among groups and individuals; includes things like trust in others, reciprocity, and group membership.

Social capital refers to the existence of intangible factors that create networks and linkages among groups and individuals. Social capital includes things like trust in others, reciprocity, and group membership that support inclusion and participation in the group (Kawachi et al. 1999; Baron et al. 2000). In the context of anthropogenic change and its impact on health, we should keep in mind that it may be more feasible to change the social environment to support better health for individuals, groups, and communities than to change the structures of society. This is the motivation behind a number of public health programs, such as the Social Inclusion initiative of the Australian Government that addresses a number of important health issues, including supporting those who are unemployed, those who live in the areas of greatest disadvantage, and closing the gap between Indigenous and non-Indigenous health. The aim of this initiative is to assist vulnerable groups by reducing disadvantage through the creation of social capital (Australian Government 2010).

Changes to personal behaviour

Another kind of anthropogenic change that may have an effect on health is related to the personal behaviour of individuals. What people choose to do, or are able to do, is closely related to developments in technology, economic status, where they live in the world, and many other factors. It is perhaps not surprising that individual behaviour today is very different from what it was in the past, but we should be aware that the things we do have the potential to affect our own health. Further, when many people change their behaviour in some way, this may affect the health of the whole community or population.

One example of change in personal behaviour that may have important health effects is the increasing use of household chemicals by a majority of people around the world. Every day, each of us uses a variety of chemicals, including soap, cosmetics, shampoo, cleaning products, insecticides, writing products, paint, sealants, and so forth. Each of these products has been determined to be safe if used in the recommended manner, and large safety factors are typically applied. However, household chemicals are generally not tested in combination, and we are only beginning to study their persistence in the indoor environment. That is, chemicals that have been shown to be safe individually may still interact in a way that affects health if they are used together, and certain chemicals may remain in the air or on surfaces for some time after their use. Exposure to these substances may be very significant as it has been estimated that the average person spends 85–90% of their time indoors (Farrow 2008).

Synthetic chemicals of this kind have been isolated from the air (especially from air samples taken indoors), from water, and from soil, meaning that we come in contact with them regularly from birth. This, it has been suggested, may account for or contribute to the rising incidence of asthmas and allergic conditions in both children and adults (Clegg & Richards 2007; Evans et al. 2008; Choi et al. 2010). The exact mechanism by which exposure to multiple household chemicals might lead to asthma or allergies is not known, but several hypotheses have been suggested. One possibility is that the modern idea of cleanliness, which is often expressed as a desire to remove all potentially harmful microorganisms from the living environment and a high use of cleaning products of all kinds, interferes with the normal development of the immune system. This, in turn, may contribute to the increase in allergic conditions, even though the specific physiologic effect is not known (Flohr et al. 2005; Garn & Renz 2007; Von Mutius 2007).

Another example of how changes in personal behaviour can affect health is the increasing interest in foreign travel across segments of many societies. More people seem to be interested in travelling, often to exotic locations, and, at the same time, travel has become affordable to more people than ever before (Mason 2008). We understand, however, that the diseases that are endemic in different parts of the world are very different, and newcomers to a given location may be more vulnerable to these diseases than people who live in the area in question. It is not uncommon for travellers to return home with unusual illnesses they contracted while travelling in another part of the world. A potentially serious situation may occur when the disease brought back is **vector-borne** (spread from person to person by an insect, such as mosquitoes) and a vector that can carry the disease already exists in the place where they live. This occurred in the New York City area in 1999. In that year, 19 patients came to light when they were hospitalised for a serious viral meningoencephalitis. This later was found to be West Nile Virus, a serious disease spread by mosquitoes not normally found in North America. By the end of the outbreak, 62 patients had been identified who positively suffered from West Nile Virus. It is assumed that the disease was introduced into the New York City area by a traveller to North Africa or the Middle East who may or may not have shown symptoms of the disease. A suitable vector (the Culex mosquito) was already present in New York and likely spread the virus from the original infected individual(s) to others who had not travelled outside the country themselves (Nash et al. 2001). It was later found that the virus had also spread to other species (LaDeau et al. 2007). While this outbreak of an exotic disease was limited in nature, we have seen that other diseases are becoming endemic in new areas, probably due to the movement of human beings between regions and countries. In Australia, for example, outbreaks of dengue fever in Queensland have been associated with the return of Australian forces from East Timor where the disease is endemic (Kitchener et al. 2002). The World Health Organization monitors **emerging diseases** and collects information on outbreaks of unusual diseases around the world through its Global Alert and Response Network (see <www.who.int/csr/outbreaknetwork/en>).

Vector-borne A disease spread by an insect (mosquitoes, ticks, lice, etc.) that transmits the disease to humans or other animals.

Emerging disease A disease that has not previously been observed in human populations.

See Chapter 9 on climate change for more information on vector-borne disease.

Stop and Think

Few international travellers think about the possibility that they might introduce an exotic disease into the environment when they return home. Nor do they consider the possibility that they could be the source of a disease that is not usual in the location they plan to visit. Nonetheless, this happens quite often, albeit on a small scale in most situations.

» What are the potential implications for the spread of disease if international travel continues to grow as a leisure activity?

» How might this affect Australia, keeping in mind that this country is comparatively isolated from other parts of the world?

Anthropogenic change and human health

As we have seen, people have changed various aspects of their living environment over many centuries. Conscious changes to the physical environment, first to fulfil basic needs and later to make life more comfortable and convenient, have often led to unanticipated changes in the social environment as well as in the way people live. There are situations where such changes have created new opportunities for infectious disease to take hold in human populations. An example of this is Legionnaire's Disease, a type of pneumonia, spread through modern air-conditioning systems and first recognised in the mid-1970s. However, by the end of the 20th century, the impact of changes in the living environment on chronic disease was beginning to be recognised. Ironically, when infectious disease was the main concern of public health in the late 19th and early 20th centuries, deconcentration of dwellings and separation of residential and business areas was considered an important measure to improve health. Now, however, it is exactly these characteristics of a surburban lifestyle that are seen as contributing to the rising incidence of chronic disease (Collins Purdue et al. 2003). Similarly, it has been suggested that the levels of environmental pollutants concentrated in air, water, and soil play a part in chronic disease ranging from certain kinds of cancers to asthma and allergic conditions. This is directly related to increasing population density and, with it, greater industrial activity and demand for resources. As the earth represents a single ecosystem, this kind of anthropogenic change affects everyone, regardless of where they are relative to where pollution occurs. For example, chemicals that have been banned for decades in North America are still found in water in the USA and Canada because they are carried there by the natural hydrological cycle from China, where they are still in use in the electronics industry (Arnold et al. 2007).

See Chapter 10 for a detailed discussion of the suburban lifestyle.

It is not surprising then that when we consider anthropogenic change we usually focus on human alterations of the environment that have adversely affected human health. This is due, at least in part, to the fact that we view the role of medicine and public health as creating and maintaining good health, and it seems natural to focus on those factors that may interfere with this aim. However, it is important to remember that many anthropogenic changes to the living environment have had a beneficial effect on human health and have become accepted as integral aspects of how we live. These include the treatment and management of drinking water; modern housing that protects inhabitants from the outside environment and can be heated and/or cooled as required; the use of modern agricultural processes that have greatly increased the availability and quality of the food supply; and many more. When we focus on changes to the environment that are detrimental to health, we do so in order to protect the amazing strides we have made in health and quality of life, especially during the 20th century.

Case Study 8.1   The conquest (and re-emergence) of tuberculosis

In the 19th and early 20th centruies, tuberculosis was an extremely serious health problem in Western societies. Caused by the bacterium *Mycobacterium tuberculosis*, and colloquially referred to as 'consumption' because of its symptoms, the disease affects the lungs and other parts of the body, causing weakness and wasting, impairing lung function, and eventually leading to death if not treated. The disease was so common at this time that it was often referred to as 'The White Plague', in contrast to the Black Plague (bubonic plague) that devasted Europe in the Middle Ages (Dubos & Dubos 1952).

By the second half of the 20th century, however, tuberculosis was very rare in Western societies. The occasional case was easily treated with antibiotics, but many doctors had never seen a real case among their patients, and most considered it a disease of the past. In the early 1980s, however, new cases of tuberculosis began to emerge. It is now known that this re-emergence of an old disease coincided with the beginnings of the AIDS epidemic, but this was not recognised until later. Originally, these new cases of the disease were associated with homelessness and other social factors in the modern urban environment (Daniel et al. 1994).

The conquest and subsequent re-emergence of tuberculosis in Western society is an excellent example of the impact of anthropogenic change on the nature of human health. More than 100 years ago, it was already noted that tuberculosis seemed to be more common among the poor, the malnourished, and those living in very crowded conditions where hygiene was poor. It was very much a disease of urban areas, and sufferers who could afford to do so were often advised to undergo a period of prolonged rest in a quiet, often rural, environment (Rosen 1993). German author Thomas Mann (1875–1955) wrote about his wife's experiences at a tuberculosis sanitorium in Davos, Switzerland, in his very influential 1924 novel *The Magic Mountain*.

The height of the tuberculosis epidemic coincided with a period of social reform that led to major changes in the living environment. These changes included the implementation of workers' compensation and other kinds of social insurance; the establishment of modern public education systems; concern for the quality of housing and the implementation of residency and building standards; and also increasing availability of more varied food all year round through improvements in production and distribution. By 1944, when streptomycin was discovered and led to the effective ability to treat tuberculosis with drugs, the incidence of the disease was already greatly reduced due to changes in the living environment associated with social reform (Bates 1992; Rosen 1993).

Once antibiotics were available for its treatment, tuberculosis lost some of the horror that had been attached to it but was still generally viewed as a disease of poverty and substandard living conditions. Cases tended to be treated aggressively with antibiotics, but the treatment process is a long one and was often poorly supervised. This led to widespread antibiotic resistance of the tuberculosis bacterium and gave rise to what is sometimes called 'The New Tuberculosis' (Gandy & Zumia 2002). When AIDS emerged as a new disease in the early 1980s, it became apparent that individuals whose immune system was compromised by HIV were particularly susceptible to tuberculosis, many strains of which can no longer be treated effectively with standard antibiotic therapy. Co-infection with HIV and tuberculosis is one of the most serious public health threats we now face around the world (Colebunders & Lambert 2002; Corbett et al. 2003). The history of tuberculosis in modern society is a good example of how anthropogenic change first almost eliminated a serious disease but then made it possible for it to reappear in a form that is much more difficult to address.

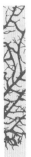

Mythbuster

It is easy to get the impression that anthropogenic change is always detrimental to health. The negative effects of human activity tend to receive a great deal of media attention and are often sensationalised. In fact, there have been many improvements to human health that are a direct result of the way people change their environment. The modern workplace is much safer than in the past due to innovations in machinery and processes, our food supply is less likely to make us sick because of changes to production and distribution and the enforcement of quality standards, our homes are safer from fire and protect us better from heat and cold due to improvements in technology and building practices as well as building regulations, and there are many more examples.

Summary

Anthropogenic change is change caused by human beings. People have been changing their environment since prehistoric times to meet their own needs and improve quality of life. Some of the earliest changes centred on agriculture and the built environment. These activities brought human populations into contact with animals and microorganisms and also new diseases. The changing nature of work has also created new risks to health. Changes to the physical environment can also change the social and cognitive environment. Some of these changes are associated with mental and emotional health issues in modern populations. Urbanisation may be the underlying cause for a range of health problems experienced around the world, including isolation, rage, and lack of social connections. Individual choices, about international travel or use of chemical products, can also affect the health of individuals, as well as of the community as a whole, as part of a larger pattern of new behaviour.

A number of previously unknown conditions are directly related to changes made by humans to their living environment. Examples include sick building syndrome; Legionnaires' Disease, a bacterial pneumonia often spread by air-conditioning systems; the spread of certain vector-borne diseases; and so on. Suburban living, providing more space and separating residential and business areas, may contribute to the burden of chronic disease. Nonetheless, many of the changes people have made to their environment over the centuries have been very beneficial to health and have become integral parts of our lifestyle and support our expectations for health.

Tutorial exercises

1   The pace of anthropogenic change has increased since the middle of the 20th century largely due to changes in technology that allowed for change in the living environment. List the innovations you think might have had the greatest impact on health (e.g. the automobile, electricity) and look up when they became widely available in Western societies. What can you conclude about anthropogenic impacts on health using what you know about changes in health since the end of the 19th century?

2   A number of new diseases have emerged during the 20th century that have been associated with human beings moving into new areas or engaging in new activities. Is this a result of anthropogenic change? Explain.

3   What are some examples of anthropogenic change that have been beneficial to health?

Further reading

Barnes, E. (2005). *Diseases and human evolution*. Albuquerque, NM: University of New Mexico Press.

Frumkin, H. (ed.) (2010). *Environmental health: From global to local*. San Francisco: John Wiley & Sons.

Hassan, R., Scholes, R., & Ash, N. (eds) (2005). *Ecosystems and human well-being: Current state and trends*. Washington, DC: Millennium Ecosystem Assessment.

Link, K. (2007). *Understanding new, resurgent and resistant diseases: How man and globalization create and spread illness*. Westport, CT: Praeger.

Websites

<www.who.int/csr/outbreaknetwork/en>

The World Health Organization monitors the appearance of new diseases around the world and makes available surveillance and epidemiological information about these conditions through its Global Alert and Response Network.

<www.cdc.gov/ncidod/EID/index.ht>

The US Centers for Disease Control and Prevention (CDC) publishes a monthly report on new diseases and health conditions called Emerging Infectious Disease.

<www.who.int/globalchange>

Climate change has been suggested as a major type of anthropogenic change that has the potential to affect human health. The World Health Organization Report on Climate Change and Human Health summarises current views on this topic.

9

Climate change: Drivers and health impacts, mitigation, and adaptation strategies for the health sector

Glenda Verrinder and Adrian Verrinder

TOPICS COVERED

This chapter covers the following topics:
- what the terms 'climate change' and 'global warming' mean
- the 'probable' causes of climate change and global warming
- the difference between 'probable' scientific truth and the 'absolute' truth demanded by climate change deniers
- the likelihood that climate change/global warming will bring about more intense and more frequent weather events
- the health impacts of climate change/global warming: health sector responses to scenarios resulting from climate change

KEY TERMS

Adaptation

Climate

Climate change

Climate change literacy

Global warming

Greenhouse gas

Mitigation

Primary prevention

Secondary prevention

Vulnerability

Introduction

There is mounting evidence that anthropogenic **climate change** is having, and will increasingly have, an impact on human health. Haines (2009, p. vii) contends that 'climate change appears to be more rapid, more serious and more dangerous than it was thought, even two or three years ago'. Health professionals will be affected individually, as family members, as community members, and as professionals. Unprecedented events around the world such as heatwaves, cyclones, floods, and drought have stretched services to the limit and beyond in recent times. These events have highlighted the need for health professionals to have a firm understanding of the evidence and implications of climate change. Paramedics, nurses, social workers, occupational therapists, psychologists, medical, public health, health promotion, and environmental health practitioners, and others in the health sector will be at the front line of professionals responding to the health impacts of climate change.

To ensure best practice, health professionals are required to understand evidence. We use evidence to determine what the health issues are, what contributes to that problem, and the magnitude of the problem. We also use evidence to determine the best course of action and whether that course of action was effective. Once, health professionals learnt about how the body and mind worked and applied their knowledge and skills to the care of individuals. Evidence about the social determinants of health then emerged and once again health professions applied this evidence to their work with individuals and communities. Now, there is evidence about the impact of climate change on health, and professionals will be obliged to apply their knowledge and skills to individuals and communities within this context. McMichael and colleagues (2003, p. 2) write:

> Our increasing understanding of climate change is transforming how we view the boundaries and determinants of health. While our personal health may seem to relate mostly to prudent behaviour, heredity, occupation, local environmental exposures, and health-care access, sustained population health requires the life-supporting 'services' of the biosphere. Populations of all animal species depend on supplies of food and water, freedom from excess infectious disease, and the physical safety and comfort conferred by climate stability. The climate system is fundamental to this life-support.

This chapter focuses on climate change and human health. It will be presented in two parts. In the first part, the science of climate change is presented with the aim of improving the **climate change literacy** of health professionals. Griffiths and colleagues (2009) argue that this is essential for all health professionals now. In the second part, some of the impacts of climate change on human health will be presented along with case studies to illustrate the roles that some health agencies are already playing to mitigate, and adapt to, climate change.

Planetary climate change and human adaptation

The earth's **climate** has always been changing. The history of the planet for millions of years is a story of perpetual climate change. Over the millennia the planet has changed from a partial frozen snowball to one where even the polar regions

Climate change A variation in climate that is attributable to either natural environmental changes or stemming from human action (anthropogenic change).

Climate change literacy General knowledge or awareness of the concepts, cause, and effects of climate change.

Climate The average weather, encompassing natural variability and extremes.

had tropical weather and back again. These ancient climate changes had natural causes in the periodic tilt and wobble of the earth and variations in its orbit around the sun.

The earth's gaseous atmosphere, liquid oceans, and solid crust can soak up a lot of heat and hold it there. The oceans provide an enormous heat sink. It is fairly hard to heat up water and once warmed it holds its heat very well. The atmosphere is rather more skittish and heats up and cools down on a daily and seasonal basis, while the sea temperature stays relatively constant.

Stop and Think

The atmosphere helps to stabilise the temperature by absorbing and retaining heat. The moon has no atmosphere.

» Find out the temperatures for (1) the illuminated side of the moon and (2) the dark side of the moon.

» What are your conclusions about the effect of a gaseous atmosphere on temperature stabilisation?

Heat is essentially an outward manifestation of how rapidly the atoms or molecules are moving and banging into each other. Hot things warm up cool things.

In the last hundred thousand years or so, humans have had to endure a series of ice ages and our ancestors adapted to them in various ways. The adaptations of fire and warm clothes made it possible to survive on the edge of the ice sheets that covered northern Europe and Asia (Verrinder 2000, 2010; McMichael 2001).

The last ice was coming to a close 12,000 years ago, the glaciers were melting, the river flats were flooding with the nutrient-rich waters and stone-age humans had enough computing capacity in their brains to work out that if you buried certain parts of plants they would grow again. The dramatic adaptation after the last ice age was the domestication of grasses—wheat, barley, rice, maize—and the domestication of some animals—sheep, goats, cows, and later, pigs. Farming was an adaptation to climate change, an adaptation that slowly swept the world, arriving in Australia just a couple of hundred years ago. It remains to be seen whether farming is sustainable in the long term. Hunter-gatherers were far less damaging to the earth's natural resources (Verrinder 2000, 2010; McMichael 2001).

The increasing use of fossil fuels

In the 1700s, engineers in Europe worked out a way to convert *heat* into *work*. By heating boilers of water, they could force steam into a cylinder containing a piston, pushing the piston back, and with a connecting rod rotate a wheel. The rotating wheel was used to run any kind of factory machine they could think of: spinning machines, weaving machines, bellows to drive blast furnaces to make molten iron and steel and cast it into whatever shape they wanted. Later in the 1800s, they worked out how to make hydrocarbons explode inside the cylinder and drive a piston back and forth—the 'internal combustion' engine is found in all kinds of applications in the 21st century (Verrinder 2000, 2010).

But where can you get a supply of heat? From fossil fuels: hydrocarbon compounds (comprising primarily of hydrogen and carbon) had been buried in the earth as part of the decomposition of prehistoric forests that have covered the earth periodically (Solomon et al. 2007; Verrinder 2000, 2010).

The carbon cycle

In a natural ecosystem, carbon dioxide and water are taken up by green plants, and by extracting energy from the sun plants manufacture high-energy carbohydrates and liberate spare oxygen into the atmosphere. This is the source of oxygen in the air. Animals directly or indirectly consume the carbohydrates and with the oxygen perform a cool burn that extracts the energy and liberates carbon dioxide and water which ultimately get taken up by green plants. Some of the green plants die and get buried before they decompose and contribute to the fossil fuels—gas, coal, oil—all still containing the energy extracted from the sun in the prehistoric forests (Verrinder 2000, 2010).

The carbon *cycle* just described essentially determines the amount of carbon dioxide and oxygen in the atmosphere—well, it does within certain limits. If there is an increase in carbon dioxide, green plants will take up more of it and store the carbon and the sunlight in the structure of a massive tree, for example. The big trees are essentially acting as carbon sinks (Liggins 2009; Verrinder 2010).

But in the last 250 years, we have been using increasing amounts of fossil fuels; we burn them to extract the heat to turn the wheels of industry and have been increasing the man-made contribution of carbon dioxide to the atmosphere. In addition, our farming practices have involved taking out long-lived trees (the carbon sinks) and growing annual grasses (wheat, rice, maize etc) which have a very limited capacity to absorb carbon dioxide. One of the physical properties of carbon dioxide is that it absorbs heat.

Farming domestic animals in large quantities, primarily herbivores, produces flatulence, notably methane, another gas which absorbs heat. So, the concentrations of carbon dioxide and methane have been increasing in the last 250 years and it is the capacity of these gases to absorb heat that is *probably* warming the planet (Solomon et al. 2007).

Evidence and probabilities

We say 'probably' because science deals in terms of probabilities rather than absolute truths. The vast majority of climate scientists estimate that there is a 90–95% probability that the globe is warming and that it is *probably* due to the man-made increase in heat-absorbing (aka 'greenhouse') gases (Solomon et al. 2007; Liggins 2009).

Climate change deniers prefer to deal in *absolute* truths. They assert that because the scientist's predictions cannot be *absolutely* accurate, there is no truth in *anything* the climate scientists have to say.

Being absolutely accurate is a difficult task in science. We are dealing with complex systems. But just to demonstrate one source of uncertainty about climate-change predictions, consider the following example. We know that sea temperatures worldwide have increased a bit over the last 100 years and that, quite naturally, this has increased evaporation, so at any one time there is more water vapour in the atmosphere. If it forms high clouds the water vapour will reflect the heat of the sun. If it forms low clouds the water vapour will absorb the heat of the sun. The actual increase in heat will depend on the proportions of water vapour that form high and low clouds. The exact proportions are hard to predict. The various climate models can and have predicted heat absorption to within plus or minus 5% (Solomon et al. 2007). That's pretty accurate but not absolutely accurate. Climate-change deniers cloud the debate by using this lack of absolute accuracy to lobby the public on behalf of the fossil fuel industry among others.

'Climate change' as a term is itself a euphemism coined to replace the term 'global warming'. **Global warming** as a term though can be misleading. It is demonstrable that the earth is, on average, warmer than it was 100 years ago (as evidenced by

Global warming
The rise in global temperature observed during the 20th century and projected to continue into the future.

Case Study 9.1   Unexpected results

Britain ranges from 50 to 60 degrees latitude north, as, obviously, does northern Europe (Melbourne is only 38 degrees south). Northern Europe is kept relatively warm by the Gulf Stream, a current of warm water running from the Gulf of Mexico across the Atlantic Ocean and up the coast of Europe. It has only been in existence since the end of the last Ice Age (about 12,000 years ago).

If the Gulf stream faltered (some pundits have predicted this as a possible result of excessive melting of the Greenland glaciers), temperatures in northern Europe could become comparable with those of northern Canada. Find out what the winter temperatures are in Canada at latitudes 50–60 degrees north and predict what would happen to agricultural production in northern Europe.

» *An example could be the Canadian City of Saskatoon, roughly the same latitude as Cambridge (UK) and Berlin (Germany).*

the sea temperatures, insect migration, earlier fruit blossoms, and the receding glaciers) but what is just as important is what this heat *does*. The first law of thermodynamics states that 'heat is work and work is heat' so the absorbed heat is available to do work. In effect the extra heat gives rise to *more energetic* weather patterns. The Intergovernmental Panel on Climate Change technical reports (Solomon et al. 2007) claim that this means more climatic extremes, more heatwaves, more energetic and more frequent cyclones, hurricanes and tornadoes—all rotating low-pressure systems driven by atmospheric and oceanic heat. More cold systems occur too, as snow storms and freezing air are driven further towards the equator by the sheer energy of the Arctic and Antarctic weather systems.

The amount of extra heat held by the oceans causes it to expand, so sea levels are slowly rising. This is nothing new. At the end of the last ice age the combination of melting glaciers and thermal expansion caused a sea level rise of 100 metres, flooding the English Channel and Bass Strait, and inundating what is now the Persian Gulf. This might have been the historic event that was later recorded as Noah's Flood.

Key messages about climate change

The six key messages from 2500 scientists from 80 countries who met in Copenhagen in 2009 were about climate trends, social disruption, long-term strategies, equity, meeting the challenges, and the consequences of inaction. Briefly, the view of the scientists was that

- Climate change is having, and will have, strongly differential effects on people within and between countries and regions, on this generation and future generations, and on human societies and the natural world.
- Poor nations and communities are particularly at risk socially and economically.
- Changes already observed in the climate may accelerate.
- Delay in initiating mitigation actions significantly increases the long-term social and economic costs of both adaptation and mitigation.
- We already have many tools and approaches to deal effectively with the challenges of climate change (Climate Change 2009).

Stop and Think

» Think about the community in which you live. What impact do you think a changing climate has had on this community in your lifetime?

Environmental determinants of human health

Global warming is measurable and real. The threats to health are direct and indirect. Human health is affected in floods, landslides, heatwaves, water shortages, and exposure to pollutants. Increased frequency and intensity of heat events, more frequent energetic weather events, and changes in arbovirus disease patterns are predicted (WHO 2005b). What effects can this have on human health and what can we do about it?

Heat and cold

Heat can kill. Human bodies strive, through homeostatic mechanisms, to keep their internal temperatures at 37° Celsius. The slow burn of carbohydrates, hydrocarbons, and oxygen give off heat proportional to the amount of work done by, for example, muscle tissue. This generated body heat is lost to the environment through the skin, through exhaled air from the lungs, and through the evaporation of sweat. Evaporation is particularly effective because in order to convert liquid water to water vapour heat has to be extracted from the skin.* When the ambient temperature is above 37° Celsius, body heat cannot be lost to the environment from the skin or the lungs—heat cannot directly flow from a cooler to a hotter body (the second law of thermodynamics). The only effective cooling mechanism is by the evaporation of litre upon litre of body water, leading eventually to dehydration. That water must be replaced. In really hot environments the body cannot keep up the pace; you only have so many sweat glands and in older persons their sweating ability is reduced by 50% simply because they have fewer functioning sweat glands. Body temperature starts to rise above normal and as the body temperature rises the homeostatic mechanisms start to fail, the cooling mechanism itself is compromised, and the body temperature soars. Nausea and vomiting are common; cramps and muscle spasms are the characteristic symptoms of 'heat-stroke' leading to a point of no return: death by hyperthermia. In extremis, it is very difficult to restore the homeostatic cooling mechanisms once they have gone awry.

Cold can kill too. When faced with freezing ambient temperatures, the human body tries to adapt. It stops sweating, and redirects blood away from the skin, limiting loss of heat by radiation.

Stop and Think

*If you don't believe this, select a 37°C day, leave water out in a bucket until it reaches 37°C, then, sitting outside under a shady tree, sponge your 37°C body down with the 37°C water. You will feel the cooling effect of 37°C water evaporating off your body and drawing heat from your skin.

Glenda Verrinder and Adrian Verrinder

It does this by dramatically constricting the peripheral arterioles, limiting the flow of warm blood to the skin and the extremities. It cannot do much about heat loss from the lungs—each lungful of air comes out at 37° Celsius. A further adaptation is shivering—the involuntary contraction of muscles, making the muscles work thereby generating heat, warming the perfusing blood. All that is left then are *behavioural* adaptations, such as insulating the skin from heat loss with clothes, lighting a fire, or moving about to generate muscle heat. Eventually, without intervention the core body temperature drops, the homeostatic warming mechanisms are compromised, and peripheral tissues starved of oxygen and glucose shut down and develop into frostbite (i.e. dead tissue) if the individual survives. In extremis, body heat continues to be lost through the lungs and the core temperature drops to a point which is, as they say, incompatible with life.

Vulnerable populations

Vulnerability Limited access to resources to adapt to changing conditions.

Vulnerability at the individual level is influenced by biological aspects such as age and sex, social aspects such as social connectedness, and environmental aspects such as geographical location. Children, older people, and people who are poor are more vulnerable to global warming.

Vulnerability at the population level means limited access to resources and infrastructure in order to adapt to changing conditions. Some groups do not have the resources for adequate responses to environmental determinants of health (Verrinder 2011).

Older persons are more vulnerable to heat and cold primarily because their homeostatic mechanisms for maintaining body temperature are just not as effective as those of younger people. Their bodies are slower to detect changes in ambient temperature and their physiological mechanisms are slower to respond. They also have less effective 'effector' mechanisms—fewer sweat glands, fewer cutaneous capillaries to bring the actual body temperature back to the set point (i.e. 37°C). In addition, they may not have the money for coolers and heaters, all of which consume energy and are expensive to run. They may not have adequate clothing. In developing countries, they may not have access to reasonable shelter or even clean water for rehydration in the heat.

Babies and toddlers are vulnerable too; having a relatively large surface-area-to-volume ratio they tend to gain or lose heat more rapidly than adults. Hence, the warning is given by governments not to leave children in cars on hot days. Poverty and relative deprivation again are hugely important. If you are relatively wealthy you can protect yourself from the heat and cold (Verrinder 2011).

See also Chapter 1 on climate change as a determinant of health.

Flood and famine

As well as the short-term effect of extreme hot and cold spells, there are indirect environmental effects on health. Clearly, the environment is affected by the amount of heat in it. Sea level rise has already been mentioned, and more severe storms will and do result in inundation of land by salt water. This is compounded when cyclones combine with high tides. Cyclones, as mentioned before, are rotating systems of atmospheric low pressure. Normal atmospheric pressure presses on the planet all the time with a pressure of 15 lbs per square inch (10.9 tonnes per square metre) and keeps the ocean 'in place' as it were. A low-pressure system releases some of this pressure and the sea rises proportionately. A combination of a king tide and a low-pressure system along with the accompanying high-velocity onshore wind can devastate low-lying agricultural land.

Sea temperature too will have an effect on the amount of rain that falls on landmasses. For example, the floods that devastated Queensland and Victoria in late 2010 and early 2011 were caused by water that evaporated off the bodies of tropical water to the north of Australia; the moisture was pushed down to the south of the continent by the energy in that system. The temperature of the northerly bodies of water was only a third of a degree Celsius warmer than normal, but that much water had that much more heat in it; it had the energy to work its way thousands of kilometres to the south.

These floods followed years of drought, caused in part by the sea temperatures to the north of Australia being a third of a degree cooler than they had been before 2011. Floods carry their own problems with environmental diseases, particularly diseases of the gut. Western societies expend a tremendous amount of money and energy to separate drinking water from sewage. Floods just slosh it all back together again. Water-borne diseases on the move include cholera, vilnuficus, cryptosporidium, and naeglaria. For a fuller account, see *Global warming and the political ecology of health* (Baer & Singer 2009).

What kind of agriculture is possible in this sort of climate? Will Australia be able to feed itself? Will other less 'developed' countries be able to feed themselves? In the event of a disaster, will they be able to afford to import enough food to keep them going in the recovery period?

If global warming—more energetic weather—means more frequent, more violent climatic events, then more heat and more frequent floods are obviously going to affect food production.

Vulnerable populations

Again, relative wealth plays a big part. If Australia cannot grow enough wheat it *currently* has the necessary wealth to import all its nutritional needs. It is much harder to recover from environmental devastation in 'developing' (i.e. poor) countries such as low-lying parts of Bangladesh. There is also a lack of available money to build protective infrastructure.

Sub-Saharan Africa has been subject to flood and famine for the last thirty years. This has brought about a dramatic reduction in the carrying capacity of that land and precipitated wars over the scarce resources. Humans are already fighting and killing over the resources of water and arable land.

Again, older persons and children are among the most vulnerable. Children are particularly prone to nutritional diseases such as kwashiorkor (lack of protein) and diseases caused by lack of vitamins and lack of essential minerals such as iodine and iron. If they do not die of malnutrition, the lack of iodine alone will lead to mental retardation, which itself may have a considerable impact on the effectiveness of the workforce in later years.

Arbovirus diseases

Disease-carrying insects, the vectors for a diverse range of human diseases from malaria to dengue, are very sensitive to environmental conditions. These vectors love warm, watery environments and are prolific breeders. Malaria is one of the biggest killers on the planet; if and when the warm wet tropics move north and south into previously temperate zones, the mosquitoes will come with them. Even if it just warms up and gets no wetter, the warmth will encourage mosquitoes to breed in the lakes and dams we use for irrigation. Not only will they head north and south, they will head up mountains and higher country as *it* warms.

Vector-borne infectious diseases also include Ross River Fever, West Nile Fever, Rift Valley Fever, Hanta, plague (the 'Black Death'), encephalitis, Yellow Fever, and Lyme Disease (Baer & Singer 2009).

Mythbuster

The International Panel on Climate Change is the best known group of scientists who have been studying climate change for more than 20 years. This panel conducts systematic reviews on climate change, meaning that only those research projects that are scientifically sound are used to advise international bodies such as the World Health Organization and national governments. For more information about this panel go to: <www.ipcc.ch>.

The CSIRO (Australian Commonwealth Scientific and Research Organisation) advises the Australian Government on climate change in Australia. For more information go to: <www.csiro.au>.

Both organisations have stated that

- climate change is happening; and
- will continue worldwide; and
- human activities are changing the climate (anthropogenic change).

» *If so many scientists have demonstrated that anthropogenic climate change is probably real, what is the basis of the climate change deniers' claims that it is not? For an analysis of climate change deniers see Climate change deniers: Heads in the sand (Washington & Cook 2011).*

In Australia, there are changing patterns of vector-borne disease (Tong et al. 2008). In Australia, Ross River virus and Barmah forest virus cause debilitating diseases and Murray Valley encephalitis can cause death.

There are people who are more vulnerable than others to arbovirus disease: those who cannot protect themselves well, such as outdoor workers, or those who cannot afford protective clothing or to screen insects from their homes.

Mental health/illness

There is a growing literature on the impact of weather and mental health/illness. Walker and colleagues (2011) draw attention to the impact of climate change on mental health. In their systematic review of literature, three themes are identified: the direct effects of extreme weather events; the impact on vulnerable communities; and the emotional stress caused by the awareness of global climate change.

In extreme weather events people can lose family members and friends, neighbours, their house, and their jobs. Communities change irrevocably. Loss of income, involuntary separation, and loss of services have all had an impact on the mental health of the people in communities.

A further loss of people, services, skills, and volunteers to run community organisations is often the result of short- and long-term changes in the weather. Furthermore, service providers believe people do not attend to their health needs because of the 'misplaced need to be stoic' (Alston & Kent 2004, p. 56).

There are health impacts of aesthetic and cultural impoverishment due to degradation of the environment as well (Alston & Kent 2004; WHO 2005b; Talbot & Verrinder 2009). Conversely, involvement in conservation and nature-based activities not only benefits the ecosystems in which people live, but also enhances community cohesion and improves mental health and well-being (Burgess et al. 2007; Ebden & Townsend 2007; Phillips & Kingsley 2007; Talbot & Verrinder 2009).

Mitigation and adaptation

Fundamentally, there are two strategies we can adopt: **mitigation** and **adaptation**. Mitigation in this context means limiting the effects by limiting the cause, while adaptation means changing our behaviour in order to limit the effects (Metz et al. 2007). In effect, the difference between mitigation and adaptation can be the difference between correcting the underlying cause of the problem and merely treating the symptoms. Fundamentally, we would like to correct the underlying cause of a problem but politically we may be forced at times to merely paper over the cracks.

In the health sector, mitigation is understood as **primary prevention**. Broad issues that have an impact on the health of a population, such as poverty, discrimination, or polluted environments, are targets for primary prevention. **Secondary prevention** is understood as strategies that enable populations to deal with risks and threats. In the health sector, policies that enable communities to adapt to the social and mental impact of drought or cope with higher than normal temperatures, wildfires, water scarcity and other problems of climate change are examples (Verrinder 2011).

Mitigation Taking action to reduce greenhouse gas emissions.

Adaptation Taking action to minimise the current and expected impacts of climate change.

Primary prevention Inhibiting the development of disease.

Secondary prevention Strategies that enable populations to deal with risks and threats.

Mitigation

Prevention is obviously better than treatment: there is less illness, less disability, and ultimately it is cheaper for individuals and societies. But to mitigate global warming is a difficult task; it means all the nations of the world agreeing, verifiably, to reduce emissions of carbon dioxide. Ultimately, it means signing an enforceable pact or treaty. Many nations are extremely reluctant to do this. The USA has been reluctant to sign many international pacts on principle. It has refused to sign the Kyoto Protocol, for example. Individual states in the USA on the other hand, like California, *have* unilaterally set themselves targets on greenhouse gas emissions, as has the European Union. Gro Harlem Brundtland (2011), former Prime Minister of Norway and Special Envoy on Climate Change to the UN Secretary-General, offers three pieces of advice to political leaders:

> The most important challenge for today's political leaders is to safeguard the human environment so that our species can survive on this planet. I think the following three points are particularly relevant for any leader wanting to strike a balance between the pressing needs of today and the decisions necessary to secure our long term survival.
>
> 1   Base your policies on sound scientific knowledge;
> 2   Seek global cooperation;
> 3   National and global redistribution is needed.

Her last point refers particularly to tackling climate change and poverty globally at the same time.

Stop and Think

» What international treaties to reduce adverse impacts on the environment has Australia signed?

Fossil fuels

The challenge is to reduce the extraction of energy from fossil fuels. Burning fossil fuels always results in the release of carbon dioxide into the atmosphere. Many suggest that we need to put a price on carbon (see e.g. Bruntland 2011). A technological fix would be to bury the CO_2 underground (geo-sequestration), which is technically feasible at least in small amounts and for which millions are being invested in research. It may be just tokenism (see below). Converting power stations from coal and oil to methane would help. Methane (CH_4) has only half the amount of carbon compared to the very long chain hydrocarbons found in coal, oil, and petrol. This would reduce emissions but could not actually reduce the amount of atmospheric CO_2.

Biofuels

The idea here is to sequester atmospheric CO_2 into biological material from palm oil, trees, and so on, and then burn it to extract the energy. This is really a zero sum game which by itself could not actually reduce the amount of CO_2 in the atmosphere. In addition, biofuels take up valuable agricultural land more useful for growing food. There are only 12 billion hectares of useful arable land on the planet (Rees & Wackernagel 1994).

Nuclear

If you purify a specific uranium isotope it gets hot; you can use it to boil water and blow the steam past a turbine, thereby generating electricity. To make it safe you have to embed a lot of energy (see embedded energy below) in the infrastructure. The specific uranium isotopes are highly radioactive, hence toxic, and have been known to explode if there are enough of them in one place ('critical mass'). This is the basis of nuclear bombs. The waste products at the end of the process are also radioactive and remain so for thousands of years. However, nuclear power has been touted as a realistic alternative to fossil fuels but many are exceedingly wary of the nuclear option. Following the nuclear disaster in Fukuyama, Japan in 2011, ongoing global opposition to nuclear power has been vindicated. Would you volunteer to live next to a nuclear dump site or power plant?

Wind and solar

Environmentalists are keen on wind power converting wind into electricity by means of propeller-driven generators and solar power—converting sunlight directly into electricity using semiconductor solar panels. Both these technologies require manufacturing the energy-extracting machinery on an industrial scale; this itself takes energy. Will the energy used to manufacture the equipment (and this energy is generally supplied by fossil-fuel-powered power stations) enable more energy to be extracted from the wind and the sun than was embedded into the equipment during manufacture?

Embedded energy

It is not that easy to calculate embedded energy; technically it should include every energy input involved in the process from its inception to its disposal. That would include the energy in the breakfasts of the factory workers, but approaching it from the other end, ultimately the embedded energy is reflected in the *cost* of an item. Remember that the 'alternative energy' industry is also highly subsided; a $10,000 price tag may well represent $20,000 worth of energy. No one knows if any of these strategies is sustainable.

Tokenism

What we do know, however, is that politicians and governments often want to *look* as though they are doing something. They are, they say, 'addressing' the problem. They may invest $50 million into research on geo-sequestration, they might subsidise solar hot water services or solar panels. Such policies are all carefully balanced to appeal to sections of the population and to keep governments in power.

Mitigation of the root cause

It is unlikely that the nations of the world will agree to limit **greenhouse gas** emissions in the near future. There will be plenty of tokenism and a fair bit of 'muddling through'. Individual countries are developing wind, solar, and nuclear options but the globe continues to warm.

Greenhouse gas A gas that contributes to trapping heat in the atmosphere, warming the earth. These gases are both naturally occurring and released into the atmosphere by humans.

Adaptation

Adaptation while holding out hope for mitigation at some point in the future seems, sadly, to be the pragmatic course for the health professions. Adaptation may be defined as modifying behaviour to fit new conditions. There is some scope for *second-order* mitigation—*preventing* heat stress and cold stress rather than treating it, for example. Immunising against water-borne and vector-borne diseases and maintaining sanitary engineering come what may are further examples of second-order mitigation.

Adaptation may be at the level of a health practitioner but more importantly *organisational adaptation* is a key determinant of healthy outcomes. Organisational adaptation also offers the opportunity for individual practitioners and groups of practitioners to have some input into the process.

Agricultural adaptation

Australia already has undergone a considerable process of adaptation in terms of irrigation. Recognising the seasonal and annual variability in rainfall in the dry continent of Australia, in the late part of the 19th century and the early and middle parts of the 20th century, vast amounts of money were invested in water infrastructure. The strategies generally involved holding the water back in the headwaters (Lake Hume and Lake Eildon are good examples). The water can be released to irrigators to irrigate the flat country of the Murray-Darling basin. This irrigation water was provided to farmers. A popular practice was to flood-irrigate whole paddocks to grow grass to feed beef or dairy cattle. As the price of water increased to more accurately reflect the actual cost of delivering megalitres of water, more precise methods of water application, such as drip irrigation, have been adopted. This process is continuing.

In the last 15 years, a period of prolonged drought, water allocations have been far less than in 'normal' years. This too has driven a more efficient use of water.

More efficient use of water has its problems. The more accurately water is applied to the roots of the plants rather than flooding the paddock, the less run-off there is back into the river system. The rivers themselves need an environmental flow in order to remain ecologically healthy. There is evidence that in extended drought years the over-allocation of irrigation water pushed river systems close to ecological collapse.

Irrigation itself leads to other problems too, primarily salinisation, that is, the accumulation of salt in irrigated soils. This has to be a consideration in the allocation of irrigation water in the future.

Over-allocation of water in the past has led to problems too. In 'normal' years 'normal' allocations may be sustained, but in drought years—and more drought years are predicted—the system simply cannot meet the allocations. So, farmers dependent on irrigation become vulnerable, as do the communities in which they live. Irrigation towns and cities are dependent to a large extent on the income generated by the farming industries in their area. Loss of some population from irrigation country towns is as inevitable as the slow depopulation of dry-farming country towns over the last 50 years.

Ultimately, difficult decisions will have to be made as to how much water is to be stored, how much is allocated, how efficiently water is used, and how much population this infrastructure can support.

Crop selection is another matter. What crops will be viable in the face of progressive global warming? Currently, Australia grows more or less what farmers and corporate interests deem profitable. Some are upstream 'water-guzzlers'. Will growing cotton be viable given the amount of water it requires? Is the current occupation of irrigated land by wine grapes viable? Is food a priority?

See the case study on food security in Chapter 10.

These decisions will have to be made and implemented. The market alone cannot ensure that Australians have an affordable healthy diet with all the vitamins, minerals, essential amino acids and so on that are required to sustain health. There is a tutorial exercise recommended at the end of the chapter to help readers explore this issue further.

Health sector adaptation

There is a great deal the health sector can do to promote, protect, and maintain the health of populations within the context of climate change. A full range of strategies are available from mitigation to adaption (Talbot & Verrinder 2009; Griffith et al. 2010; Walker et al. 2011). Mitigation clearly means working on reducing greenhouse gas emissions. This can be done at the organisational and individual levels.

Ebi and Semenza (2008) suggest that it will remain vitally important to address social, cultural, environmental, political, and economic determinants that increase vulnerability. They propose a health planning cycle of community outreach, situation analysis, asset mapping, stakeholder involvement, intervention implementation, and evaluation. Talbot and Verrinder (2009) concur and, further, propose integrated health promotion strategies such as policy development at the local

Case Study 9.2   Healthcare organisations reduce greenhouse gases

The Green Star—Healthcare v1 tool is available specifically for use by healthcare agencies such as hospitals, community health centres, diagnostic centres, aged care facilities, and mental health facilities (Green Building Council of Australia). Healthcare organisation projects are awarded a Green Star rating based on accumulating credit points in various categories including, but not confined to, energy and water conservation, transport policies and facilities of the organisation, recycling of materials, land use management, patient and staff access to clean and healthy indoor and outdoor areas, and disposal and reduction of trade wastes. Governments are supporting initiatives such as these, for example, Greening Victoria's Hospitals program (Sustainability Victoria).

level, building capacity of organisations and communities through education, providing information through social marketing, and monitoring the impacts of climate change in communities. In Chapter 7 in this book, Hulme Chambers and Walker have linked health promotion and climate change. As they point out, health promotion has a wellness focus that assists people to maintain and improve their health rather than simply focusing on factors that cause disease. They use the Ottawa Charter for Health Promotion as a conceptual framework to address health issues.

See the case study on climate change in Chapter 7.

Health impacts will be different in different communities and at different times. Evidence, information, and practical examples for the health sector are already apparent.

Heat/cold

Extreme heat events globally have killed thousands of people. In Australia, the health impact of the heatwave in Victoria in 2009 stretched health sector resources. For example, compared to the January–February period the previous year there were 25% more emergency ambulance dispatches and more Medical Deputising Service calls. More cardiac arrests were reported as well as heat stress, heat stroke, and dehydration. There was a threefold increase in deaths on arrival to Emergency Departments compared to the same period in 2008. Seventy per cent of these were over the age of 75 (State of Victoria 2009).

Ideally, no one should be exposed to extreme heat or cold at home or in the workplace. Outdoor workers, however, are frequently exposed to environmental temperatures above 30°C. Indoor workers are frequently exposed to similar temperatures, especially if they work in uninsulated iron sheds or factories. Even some office workers are exposed to extreme temperatures. It is generally recognised that temperatures above 26°C may lead to the early stages of heat stress.

See the case study on the Victorian heat planning strategy in Chapter 10.

Arboviruses

The impact of arboviruses can be ameliorated by insect (e.g. mosquito) control measures. Responses to mosquito-borne disease are practised now in some areas of Australia through local government. These responses may change as disease patterns follow climate change. These viruses can lead to debilitating illness and in some cases death. The following case study is an example of a local government response in Victoria.

Case Study 9.3   Monitoring arbovirus

Where local governments are situated in areas of high mosquito activity, many of them monitor mosquito activity as part of both state and federal initiatives. These programs are specifically interested in vector mosquitoes (i.e. those species of mosquitoes that are known to carry or are capable of carrying arboviruses); however, at local government level the program will also include education about living with nuisance mosquitoes.

There are three main sources of water that will enable mosquitoes to become a problem or nuisance. These are irrigation, heavy rains/floods, and domestic watering. Mosquito monitoring programs are scoped to include all these sources, though the manner in which each problem is dealt with varies. In Victoria local government have specific powers for the 'Prevention of mosquito breeding' under the Public Health and Wellbeing Regulations 2009. In addition, and most states have similar legislation, there is scope for dealing with mosquito problems under the nuisance provisions of the *Public Health and Wellbeing Act 2008*.

The mosquito-monitoring programs have four major activities:

Education—This is multifaceted. The broadest education programs are for the general public and are aimed at ensuring the public minimise their contact with mosquitoes or are suitably protected at times when this cannot be avoided. More specific education is provided to individuals and organisations about minimising situations that allow mosquitoes to breed. This sort of education is around maintenance of waterways/ponds/dams and appropriate use of water (particularly irrigation methods).

Site detection and evaluation—This part of the program is about finding the breeding sites, determining what species are breeding in them, and treating the site as appropriate. It is critical that organisations keep a register of these sites and have a maintenance program or works program (the best method of control is to remove the site if possible).

Monitoring—The major part of this is setting traps during the breeding season (normally November to March in Victoria). These traps are set up at the same sites every year. The mosquitoes are identified (the number of each species is individually counted) and the vector species are crushed and tested for the presence of arboviruses. This forms part of an early warning system for an outbreak of disease and provides data for ongoing research. Traps may also be set in areas of high activity or where complaints are received.

Blood sample testing—This is where samples of blood are taken from animals and tested for the presence of arboviruses. This is the second part of the early warning systems and ongoing data collection for research. Most of this testing is done through sentinel chickens (flocks of chickens that are stationed in the high-activity areas and tested weekly). Samples may also be collected and tested periodically from horses, pigs, and kangaroos, which are all potential disease hosts.

Each state collects, collates, and reports on the information at the end of each season. This data is then also reported to the federal Department of Health and Ageing's 'Arbovirus and malaria surveillance program'. This program is a joint federal, state, and territory initiative, which has been created to assist health authorities in the reduction of arboviral and malarial diseases by:

◊   rapid and greater dissemination of national arbovirus and malaria surveillance data
◊   transfer of interpretations of this data and support information between health authorities
◊   aiding early recognition of unusual mosquito, arbovirus, and malaria activity
◊   provide access for the general public to arbovirus and malaria surveillance information
◊   increasing public awareness of the potential mosquito-borne disease risks in their region. (Australian Government Department of Health and Ageing, *Arbovirus and malaria surveillance*)

The surveillance of mosquitoes and arboviruses forms one part of the broader Communicable Diseases Surveillance program and the National Notifiable Diseases Surveillance System. This again is part of the broader government policies relating to the prevention of disease and attempts to reduce the burden on Australia's hospital system.

This case study was prepared by Jeremy Draper (Environmental Health Practitioner)

Adaptation is a shared responsibility that requires building partnerships between different groups such as government organisations, businesses, communities, and individuals. Partnerships are a way of building capacity individually and collectively in adaptation responses. Case Study 9.4 is a further example of organisational approaches to adaptation to climate change within the health sector. As we have said, organisational adaptation offers the opportunity for individual practitioners and groups of practitioners to have some input into the process.

Case Study 9.4   Climate Change and Primary Healthcare Intervention Framework

The Climate Change and Primary Healthcare Intervention Framework emerged from a partnership between the South East Healthy Communities Partnership and La Trobe University. Sixteen agencies teamed up with the aim of finding out what primary healthcare agencies needed to know about climate change and its health and social effects, and to develop agency priorities and work programs.

- The strength of the partnership enabled the agencies to develop their first climate change adaptation strategic plan. The objectives were to build community resilience to learn and adapt to environmental changes, minimise adverse impacts on health, and embed climate change responses in service delivery. This plan focused on vulnerable groups in their communities such as older people and those with chronic conditions, as well as staff of the agencies. The development and dissemination of information about adaptation to climate change was a key strategy in creating a supportive environment for change in the agencies and community at large. Storylines were also developed. For example, using temperature as a storyline, the effects, responses, and scale of increased hot days were identified. Who might be most affected in a heatwave, which agencies would be involved in the response, and the impact of those responses to minimise the effect were documented.

This case study was prepared by Assoc. Professor Rae Walker in collaboration with the South East Healthy Communities Partnership

---

🐧 Summary

Human health is determined by the relationship between humans and their environment. When the relationship between humans and their environment changes, particularly when the change is rapid, health is fundamentally affected. These impacts can be direct or indirect, short term or long term, negligible or devastating.

The evidence is clear. The climate is changing and further, there is a significant risk of abrupt and irreversible climatic shifts. Societies are highly vulnerable to even modest levels of climate change, with poor nations and communities particularly at risk.

Health professionals are, and will continue to be, affected individually, as family members, as community members, and as professionals. The health sector is required to work in partnership with other sectors to implement mitigation and adaptation responses to protect the health of humans in the face of a rapidly changing climate.

🖉 Tutorial exercises

1 Are we facing a global food crisis? Watch the SBS documentary *The future of food*, <www.sbs. com.au/documentary/program/thefutureoffood>. Thinking about the documentary and the discussion in this chapter, what are the probable implications for Australia?

2 Arbovirus surveillance: In Australia, mosquito-borne diseases (arboviruses) are notifiable diseases, meaning that cases of the diseases must be reported by health practitioners to the national and state government surveillance systems. Ross River virus disease is the most common mosquito-borne disease in Australia. Rainfall, temperature, and high tides are determinants of Ross River virus transmission, but the nature and scale of the relationship between disease, mosquito density, and climate variability varies with geographic location and socio-economic conditions (Tong et al. 2008).

   What do you think will be a likely outcome of the higher-than-average rainfall and temperatures in south-eastern Australia in 2010 on the prevalence of mosquito-borne diseases?

   Information on the *HealthInsight* page may help you in your discussion: <www.healthinsite. gov.au/idol_templates/idol_search_results.cfm>.

3 A Socratic dialogue is a method for using evidence in homing in on the truth. The method is as follows:

    1 Locate a *statement* confidently described as common sense.

    2 Imagine for a moment that despite the confidence of the person proposing it, the statement is false. Search for situations or contexts in which the statement would not be true.

    3 If an exception is found the statement must be false or at least imprecise.

    4 The initial statement must be nuanced (subtly changed) to take the exception into account.

    5 If one subsequently finds exceptions to the improved statements the process should be repeated. The truth insofar as a human is able to attain such a thing lies in a statement which seems impossible to disprove. It is by finding out what is not that one comes closest to understanding what it is. (Alain de Botton 2001)

   Obviously, a Socratic dialogue is a group exercise—a structure for a discussion which hopefully will lead to a definitive statement.

   So, have a go: take the statement 'Humans have little effect on the environment in which they live' (step 1) and proceed through steps 2 to 5; keep repeating the process until you arrive at a statement which seems impossible to disprove.

Further reading

Baer, H., & Singer, M. (2009). *Global warming and the political ecology of health*. Walnut Creek, CA: Left Coast Press.

Griffiths, J., Rao, M., Adshead, F., & Thorpe, A. (eds) (2009). *The health practitioner's guide to climate change. Diagnosis and cure*. London: Earthscan.

Martin, J., Rogers, M., & Winter, C. (eds) (2009). *Climate change in regional Australia: Social learning and adaptation*. Ballarat, Vic.: VUURN Press.

Talbot, L., & Verrinder, G.K. (2009). *Promoting health: The primary healthcare approach*, 4th edn. Sydney: Elsevier.

Websites

<www.climatechangeinaustralia.gov.au/pastchange.php>

This is the website about climate change in Australia.

<www.latrobe.edu.au/news/articles/2009/article/tim-flannery-talks-with-robert-manne>

This is a 2009 'Climate Change and sustainability' Podcast, La Trobe University conversation series. Tim Flannery talks with Robert Manne, 15 June. It is about 40.54 minutes.

<www.climateinstitute.org.au>

This is a climate change health check 2020 of Climate Institute of Australia (Horton & McMichael 2008).

<www.ipcc.ch/ipccreports/ar4-wg3.htm>

This website contains Intergovernmental Panel on Climate Change Assessment reports.

<www.sustainability.vic.gov.au/www/html/2482-wider-sustainability-initiatives.asp>

This website is about Sustainability Victoria.

<www.health.vic.gov.au/chiefhealthofficer/downloads/heat_impact_rpt.pdf>

This website contains information about the Victorian Government Department of Human Services report: *January 2009 heatwave in Victoria. An assessment of health impacts.*

<www.who.int/globalchange/ecosystems/ecosystems05/en/print.html>

This is the WHO paper on ecosystems and human well-being: Health synthesis. Millennium Ecosystem Assessment.

<www.who.int/mediacentre/factsheets/fs266/en/index.html>

This website contains WHO climate change and health Fact Sheet No. N266.

More information on mosquitoes

<http://medent.usyd.edu.au/index.htm>

This site is the most comprehensive in Australia and includes details on how to identify mosquitoes, how to treat sites, education resources, and hundreds of photos.

<www.health.gov.au/internet/main/publishing.nsf/Content/health-arbovirus-important.htm>

Australian Government Department of Health and Ageing produce details of arboviruses important to Australia.

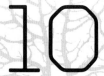

10 Health and the living environment

Cameron Earl, Jaco Terblanche, and Emma Patten

TOPICS COVERED

This chapter covers the following topics:
- public health issues associated with the living environment
- the positioning of the local government to deal with these issues
- environmental health, town planning, emergency management, and health promotion responses to these issues within the local government context

KEY TERMS

Emergency management
Environmental health
Health promotion
Living environment
Local government

Municipal health and well-being plans
New urbanism
Town planning

Introduction

The **living environment** in Australia has become increasingly urbanised, more populous, and much more complex (CDH&AC 1999). Australia evolved from a continent inhabited by hunter-gatherers, through to first European settlement, to what we know today as the urban areas of Australia. One characteristic has, however, not changed since European settlement—the high level of urbanisation. By the end of the 19th century, Australia's urbanisation was among the highest in the world, with 49% living in urban settlements, which in 2005 rose to 88.2%, and is forecasted to be 89.9% in 2015 (Forster 2009; Corcoran et al. 2010).

The Australian urban form has changed with the changing **town planning** paradigms. With the arrival of Europeans, the settlements were military and prison-style camps, highly ordered and controlled. These gave way to urban areas with grid street patterns, and in the late 19th century and early 20th century two planning movements—the City Beautiful and Garden City movements—added civic centres, boulevards, parklands, and green belts, of which Canberra is a prime example (Freestone 2010). However, Australia followed the global trend to a sprawling, decentralised, and car-dependent settlement form (Forster 2009). This sprawling settlement form has been questioned for its social impact, long-term economic viability, environmental sustainability, and ongoing implications for **environmental health**. This has led to the formulation of a number of theoretical concepts for a more sustainable urban form, such as Smart Growth and **New Urbanism**.

Historically, urban environments have been synonymous with health hazards attributed to the consumption of unsafe drinking water, inadequate basic sanitation and waste disposal, occupational injury hazards, and the prevalence of disease vectors (Stoneham 2003). Table 10.1 outlines a number of these factors associated with the living environment. Over time, the priority and risk in these factors have changed as we have developed the technology and infrastructure to manage them. However, new environmental health hazards have arisen, and they are more complex, often with delayed health effects. These new hazards are the result of development activities occurring without sufficient safeguards and the unsustainable consumption of natural resources (CDH&AC 1999; Stoneham 2003).

Examples of these hazards are water pollution generated from residential areas, industry, and intensive agriculture; urban air pollution resulting from transport and electrical power generation; hazardous waste accumulations; chemical and radiation hazards resulting from introduction of new technologies; emerging and re-emerging infectious disease hazards; deforestation; land degradation; and global climate change (Yassi et al. 2001). These changes are contributing to a range of health conditions including respiratory and cardiovascular diseases, physiological and neurological disorders, and numerous cancers (CDH&AC 1999). Notably, the phenomenon of urban sprawl has added another dimension to these hazards (Frumkin 2002). In terms of responding to these issues within the local living environment, **local government** (LG) is very influential. This chapter focuses on the living environment and discusses how environmental health, town planning, emergency management, and health promotion have responded to these issues within the local context.

Living environment
The surroundings in which we live, work, and participate; everything that is external to the human body that incorporates social, cultural, and political processes, built and natural elements, and the interaction of these as one ecosystem.

Town planning
The direction of the development and use of land to serve the economic and social welfare of the community, as well as to protect and enhance the natural environment.

Environmental health
The assessment, correction, control, and prevention of those aspects of human health, including quality of life, that are determined by physical, chemical, biological, and psychosocial factors in the environment.

New Urbanism
An urban design movement that is scaled for the pedestrian, yet capable of accommodating public transport and cars; it contains a range of housing and job types, with a high-quality public realm, and is strongly influenced by urban design standards prominent before the rise of the car.

Local government
Australia has three tiers of government, with local government being the closest to the people, providing local public services such as rubbish collection and immunisation, and facilities such as parks and community buildings within a particular area.

Table 10.1   Environmental health factors associated with the living environment

Biological Factors	Chemical Factors	Physical Factors	Social Factors
Infectious agents associated with: • Water (e.g. giardia) • Food (e.g. salmonella) • Air (e.g. influenza) • Soil (e.g. tetanus) • Zoonoses (e.g. Q-Fever) • Vectors (e.g. mosquitoes) • Pests (e.g. head lice) • Infectious wastes (e.g. hepatitis B)	• Indoor air pollutants such as asbestos and lead • Outdoor air pollutants such as ozone and particulates • Hazardous wastes (e.g. Cytotoxic drugs from hospitals)	• Noise • Overcrowding • Housing type and quality • Light • Motor vehicle accidents • Pedestrian injuries and fatalities • Low connectivity (e.g. isolation) • Heatwaves • Heat island effects • Natural disasters (e.g. fires, floods) • Radiation hazards (e.g. UVR) • Occupational hazards (e.g. trips and falls) • Limited open space	• Neighbourhood quality (e.g. safety) • Motor vehicle dependency • Loss of social capital (e.g. community participation in decision-making) • Anti-social behaviours (e.g. road rage) • Lack of physical activity • Social stratification (e.g. income inequity) • Cultural diversity (e.g. values and behaviours)

Source: Adapted from CDH&AC 1999; Yassi 2001; Cromar et al. 2004

Health promotion
The process of enabling people to increase control over, and to improve, their health.

Emergency management
A systematic approach based on science and undertaken by experts. It focuses on planning, organising, directing, and controlling emergency situations and it is collaborative and intersectoral in implementation.

Local government

Local government has a direct mandate to contribute to healthy, safe, and enjoyable environments at the local level (CDH&AC 1999). LG is the closest form of government to the people and has detailed knowledge of their communities and the environment in which they operate (Eggleston & Koob 2004). In the post-Second World War period, LG increased their traditional roles of 'roads, rates, and rubbish', adding urban design functions, local development control, enforcement of building and health standards, recreation and sports facility management, welfare services, and local economic development. Direct contributions to public health occur through myriad operational activities including town planning processes, **health promotion** activities, and environmental health functions such as food safety and **emergency management** (National Public Health Partnership 2002). A range of statutory instruments create the structural framework for public health roles for LG.

In Victoria, the *Food Act 1984* is an example of important legislation that provides Environmental Health Practitioners (EHPs) with statutory authority to assess, approve, register, and monitor all food premises within each LG area. The *Planning and Environment Act 1987* similarly provides the mechanism for town planners to shape our cities, towns, neighbourhoods, and industries, and manage the natural environment. Additionally, LGs are required to develop and implement **Municipal Health and Well-being Plans** (MHWP), so strategic planning and decision-making considers impacts on health using the social model of health, to fulfil obligations under the *Public Health and Wellbeing Act 2008*.

Natural emergencies are significant public health problems within the living environment; emergency management is the strategically planned response to these, with LG playing a critical role. A wide range of emergency situations can impact on the living environment: infrastructure disruptions (e.g. power and transport), bushfires, extreme weather events (e.g. heatwaves and tsunamis), chemical-biological-radiological-nuclear events, and direct public health threats (e.g. HIV/AIDS and SARS) (Cole & Buckle 2004). The impact of these events can be anticipated and significantly ameliorated by appropriate planning and preparation (Kizer 2000; Dover 2004).

The remaining sections within this chapter cover the role of LG in responding to health challenges within modern urban environments and focus on environmental health, town planning, emergency management, and health promotion responses.

Municipal Health and Well-being Plans
Planning documents designed to ensure that LG strategic planning and decision-making considers impacts on health using the social model of health perspective.

Environmental health responses

'Environmental health' is the modern term for what was known as 'sanitation' in the 19th-century movement where the idea of public health originated (CDH&AC 1999). Sanitation aimed to control diseases that resulted from the prevailing unsanitary conditions (Gochfield & Goldstein 1999); through the provision of safe drinking water and removal of liquid and solid waste, the movement brought about significant reductions in premature morbidity and mortality (CDH&AC 1999). It is from these beginnings that the current discipline of environmental health has evolved.

Environmental health practice focuses on those aspects of human health and quality of life that can be affected by physical (e.g. noise control), chemical (e.g. air pollution), biological (e.g. food borne illness prevention), and social factors (e.g. public safety) within the environment (CDH&AC 1999). Similar to public health practice, environmental health practice is evidence-based and is collaborative in nature, relying heavily on the support of a wide variety of disciplines (Brown 2001; Goldman 2004). However, it is environmental health practitioners who are tasked with the delivery of environmental health programs at the LG level. It is their role to evaluate local environmental health issues and guide the management processes (CDH&AC 1999).

MacArthur (2000) considers that the greatest gains for environmental health are the consolidation and enhancement of action at the local level. EHPs working for LG generally focus on noise, air, and water pollution; food safety; liquid, solid, and hazardous waste disposal; and reducing the impacts of emergencies such as bushfire and floods (Bell 2002). These hazards more often directly translate into a health condition such as someone drinking contaminated water and contracting a gastrointestinal disease (Stoneham 2003). These are understood and supported by well-documented management and legislative approaches, but less is known about contemporary issues. As previously stated, new hazards are more complex and tend to have long latency periods with links to individual physiology, urbanisation, and environmental degradation (Stoneham 2003). Examples of contemporary hazards are community exposure to solar ultraviolet radiation (UVR) or asbestos fibres, both of which can result in cancer later in life (CDH&AC 1999). Also, the prominence of climate change impacts has required EHPs to consider working towards achieving the goals of ecologically sustainable development (Gochfield & Goldstein 1999; Brown 2001); the most common work at the local level is in food safety.

See Chapter 9 for more discussion of climate change and health.

Stop and Think

» New environmental health hazards are more complex and tend to have long latency periods; exposure to UVR and asbestos are two examples. Discuss the difficulties of communicating risks about these hazards to the community. How does this impact on the work of LG?

Food-borne illness can result in significant societal costs and have major implications for the food industry through lost earnings, lawsuits, and damaged consumer confidence (O'Brien et al. 2002). The total annual cost of food-borne illness in Australia is $1.249 million per annum (Commonwealth Department of Health and Ageing 2006). Dalton and colleagues (2004) analysed food-borne illness outbreaks in Australia from 1995 to 2000 and reported that 94% (202 out of 214) outbreaks reviewed were associated with restaurants and commercial caterers. The review also showed that bacterial diseases such as salmonella were responsible for 61% of outbreaks, 64% of cases, and 95% of deaths. The most frequently implicated foods were meats (in particular chicken), fish, seafood, salads, sandwiches, and eggs (Dalton et al. 2004).

Food safety requires a whole-of-industry approach to be successful. Included in this is a quality control approach that covers the production of raw materials, food processing, storage and transport, food preparation, and finally consumption (Yassi et al. 2001). The food industry is guided by the requirements of the National Food Safety Standards (FSANZ 2002). Similarly, achieving food safety is a whole-of-government responsibility. EHPs work directly with each food business to improve food safety standards and then ensure that suitable standards are maintained. LG EHPs use processes provided within the food legislation in each state and territory to pursue positive changes (e.g. the *Food Act 1984* in Victoria). These processes include registering food businesses, conducting on-site assessments and audits, investigating food-borne illness outbreaks, issuing on-the-spot fines, or in extreme cases initiating legal action through the courts. The investigation of food-borne illness outbreaks is a particularly interesting and challenging part of working as an EHP.

Case Study 10.1   EHPs and a food-borne illness outbreak investigation

Two gastroenteritis outbreaks occurred in two separate aged care facilities in Melbourne in November 2009. The first outbreak affected 22 out of the 71 residents at the first facility and onsets occurred over a two-week period. The second outbreak affected 20 out of the 60 residents at another facility and, like the first outbreak, the onsets occurred over 13 days.

EHPs investigated both outbreaks:

- All affected residents were put in isolation and staff donned aprons and gloves when working with these residents and washed their hands to limit the spread of the disease.
- Faecal samples were taken from the affected residents and *Salmonella* was identified as the cause. This organism
  - adheres to the walls of the small intestine, grows, then releases enterotoxin
  - usually needs a high infective dose
  - causes illness 8 to 72 hours after ingestion of the contaminated food
  - is associated with symptoms such as abdominal pains, nausea, and watery diarrhoea, sometimes with mild fever, vomiting, and headaches which usually last for 2–5 days
  - can affect all age groups but symptoms are most severe in the elderly, infants, immuno-suppressed, and the infirm
  - is typically associated with animal foods such as meat, eggs, and milk, and foods contaminated from the environment.
- The spread of onsets over a fortnight in both outbreaks suggested ongoing low-dose contamination of foods and/or kitchen equipment. The following are suggested methods of preventing or minimising the growth of *Salmonella*:
  - keep perishable foods cold or hot
  - wash vegetables and fruit well if eaten raw
  - prevent cross-contamination
  - practise good personal hygiene
  - wipe up meat and vegetable residue
  - keep kitchen sponges and clothes clean, dry, and replaced regularly
  - ensure that people recovering from gastric illness do not handle ready-to-eat foods.
- EHPs interviewed the affected and unaffected residents to determine their food intake in an effort to find the contaminated food source and assessed the kitchens at both premises for compliance with the requirements of the National Food Safety Standards.
- A specific food source was unable to be identified for either outbreak.

Source: This case story has been adapted from the *Victorian Infectious Disease Bulletin* 13(1) 2010, and <www.Safefood.net.au>

Town planning responses

Australia has followed the global trend in a sprawling, decentralised, and car-dependent settlement form commonly referred to as 'urban sprawl' (Forster 2009). Evidence shows that this type of settlement results in adverse impacts on local social, economic, and environmental conditions (Frumkin 2002).

Urban sprawl generally has the following characteristics:

- A land-use pattern with single-use rather than mixed-use developments; with bland and stereotyped housing subdivisions (also referred to as 'McMansions', 'Cookie Cutter', or 'Lego Land' housing). The retail sector is mostly characterised by shopping malls or 'big-box' retail

Figure 10.1 Big-box retail centre in Griffith NSW—a design that can be seen anywhere in North America or Australia, that bears no relation to place

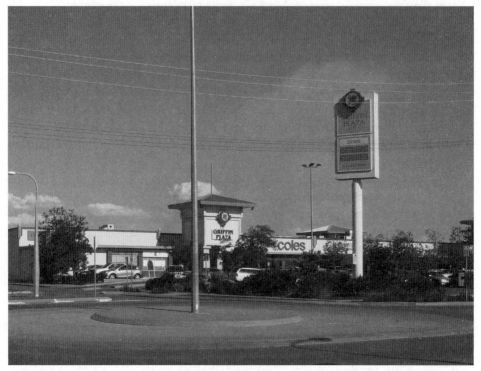

Source: Photo by J. Terblanche

centres, with expansive parking lots in front, with no connection to the local history or place (see Figure 10.1).

- Large single-use tracts compared to neighbourhoods with discernible centres.
- Branched street patterns such as collector roads with loops and culs-de-sac running off these, rather than well-connected grid or hybrid road systems.
- Sprawling and low-density usage.
- The design of streets for cars rather than pedestrians, such as wide and bland higher speed roads, instead of narrower and slower roads that are safer for pedestrians and cyclists.
- Civic uses (schools, churches, council buildings) that are disconnected in space, connectivity, and architecture, compared to being accessible and fostering a sense of place and pride in a community (Duany et al. 2000; Steuteville & Langdon 2003).

Environmental impacts of urban sprawl include lower air quality linked with vehicle travel behaviour, detrimental impacts on local hydrology, or the loss of farmland to make way for housing developments. Public health impacts include a reduction in physical activity by unconnected, pedestrian-unfriendly, and dangerous streets, and significant distances between work, school, home, and recreation. Mental health impacts can occur due to long periods of commuting, aggressive driving, and antisocial behaviour such as road rage, as well as vehicle and pedestrian accidents (Frumkin 2002). There are also other general impacts such as creating unsustainable financial situations for local and state government, and access problems for emergency services (Duany et al. 2000; Trowbridge et al. 2009). This has led to the formulation of a number of theoretical concepts for a more sustainable form of urban settlement, such as Smart Growth and New Urbanism.

Smart Growth is mostly associated with levels of government and policy documents, especially in the USA (Ganapati 2008). New Urbanism has emerged to be a global urban design movement primarily driven by the Congress of New Urbanism (USA), with the first New Urbanist style towns appearing in the early 1980s. The features of New Urbanism that are the most important in the Australian context are:

- *Creating a centre in towns, where you can work, live, and shop*. This centre must be identifiable, and considered the 'heart of the community' with a mixture of residential, commercial, retail, and civic uses (Dover & King 2008). These places should facilitate both organised and spontaneous pedestrian gatherings, where all members of the public feel welcome (Oldenburg 1999). In Figure 10.2, it can be seen that urban sprawl would not have a community hub or centre, unlike a New Urbanist town. Alternatively, with urban sprawl developments the retail uses will often be separated from residential areas in long strip developments or shopping malls.
- *Enhancing the walkability of urban areas through interconnected street grids*. Narrower grid roads provide the pedestrian or cyclist with a variety of routes, normally of a shorter distance, with vehicular loads spread over a number of routes in the grid system. In Figure 10.2, there are limited ways to move within a sprawl development, compared to a variety of shorter routes in an urbanist development.
- *Creating pleasant and safe walking environments, and good street landscaping*. As can be seen in Figures 10.3 and 10.4, in sprawl developments roads are normally wide with houses set well back from the road (Hall & Porterfield 2001). In New Urbanist developments the roads are normally narrower, slowing down vehicular traffic and limiting the impermeable road surface (refer to Figure 10.5). Limiting impermeable road surfaces helps reduce urban runoff volumes and stormwater pollution. Street trees planted close together and overhanging roadways help to catch rainwater, reduce solar heating of roads, and increase visual amenity (Girling & Kellet 2005). Residential buildings should have limited setbacks, face the opposing building, have low plantings to define the lots, and windows, balconies, and porches facing the street. The use of

Figure 10.2 Urban sprawl in a curvilinear layout (left) and New Urbanism in a modified grid layout (right)

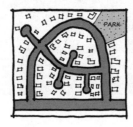 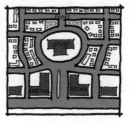

Source: Diagrams produced by J. Terblanche

Figure 10.3 Section of an urban sprawl residential street (top) and a New Urbanist street (below)

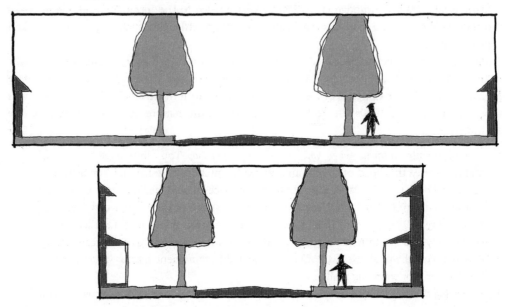

Source: Diagrams produced by J. Terblanche

Figure 10.4 Urban sprawl in Griffith (NSW) with wide roads and large setbacks, and the streetscape dominated by driveways and garages

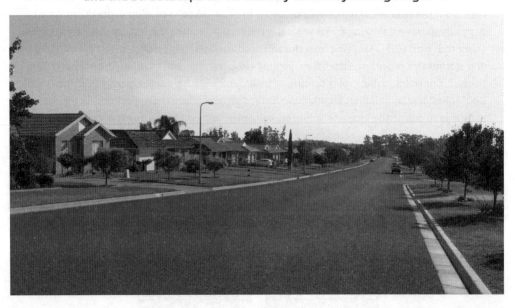

Source: Photo by J. Terblanche

Figure 10.5 New Urbanism in Mawson Lakes, Adelaide, with narrow roads and small setbacks

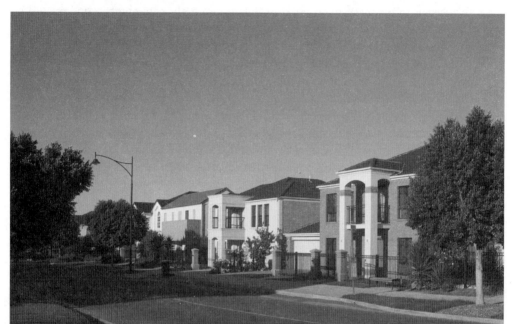

Source: Photo by J. Terblanche

laneways is promoted to prevent garages and driveways impacting on passive observation from the houses and the overall streetscape. Commercial streets utilise the same principles, with at least half the frontage recommended to be transparent storefronts, loading areas, residential parking in back laneways, offices and residences above the ground floors, and no parking permitted in front of buildings (Gindroz 1999).

- *Mixed uses are recommended even for the residential areas to improve the safety of the area, and to provide a variety of housing choice* (Dover 1999; Gindroz 1999). Land uses are usually integrated within New Urbanist developments (see Figure 10.2). Alternatively, urban sprawl districts normally have a single land use, where there are no retail or civic uses integrated within the residential areas. A New Urbanist district would include civic precincts, medical precincts, educational campuses, noxious industries, depots, and terminals, and entertainment zones. Regardless, all district types benefit from being well connected with a transit system to neighbourhoods (Duany et al. 2000).

- *Transit Oriented Development* (TOD). New Urbanists and Smart Growth proponents have embraced TODs. From its inception, TODs have been called a return to the 'streetcar suburb', with residences being within walking distance from stations (Poticha 2008). These residential areas would provide compact development, mixed land uses, and have a focus on pedestrians, in combination with public transport (Freilich 1998).

- *Creating a good public realm, with good civic buildings, good parks, and having these easily accessible.* Civic spaces such as squares, boulevards, and parks must be large enough to be seen by people in the space, to denote their importance to the community (Gindroz 1999). These spaces should relate to their purpose, history, and context, and should be designed taking into account the local climate and topography (Kelbaugh 1999). They should be located in a well-used area, and should be sensitive to the historical built form (Dover 1999).
- *The protection and responsible utilisation of all open spaces, which range from wilderness to farmland, is of paramount importance.* Farmland should be protected through exclusive agricultural zonings, such as Rural Conservation Zones and Farming Zones. An urban settlement should not be allowed to sprawl uncontrolled into agricultural areas, but should be controlled by an Urban Growth Boundary (Duany et al. 2000; Congress for the New Urbanism 2004).

Stop and Think

» As growth of urban areas is inevitable, local residents may choose to utilise roadside and street reserves to develop gardens for individual and community use. What land-use issues need to considered in supporting these types of gardens?

Case Study 10.2   New Urbanism in action, Mawson Lakes, Adelaide

Mawson Lakes is a 600-hectare greenfield development located 12 km north of the city of Adelaide. It was developed as a joint venture between the South Australian Government and the private sector. It is estimated that in 2011 there will be 11,000 residents living in 4000 homes, with employment of 7000 workers and 7500 students (Delfin Lend Lease n.d.; Hurlimann & McKay 2006).

Mawson Lake has a modified grid layout, with generally good accessibility. The central section of the development is a town centre, adjoining a small lake. The town centre contains the school, businesses, a community centre, a campus of the University of South Australia, and is easily accessible by a transit interchange. The parking in the town centre is mostly in the middle of the blocks and with businesses built up to the sidewalk, creating a pedestrian-friendly and vibrant streetscape.

The development contains a range of housing choices, from 'high end' single residences down to one-bedroom flats and loft-type accommodation. Residences are mixed throughout the development, with no one type of residence being exclusive to any district. As the development has aged care facilities as well as childcare centres, it caters for various age groups. The development deviates from the New Urbanist model slightly in that back alleys are generally not used in the development, with most garages still on the street front but not a dominating feature.

Mawson Lakes is well connected for the pedestrian or cyclist, which contributes to creating a healthy environment. It has footpaths and cycle routes criss-crossing the development, with these paths leading to meaningful destinations such as recreational facilities, businesses, and educational facilities. As the roads are narrow, vehicular traffic is generally slow-moving and together with small setbacks (placing houses close to the street) this creates good passive observation and a safe pedestrian environment. The routes will generally be well shaded as street trees mature, providing shelter from the sun.

Figure 10.6   Town centre in Mawson Lakes, Adelaide

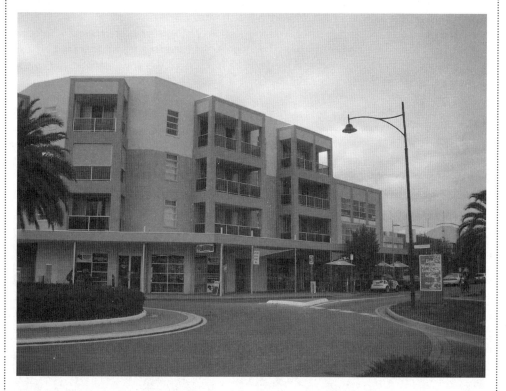

Note the housing integrated with the retail in a mixed use development.

Source: Photo by J. Terblanche

Emergency management responses

Emergencies and disasters rarely conform to jurisdictional boundaries, and local government is an important stakeholder for local emergency response (Eggleston & Koob 2004; Queensland Health 2005). Emergency management is similar to public health in that it 'is a range of measures to manage risks to communities and the environment' (Salter 1998, p. 28). Emergency management is a systematic approach based on science and undertaken by experts; it focuses on planning, organising,

Mythbuster
The Good, the Bad, and the 'Alley'

A laneway or 'alley' in a residential area has a bad reputation—a place where a person is likely to be a victim of crime, a place inhabited by rats and stray cats, a place more suited to Dickens than today's society. So, why would New Urbanists start using alleys behind houses in residential areas again?

Back laneways are being used in New Urbanist developments for a number of reasons:

- Garages are put at the back of houses. This has a positive impact on the streetscape, and creates limited vehicle crossings (from driveways) over the footpaths or shared paths, which increases pedestrian safety and comfort in the streets.
- All the services (electrical, gas, telecommunication, water, sewer, stormwater, garbage collection) can be put in the laneway. This leaves the road free from services, with less disturbance for its maintenance; a road can be made narrower for aesthetic and safety reasons, and more trees can be planted in the road with less interference with underground services.
- Back laneways can be made safe by the increase in passive observation, adding accessory dwelling units or studios on top of the garages, and by having a clear street-to-street view down the laneway.

Figure 10.7   A laneway in Griffith NSW (left) compared to a laneway in a New Urbanist development in Adelaide

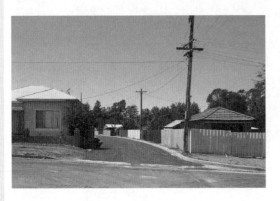
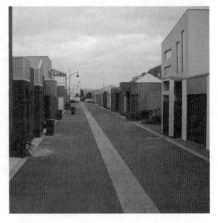

Note the laneway on the right has accessory dwellings and a street-to-street view to facilitate better passive observation.

Source: Photos by J. Terblanche

directing (leading), and controlling emergency situations (Cronan 1998) and is collaborative and intersectoral in implementation (Krimm 1998; Salter 1998). LGs have a key role in the response to and recovery from an emergency or disaster event, usually in a broader state, territory, or even national context. The benefits that LG provide include experience with essential services, infrastructure, and risk management, and possession of good local knowledge (Eggleston & Koob 2004). The Australian

Local Government Association (2006) indicated that LG undertake the following emergency management activities:

- conduct risk assessments
- encourage community safety
- undertake works to reduce local risks in partnership with federal and state government
- facilitate local emergency management arrangements in partnership with emergency management agencies
- respond to emergencies where the consequences are within their resources
- support state or Commonwealth government activities during emergency responses
- assist local residents during their recovery from an emergency
- assess the impact of an emergency
- provide leadership where long-term strategies for local community and economic recovery are needed.

Other frontline agencies in Australia providing emergency responses include the Defence Forces, State Emergency, Fire, and Ambulance services (including voluntary services) and Police Services (Abrahams 2001). These organisations are supported by a federal and state emergency management system. Within these systems there is a framework for the provision of financial assistance and strategic guidance through the Counter-Disaster Task Force, National Emergency Management Committee, Emergency Management Australia, and state and territory emergency management organisations (Angus 1998). The public health sector also contributes to emergency management. These roles carried out by the public health sector include routine surveillance, provision of immunisation programs, environmental controls, and medical care systems (Shoaf & Rottman 2000). The peak emergency management agency in Australia is Emergency Management Australia. This has a variety of functions and responsibilities including education, training, research grants, and planning and operational support (EMA 2001).

Traditionally in Australia, emergency management policy has been based on what is known as 'the comprehensive approach'. This approach has been more commonly expressed as prevention, preparedness, response, and recovery (Crondstedt 2001). At the core of this policy are legislative and regulatory arrangements guiding the actions of these emergency service agencies and the community (EMA 1996). In recent times, there has been a shift towards the use of risk management models to improve community safety and further reduce the impact of disasters (Parkes 2000; Crondstedt 2001). Within this shift, there has been a swing away from response management and reactive approaches undertaken by single agencies to a more proactive and collaborative approach incorporating risk management (Salter 1998). This has meant that the focus of emergency services has moved from a focus on the hazards to the reduction of vulnerability in the community (Pagram 1999). An excellent example of this approach is the heatwave planning that LG are involved with in Victoria.

Stop and Think

» Emergency management now has a strong focus on reducing vulnerability within communities. Give examples of these vulnerabilities.

Case Study 10.3   Heatwave planning in Victoria

In Victoria in recent years there have been a number of heatwave events that have increased the incidence of mortality and morbidity (Victorian Department of Human Services 2009). Consequently, Victorian LGs have been encouraged to develop Heatwave Plans. These plans should

- have a threshold temperature when the plan is activated (e.g. 38°C)
- be collaboratively developed and implemented (partners include community health centres, aged accommodation and services, and emergency services such as the ambulance and SES)
- identify vulnerable population groups (e.g. older people, children under 5 years, people with pre-existing medical conditions such as heart disease or diabetes, homeless people, outdoor workers)
- include a range of activities to be carried out before a heatwave (e.g. developing a register of vulnerable groups, promoting awareness of heatwaves through the local media, providing training to increase preparedness, preparing cooling centres) and during a heatwave (e.g. increasing the number of emergency services and medical personnel on duty, activating a 'heatline' telephone service, rescheduling outdoor events).

Source: Victorian Department of Human Services 2009

Health promotion response

Public health problems and priorities change over time, and as such require flexible and appropriate responses. Municipal Health and Well-being Plans enable local governments to identify and assess current local community health priority areas, and guide LG actions towards promoting and improving community health outcomes. *Environments for Health* is the framework used for this type of planning; it considers the impact of factors originating across any or all of the built, social, economic, and natural environments on health and well-being (Municipal Association of Victoria 2007). MHWPs draw on a number of core public health approaches to planning:

- *Strategic local area planning*: A strategic and integrated approach to MHWPs promotes a model for integrating physical, social, and economic planning, with community participation as a key principle.
- *Social model of health*: A conceptual framework for thinking about health that recognises the effect of interrelated social, economic, cultural, and political factors and conditions that contribute to individual and community well-being. Addressing issues of disadvantage, community participation, and empowerment are key aspects.
- *Health-promoting systems*: A holistic approach ensures that the relationships between all major issues affecting individuals and families in the context of their local spaces, resources, organisations, and workforce are taken into account.
- *Focusing on health outcomes*: Utilising evidence of local community health conditions and outcomes from the Victorian Burden of Disease Study, the National Health Priority Areas,

Primary Care Partnerships, and other sources to identify current and future priority areas for consideration in planning (Adapted from Geelong Health and Wellbeing Plan 2009–2013, City of Greater Geelong 2009).

The combination of population growth, climate change, competition for land and water, economic development, and fuel production has created a number of issues identified as community health priorities at the local, national, and international levels, including food security. Food insecurity is when individuals or communities have difficulty regularly accessing safe, nutritious, and acceptable food (VicHealth 2010a). Short-term consequences of food insecurity include ongoing hunger, anxiety, and lethargy. In the longer term, food insecurity is related to becoming overweight or obese because poorer quality and low-cost foods are often higher in fat, salt, and sugar (Harrison et al. 2007). LG has a key role in communities attaining food security.

As previously mentioned, LG monitors food safety but they also manage land-use planning for food retail outlets, agricultural and horticultural activities, and provide food for those on a low income or unemployed, and during natural disasters (Yeatman 2008). For Victoria, these activities were significantly boosted by the mandating of MHWPs by the Victorian State Government with its social view of health (Yeatman 2008). Consequently, the findings of a national survey undertaken in 2007 showed that Victorian LGs performed significantly better than other states, particularly in food and nutrition activities relating to community services (Yeatman 2008) and in providing support for local produce (Yeatman 2007). This survey also showed that general managers and staff in Victorian LGs were significantly more likely to rate issues about food as important, demonstrating increased awareness of food issues as a priority area (Yeatman 2007, 2008). This comes as evidence continues to show increasing rates of overweight and obesity and related health issues (see Drewnowski & Spencer 2004). Responding to these issues (Figure 10.8) is not as simple as educating individuals and communities.

Figure 10.8 Aspects of our living environment that impact on food security

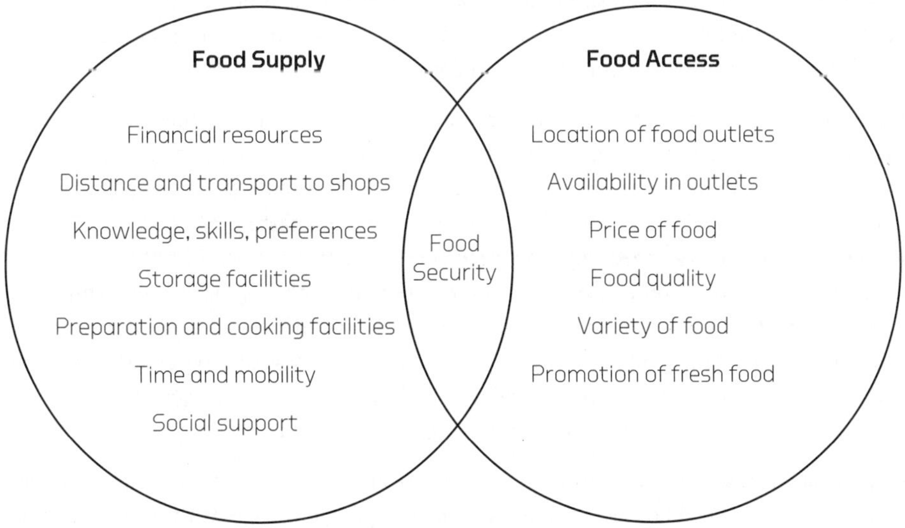

Food Supply

Financial resources

Distance and transport to shops

Knowledge, skills, preferences

Storage facilities

Preparation and cooking facilities

Time and mobility

Social support

Food Security

Food Access

Location of food outlets

Availability in outlets

Price of food

Food quality

Variety of food

Promotion of fresh food

Source: Diagram produced by E. Patten

In partnership with the Victorian Health Promotion Foundation (VicHealth), the *Food for All* program is assisting LGs to improve access to nutritious food and to influence the cultural, social, economic, and environmental barriers poor and disadvantaged communities face in eating healthily. As identified by VicHealth (2010b), there are a number of ways LGs can work to address food security, including:

- making sure there are local sources of fresh fruit and vegetables at affordable prices
- ensuring that those living in poor-quality housing have access to food storage and cooking facilities
- improving food and cooking knowledge among disadvantaged groups
- improving transport options for those without a car
- increasing community awareness of the problem of food insecurity.

One of the most popular strategies to address changing social and political living environments has been community gardening programs. Authors such as Grayson (1995) and the Marrickville Council (2007) indicated that community gardens are much more than just a local source of fresh food:

- *They increase community connection.* A sense of community is valued above the gain of access to fresh food and benefits to health. Community gardens have also provided family-friendly spaces, opportunities to meet people, and increased social bonds. Gardening is seen as an activity that bridges all cultures, bringing people from all backgrounds together to develop a shared culture of cooperation and social responsibility.
- *They contribute to greening communities and neighbourhood improvement.* Derelict or unused land has been turned into productive land with the addition of exotic food plants, native food plants, and return of wildlife. Seed saving and the reintroduction of food plant varieties increases biodiversity. Gardening skills also reduce household green waste going to landfill.
- *They contribute to reducing poverty.* Community gardens have provided a social means to addressing poverty. Individuals and communities benefit from developing horticultural skills, waste management skills, and sustainability knowledge as well as other employability skills that can be transferred to employment or further education opportunities. The gardens also provide opportunities for the establishment of small enterprises.

There are two main approaches of the community garden: allotment gardens, where individuals have rights to a defined space within a larger garden setting (e.g. Ringwood Community Garden, Melbourne); and common gardens, where individuals contribute to a complete garden and share the produce (e.g. Groundswell Community Garden, Frankston, Melbourne). The method chosen will depend on local needs and the preferences of those involved in setting up the garden. Some community gardens may also use a combination of both approaches to using the space (e.g. Collingwood Children's Farm uses both large allotments and shared gardening space). Either approach has benefits and challenges of efficiency and effectiveness of food production, associated environmental health impacts (e.g. vermin, odour), and sustainability of the garden (Grayson 1995).

There are a number of ways LG can support community gardens:

- supporting establishment of community gardens in specific communities, including childcare centres, neighbourhood houses, community centres, and open spaces within the local region
- supporting urban agriculture, such as the planting of fruit and vegetables in public spaces such as parks, gardens, and streets

- supporting home gardening through waste management and water conservation measures
- supporting food swaps, from both individual and community gardens
- reviewing land use, open space, and building policy and practices to make it easier for the above to occur (VicHealth 2010c).

Case Study 10.4   Addressing food insecurity: Manatunga community garden, Swan Hill Rural City Council

In 2007, the Swan Hill Rural City Council, Victoria, identified food insecurity as a priority community health concern. From the Community Indicators Victoria Survey (2007), 8.6% of respondents in the Swan Hill region (compared to the Victorian state average of 6%) indicated that they had experienced food insecurity in the past 12 months. The region has experienced drought, climate change, increasing prices of petrol and food, and housing stress, all of which have contributed to the experience of food insecurity (Swan Hill Rural City Council 2006). This is despite the significant production of fresh food grown locally for export markets. As a result, the Swan Hill Rural City Council was one local government area funded under the VicHealth *Food for All* program to support food security in the local community.

Inclusion of food security in the Swan Hill Rural City Councils 2007–10 MHWP was an important factor in establishing action towards food security. Improving access to food for healthy eating to enhance the health and well-being of the community, particularly those most in need, was an action area within the plan's 'promoting healthy connected communities' goal. Including food security in the plan had a number of positive outcomes for addressing food security, including:

- strengthening existing partnerships to enable a more coordinated approach to strategies
- mobilising existing program resources to address factors that impact on food security
- creating awareness of the broader determinants of food security among local service providers
- creating a foundation by which local decision-making (e.g. for land-use planning) can be made in consideration of the social model of health.

A number of strategies were undertaken to achieve this objective: establishing a local farmers' market that welcomes all nationalities and is family-friendly; creating partnerships between community services, local programs, and not-for-profit groups to support food access through education, resource support, and skill development; establishing a kitchen garden in a local school that has a high proportion of children from families at risk of food insecurity; working with an existing garden program in the local special school to provide excess produce to those in need; and supporting an existing Indigenous garden—Manatunga Community Garden—to become more productive (VicHealth 2010c).

Manatunga Community Garden has been in existence in Robinvale, near Swan Hill, for over ten years. Working with the garden community, the Council has assisted with a number of activities to increase productivity throughout the year:

- successful application for federal funding to install water tanks and a water dripper system and to purchase fruit trees to establish an orchard

- providing infrastructure support such as building products for a greenhouse to grow seedlings for more of the year, and a barbeque to cook produce on-site
- supporting community horticultural education sessions
- partnering with the Robinvale Market to sell excess produce and use the income to purchase fruit and vegetable plants and equipment. This has provided fresh fruit and vegetables to the community at accessible prices
- engaging more of the community, particularly Indigenous community members, to be involved in the garden and be provided with fresh produce for meals
- providing food for local Indigenous community cooking sessions.

Source: VicHealth 2010c; Swan Hill Rural City Council 2006

Summary

The living environment in Australia has become increasingly urbanised, more populous, and much more complex (CDH&AC 1999). Additionally, Australia has followed the global trend in a sprawling, decentralised, and car-dependent settlement form (Forster 2009). Most cities, towns, and neighbourhoods lack real centres, with these having been replaced by shopping strips surrounded by parking, removed from residential areas, or by business parks. This not only forces all residents to rely on driving and creates a thoroughly unpleasant living environment, but also does not help in creating a sense of community. It is local government that is best placed to reduce the impacts of urban sprawl by managing local town planning and discharging their environmental health, emergency management, and health promotion activities.

Human health outcomes are closely intertwined with conditions of the living environment. While many aspects of the living environment pose traditional risks to health, there are emerging conditions that are not as well understood. These require a multifaceted risk-based response guided by strategic and coordinated approaches. Local government are well placed as leaders in managing these emerging and traditional health issues associated with the living environment.

Tutorial exercises

1 Identify the Local Government Area (LGA) that you live in. Through research and observation, describe your LG's involvement in your living environment and how this is benefiting local community health.
2 How does a healthy living environment assist in the management of chronic conditions, such as HIV, heart disease, diabetes, and so on?
3 Compare the design features of New Urbanism with your current living environment.
4 What elements of an urban environment create a safe and pleasant pedestrian experience?
5 Which would be the best in a predominantly residential area—wide or narrow streets, and why?

Further reading

Commonwealth Department of Health and Aged Care (1999). *National environmental health strategy*. Canberra: Australian Government Publishing Service.

Frumkin, H. (2002). Urban sprawl and public health. *Public Health Reports*, 117, 211–24.

Gochfield, M., & Goldstein, B.D. (1999). Lessons in environmental health in the twentieth century. *Annual Review of Public Health*, 20, 35–53.

Thompson, S., Corkery, L., & Judd, B. (2007). The role of community gardens in sustaining healthy communities. Unpublished paper, Faculty of the Built Environment, University of New South Wales, Sydney.

Yeatman, H. (2008). Action or inaction? Food and nutrition in Australian local governments. *Public Health Nutrition*, 12(9), 1399–407.

Websites

<www.ema.gov.au/www/emaweb/emaweb.nsf/Page/Publications_AustralianJournalofEmergencyManagement_AustralianJournalofEmergencyManagement>

This is an Australian *Journal of Emergency Management* (the free access journal of Emergency Management Australia).

<http://communitygarden.org.au>

This is an Australian City Farms and Community Gardens Network.

<http://journal.eh.org.au>

This website refers you to the *Environmental Health Journal* (the free access journal of Environmental Health Australia).

<www.walkable.org>

This website is about making places walkable.

<http://acnu.org>

This is the website of the Australian Council for New Urbanism.

<www.cnu.org>

This website represents the Congress for the New Urbanism.

<www.transitorienteddevelopment.org>

This website provides information regarding the Transit Oriented Development (TOD).

<www.pps.org>

This is the website about the design of public places.

<www.vichealth.vic.gov.au/en/Programs-and-Projects/Healthy-Eating/Food-Security.aspx>

This website provides information regarding VicHealth food security programs.

Part 2

Social Determinants of Health, Illness, and Well-being

11

Social determinants of health: Historical developments and global implications

Bruce Rumbold and Virginia Dickson-Swift

TOPICS COVERED

This chapter covers the following topics:

- social determinants of health
- an introduction to health promotion
- how individual risk factors can determine health status
- key principles of public health
- how healthcare reform may address the social determinants of health

KEY TERMS

Equity
Social determinants
Social epidemiology
Social exclusion

Social gradient
Social inclusion
Socially inclusive society
Socio-economic status

Introduction

In every society, the health status of the population is fundamentally determined by social and cultural factors. However, national healthcare systems, particularly in developed nations, are devoted to delivering clinical services that respond to immediate health problems confronting individual citizens. The underlying social and cultural determinants, the causes of these health problems, are neglected, either because they are seen as secondary to meeting immediate needs or because they raise issues too difficult to address through the short-term policy agendas of governments driven by election cycles. These asocial clinical models also influence the healthcare systems of most developing nations through the support provided by overseas aid programs and the developed-world training given to their healthcare workforce.

This chapter traces the growth in understanding of the roles played by social factors in health, and the development of a body of evidence that identifies the factors and strategies through which

Figure 11.1 The Social Skeleton: Health, illness, and structure energy

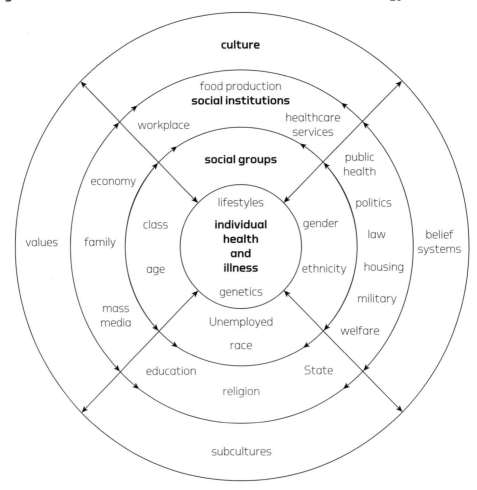

Source: Germov 2005

they might be addressed. The findings and recommendations of the WHO Commission on Social Determinants of Health, currently the most comprehensive repository of global information on social determinants, will be outlined. Findings and recommendations will be applied to Australian society and current debates about reforming the health system.

Social determinants mediate between the individual and environmental determinants dealt with in the previous ten chapters. Social experience and social structures shape both our individual capacities and the way the environment supports and challenges us. These interactions between human biology, lifestyle, and the physical and social environment all influence how we experience health and illness.

Social determinants involve much more than interpersonal support, which is often the limited meaning given to 'social' in a biopsychosocial framework. Rather, 'social determinants of health are the circumstances in which [we] are born, grow up, live, work, and age, and the systems put in place to deal with illness. These circumstances are in turn shaped by a wider set of forces: economics, social policies, and politics' (WHO CSDH 2008a, p. 1). In experiencing these determinants, we find a tension between structure and agency, between constraints (circumstances and forces) that we cannot immediately influence, and initiatives that we can take despite those constraints. Bauman (1999) observes that individual choices in *all* circumstances are limited by two sets of constraints: choosing from among what is available; and social roles or codes that tell the individual the rank order and appropriateness of preferences. People can act independently of the social structures in their lives, but the occasions on which they do so appear to be rare.

> **Social determinants**
> Social, cultural, economic, environmental, and political factors that can impact on the health of individuals.

Stop and Think

Tristan is 9 years old and he lives with his mum and his brother in a public housing flat in a high-rise inner-city housing estate. They have recently moved to the city and most of their family live in a rural town some four hours away. The flats are in quite good condition but his mum worries about the smell of the carpet and the fact that there are not many places for the boys to play. Tristan and his brother attend the local primary school, about a 15-minute walk away. They do not have a car and public transport costs are high so mum walks Tristan and his brother to school. Tristan is happy at school but lately he has been complaining of feeling he cannot breathe at times during the day and he has been coughing quite a lot at night. Tristan was diagnosed with asthma when he was 4 and has had a number of hospital admissions for asthma over the years. He takes a reliever medication when he feels wheezy and has also had a preventer prescribed some time ago but he does not use it as often as he should.

» Based on the information provided above, explore some of the social determinants of health for Tristan. Why is it that we treat people without changing what makes them sick?

Stop and Think

Often children like Tristan end up in the Accident and Emergency room of the local hospital. Frequently this leads to a hospital admission and further forms of treatment. When we take a social determinants approach to examining conditions like asthma we can begin to see that the issues that impact on Tristan's asthma can come from several places: his housing environment, the stress of moving to a new school, air pollution, lack of asthma education, just to name a few. We can treat kids like Tristan with the latest asthma drugs to get them through the acute episodes but if we do not address the social determinants (housing, transport, education, environment, etc.) then it will be difficult for Tristan to feel healthy.

Obviously, asthmatics need to follow a medication regime, but health professionals also need to be aware of those social issues that can determine a person's health. If we continue just to treat the Tristans and send them home to an environment that may be polluted, into a house that may be damp, to a family that lacks the education to follow the asthma plans, then we are actually achieving very little (and adding to the health budget quite a lot).

Often initiatives to respond to social determinants have had to run ahead of conclusive evidence, but in recent years much greater coherence has emerged, and a global consensus is taking shape. Much of the impetus for this has grown from the classic publication *The solid facts* (Wilkinson & Marmot 2003). The contributors reviewed thousands of publications and condensed their findings into ten key propositions about social determinants of health, intentionally packaged to be accessible to policymakers. The propositions are:

- *The social gradient*: Life expectancy is shorter and most diseases are more common further down the social ladder in each society.
- *Stress*: Stressful circumstances, making people feel worried, anxious, and unable to cope, are damaging to health and may lead to premature death.
- *Early life*: A good start in life means supporting mothers and young children.
- *Social exclusion*: Life is short where its quality is poor. By causing hardship and resentment, poverty, social exclusion, and discrimination cost lives.
- *Work*: Stress in the workplace increases the risk of disease. People who have more control over their work have better health.
- *Unemployment*: Job security increases health, well-being, and job satisfaction. Higher rates of unemployment cause more illness and premature death.
- *Social support*: Friendship, good social relations, and strong supportive networks improve health at home, at work, and in the community.
- *Addiction*: Individuals turn to alcohol, drugs, and tobacco and suffer from their use; but use is influenced by the wider social setting.
- *Food*: Because global market forces control the food supply, healthy food is a political issue.
- *Transport*: Healthy transport means less driving and more walking and cycling, backed up by better public transport.

These ten solid facts are key social determinants of health.

Social factors in illness

In urging policymakers to attend to social determinants of health, Wilkinson and Marmot (2003) are not introducing a new idea. Human societies have for millennia managed illness through a variety of forms of social organisation. Nomadic groups, for example, kept on the move not only to maintain an adequate and varied diet but also to maintain equilibrium with their environment. Their moving on minimised their impact on the land and ensured that food supplies would be replenished. Their life span rituals were correlated with their cyclic movement through the landscape, so that birth, growth, illness, and death were integrated into the journey. Human settlement, taking up permanent quarters, raised new problems, particularly concerning hygiene. These were handled by strategies that ranged from religious prescription (as, for example, in Judaism's rules for food preparation and for conducting social relationships) through quarantine (the social exclusion of 'infectious' people, lepers in particular) to town planning and engineering (the Romans' separation of water supply from sewage disposal, construction of public bath houses, and so forth).

Older town planning strategies broke down as new manufacturing technologies changed the use of waterways and led to the rapid construction of cheap housing as well as the overuse of older dwellings as cities expanded. Concerns about hygiene drove reforms necessitated by the Industrial Revolution, culminating in the Public Health Acts of the 1850s. An explanation of why these Acts were effective in reducing the incidence of disease came decades later with the development of germ theory. This theory led in rapid succession to the population-wide initiatives of vaccination and immunisation, a huge social experiment in its own right, and an indication of the ascendancy of scientific knowledge at the end of the 19th century. The new theory of infectious disease, reinforced by each citizen's personal experience of an immunisation needle in the arm, focused credit for the growing control of infectious illness upon clinical advances and obscured the foundation that had been laid in the hygiene acts. In many respects, this love affair of Western society with clinical practice has continued: the care of individuals is elevated, and the social context is played down. Only now at the beginning of the 21st century are we starting to understand some of the less desirable outcomes of our medical advances and to consider both their social preconditions and social impact.

In Western societies, the requirements of adequate hygiene are now assumed. They remain the responsibility of health departments, but seldom does the public see them as the core business they are—except when they fail under extreme circumstances such as the impact of cyclone, earthquake, fire, or flood. Our society's health focus continues to be on hospitals, places where health problems arrive once they become critical. Strategies to deal with potential problems earlier, through prevention or earlier intervention, are less developed and minimally funded. Our social mindset has moved away from prevention or containment to elimination or cure as a first-line response. We seem to be questioning whether we still need prevention when we can now effect cures. But increasingly we are finding that these cures often come with unwanted side effects, are not necessarily complete fixes, and are ultimately not affordable as people live longer and the costs of medical technology spiral upwards. The 'triumphal progress of medicine' stories in today's popular media tend to ignore many of these limitations, including the fact that in the end mortality remains 100%: we must all die from something.

In developing nations, the fundamental health problems caused by inadequate water supply and poor sanitation are more obvious. Western influence, however, still skews interest towards clinical approaches, and has too often created situations where a poor country's health budget has been devoted to developed-world hospital-based strategies that can benefit only a few, rather than primary

Social epidemiology
The systematic and comprehensive study of health, well-being, social conditions or problems, and diseases and their determinants, using epidemiology and social science methods to develop interventions, programs, policies, and institutions that may reduce the extent, adverse impact, or incidence of a health or social problem and promote health.

care resources or community infrastructure development that have the potential to improve the health of many.

In the latter part of the 20th century, **social epidemiology** has identified and mapped social patterns in prevalence and incidence of disease (Cwikel 2006). This evidence itself is shaped by social and cultural factors, such as the UK's interest in the effect of social class, and the USA's interest in the effect of race and gender upon health. Such divergent interests complicate comparison of the data; but nevertheless an increasing number of multinational studies and meta-analyses are identifying global themes in health and illness.

Stop and Think

» Has medical intervention in the form of immunisation been unambiguously good?

» What, if anything, might be the downside of such interventions?

Social factors in health

The heroic narrative of medical progress has dominated much of the 20th century, and it is unquestionable that the increasing effectiveness of medical treatments has rendered treatable or curable many conditions that earlier might have led to premature death. The removal of these causes has, however, resulted in a larger ageing population, placing an increased burden on the health system as death often follows upon years of disability or degenerative illness. While health planners gauge the effectiveness of healthcare by a society's increasing life expectancy, the same planners are now beginning to see it as a looming problem for the future (see e.g. the Intergenerational Report 2010 on Ageing in Australia [Australian Treasury 2010]).

As noted above, the first great social health intervention of the modern era was the Public Health Acts, and arguably the second was universal immunisation. Immunisation has certainly contained, and in some instances eliminated, infectious disease, although its preventive power was quickly challenged by its inability to respond to the great influenza pandemic of 1919–20 during which, depending on the estimate preferred, between 40 and 100 million people died worldwide. (Ten million men perished in the Great War; our continued social memory of these deaths contrasts strangely with the lost memory of many more deaths in half the time during the pandemic.)

A further major social intervention midway through the century was exemplified by the UK's National Health Service (NHS), an attempt to improve the nation's health by providing accessible clinical services funded not through an insurance scheme but by taxation revenue. It was one manifestation of the post-Second World War interest in nation-building expressed variously through the renewal of war-ravaged Europe and the emerging prosperity of the USA. The aim of the NHS was, by providing universal access to health services, to improve the health of the population to an extent where expenditure might decrease. This particular outcome was certainly not achieved, as the Black Report (1980) showed with devastating clarity—although it should be said that the NHS has achieved better population health outcomes for a much lower per capita expenditure than many other health systems, most notably that of the USA.

The NHS experiment did at least raise the question 'what is health?' as distinct from 'how can we cure illness?' This question about health became important globally. Colonialism ended, expanding global awareness brought questions about development to the fore, and emerging nations began to take responsibility for services that to this point had been an uneasy mix of traditional medicine and institutions set up by the colonisers.

In the climate of optimism and expansion that marked the postwar period, there was as yet little or no sense that resources might be finite, that wealth creation might have actual, if not ethical, limits, or that a century of industrialised progress might have consequences for the environment. (Warning voices on all these issues began to emerge in the 1970s, but had little impact on political and economic leaders who were, as today, largely immersed in their own immediate concerns.)

It is not possible in the space of a single chapter to review the huge body of evidence for social and cultural determinants of health that has been compiled in recent decades. However, there are several key studies that have established new directions in research and become models for many others. Similarly, there are a number of key documents that have given rise to many other similar national reports and policy documents. These are available in the WHO collection *Milestones in Health Promotion* (2009c), and provide the backbone of what follows here.

Health promotion as a response to the emerging evidence

Irwin and Scali (2007) identify four phases in social approaches to health after the Second World War:

- 1950s: emphasis on technology and disease-specific campaigns
- 1960s and early 1970s: rise of community-based approaches
- 1980s: neoliberalism dominates the political economic context
- 1990s and beyond: contested paradigms and shifting power relations.

1950s

The focus of public health in the postwar decade was on supporting the new clinical services that were emerging. Unlike today's public health advertisements that encourage individuals to make behavioural and lifestyle changes, the advertisements in the 1950s educated individuals about the symptoms for which they should seek expert medical advice. Another major focus was on immunisation for baby boomer children (children born 1946–64).

1960s and early 1970s

The baby boomers' entry into adulthood led to social change, with a particular interest in community. Health workers and community organisers joined forces to explore new approaches to community health. One Australian expression of this in the early 1970s was the community health movement initiated by the Whitlam Government. The focus was on creating health, not just combating illness; on community participation, not just professional activities. Australia was at this time a world leader in health promotion.

1980s

The 1980s saw the rise of neoliberal governments and a corresponding concern for economic management of the burgeoning healthcare sector. The new managerialism introduced in that decade arose to contain the healthcare costs that resulted from myriad confidential consultations between healthcare practitioners and clients. By identifying and assigning costs to various clinical interventions, and requiring practitioners to report their activities in terms of these services, managers were able to monitor and influence clinical decision-making. The new public health movement that was developing in this decade found itself caught between its social reformist vision and the realities of governance in the health sector from which funding was sought. Community health found itself reporting not in terms of community development but according to frameworks set up for health service delivery. The resulting compromise caused health promotion to lose its reforming edge and focus more on changing individual health behaviours.

1990s

The evidence-based medicine movement in the 1990s reasserted some professional control of territory by mandating best practice interventions, but clinical practice continued to balance best practice with cost-effective practice. The effect on health promotion was to intensify further the pressure to adapt to its healthcare environment—that is, to describe its work in terms of interventions and its outcomes in terms of services delivered, if not to individuals then to identifiable groups in the community, evaluated by short-term outcomes. It led inevitably to a focus on agency—what individuals could be instructed or persuaded to do—more than upon the structures that shaped or constrained those choices.

Case Study 11.1   The problem with tobacco

The first clue that smoking might be harmful came from studies that showed an exponential rise in cancer of the lung in UK men (Kenneway & Kenneway 1936, 1947). Various interpretations of this increase were put forward, until Doll and Hill (1950) concluded, on the basis of a retrospective epidemiological study, that smoking was an important factor in the production of carcinoma of the lung.

Their paper was criticised severely, so they embarked on a prospective study (Doll & Hill 1954). Their inspired choice was to investigate smoking in medical practitioners. All 59,600 men and women on the UK Medical Register were contacted, and 40,637 enrolled in the trial—34,445 men and 6192 women. All respondents were classified as current smokers, ex-smokers, or non-smokers. The group was followed for 50 years: the study closed in 2004 once all participating smokers had died and some 6000 non-smokers were still living. Doll himself was involved in the study from start to finish.

As early as 1957 the Medical Research Council endorsed the hypothesis of a cause-and-effect relationship between smoking and lung cancer. Doll and Hill's ten-year follow-up (1964) associated smoking with seven causes of death, coronary disease among them. The 20-year follow-up consolidated and extended these findings (Doll & Peto 1976), while at 22 years the pattern of mortality among the women doctors matched that of the men

(Doll et al. 1980). The 40-year review, with over 20,000 of the group having now died, found 25 causes of death associated with cigarette smoking, only one of them (Parkinson's Disease) positively (Doll et al. 1994). These findings were confirmed in the 50-year final review (Doll et al. 2004). Numerous other studies supported this longitudinal study, but no other has followed a smoking epidemic to its conclusion.

Responses to the evidence for cigarette smoking as a health determinant show strategies evolving according to the pattern outlined by Irwin and Scali (2007), beginning in the 1960s with health information encouraging young people not to start smoking and older smokers to moderate consumption. In the 1970s health promotion campaigns began advocating actively for smoking cessation. By the 1980s pressure on governments to introduce tobacco control was increasing, and restrictions on labelling, availability, and use of tobacco products were introduced. In the 1990s the focus turned to passive smoking, and controls were extended to include this aspect of health threat. At every step these strategies were resisted, both overtly and covertly, by the tobacco industry. While tobacco use has declined in developed nations, an epidemic of smoking among young women continues to cause concern. The tobacco industry has now turned its attention to increasing markets in developing countries.

While smoking among men in the USA peaked in the 1950s, the peak of tobacco-related deaths was not reached until the 1990s. Thus, in a country like China, where the smoking epidemic peaked in the 1990s, tobacco-related deaths, which are already increasing rapidly, can be expected not to peak until around 2030 (Boyle et al. 2006).

The key issues shown by this history are both the time involved in developing epidemiological evidence and the social process of reception. Only through sustained political process has regulation of tobacco products become possible. The right of the state to legislate arises from the responsibility of the state to fund the consequences of having legalised and benefited from taxation on tobacco products.

Individual risk factors and social determinants

The thrust of a great deal of epidemiological research has been to identify risk factors that relate to particular illnesses. Many of these risk factors overlap or coincide to identify a series of social behaviours that adversely affect health. Chief among these is cigarette smoking, accompanied by others such as obesity, substance abuse, and risky sexual behaviours. Health education programs seek to raise individual awareness and modify or eliminate risky behaviour. But the social underpinning of many of the risk factors is not adequately addressed. Identifying the risk factor 'poverty', for example, may not adequately represent the complex picture of deprivation that excludes people from constructive participation in their society (Harris et al. 2001, p. 259).

Identifying social determinants of health and disease is important to highlight pathways in the social production of health. The health iceberg model can help us examine the determinants of health and explore how those determinants relate to health outcomes (Talbot & Verrinder 2009). The iceberg is divided into three sections. Only the small section at the top that is visible above the waterline refers to observable states of health. These can be positive or negative and can include morbidity and mortality measures or prevalence of risk factors (e.g. cardiovascular disease [CVD]).

Figure 11.2 The iceberg

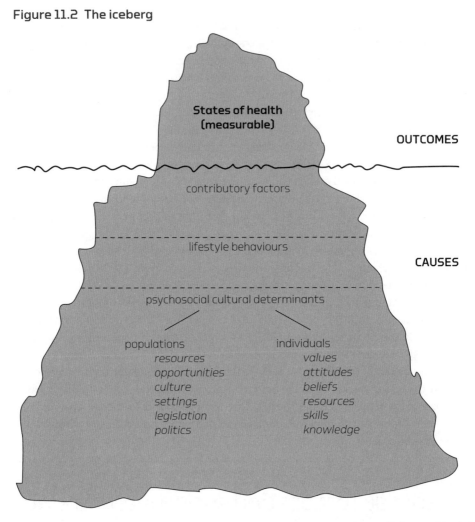

States of health
(measurable)

OUTCOMES

contributory factors

lifestyle behaviours

CAUSES

psychosocial cultural determinants

populations
resources
opportunities
culture
settings
legislation
politics

individuals
values
attitudes
beliefs
resources
skills
knowledge

Source: Talbot and Verrinder 2009

The second section of the iceberg (just below the waterline) relates to easily identifiable individual lifestyle choices and behavioural risk factors (e.g. the link between lack of physical activity and CVD). In the next section of the iceberg lie the major psycho-socio-cultural factors that influence individual and population health. At the very bottom of the iceberg are ecological and environmental factors that underpin our future health status (Talbot & Verrinder 2009).

The social gradient

The changing statistics on morbidity and mortality at population level are only part of the story. We often speak of differences in life expectancy that correspond to variations in health and disease across societies. These differences are evident between nations, and are variously attributed to differences in standard of living, in national infrastructure, and the quality of health services available. Figures like these are familiar to us.

Table 11.1 Men's life expectancy at birth in 2008

India	61
Philippines	65
Korea	65
Lithuania	66
Poland	71
Mexico	72
Cuba	75
USA	75
UK	76

Source: WHO 2008

A further important part of the story is that there are differences in morbidity and mortality within each society, and those differences appear to be a function of social position: those towards the bottom end of the social scale are on average more often sick and die earlier than those towards the top end of the scale. This is known as the **social gradient** in health. The classic example of this is the Whitehall Study II, so called because it was a major longitudinal study of mortality and social class within the British public service, whose headquarters are in Whitehall in London. It followed Whitehall I, which had been a study of men's vulnerability to CVD. Michael Marmot, who headed both studies, used categories of social class that had appeared in UK censuses since the 1930s. Class I includes professionals, class II is intermediate (managerial and technical) occupations, class IIIN is skilled non-manual occupations, class IIIM is skilled manual occupations, class IV is semi-skilled manual occupations, and class V unskilled manual occupations.

Social gradient Life expectancy is shorter and most diseases are more common further down the social ladder in each society.

Table 11.2 Life expectancy by social class 1972-76 and 1992-96, England and Wales

Social Class	Men 1972-76	Men 1992-96	Women 1972-76	Women 1996
I	72.0	77.7	79.2	83.4
II	71.7	75.8	77.0	81.1
IIIN	69.5	75.0	78.0	80.4
IIIM	69.8	73.5	75.1	78.8
IV	68.4	72.6	75.0	77.7
V	66.5	68.2	73.9	77.0
Difference	5.5	9.5	5.3	6.4

Source: Marmot 2003

Mythbuster

Providing health services to all will ensure equal health outcomes for all.

Consider Glasgow's figures for male life expectancy. These are 54 years in an inner-city suburb (well below India's average) and 82 years in an affluent suburb (well above UK's average). These differences occur in the same city, in the same country, for people potentially able to access the same health services, under the same universal insurance scheme (Hanlon et al. 2006).

Case Study 11.2   The health of 2000 San Francisco bus drivers

Among drivers over the age of 60, workplace medical examinations found the prevalence of hypertension to be 90%. A study was launched. This found that drivers complained of back pain, and then gastrointestinal and respiratory difficulties. High rates of alcohol use after work were also observed. More funding was secured and more interventions designed, but this did not solve the essential problem.

The researchers were so focused on specific diseases that they failed to recognise the fundamental problem: the job. They then investigated why the job caused so many problems. Computers devised a rigid bus schedule that allocated time depending on the number of buses available, but the computers were allocating time in a city with a bus shortage. Drivers had to get from Mission and Army Street to Mission and Geneva Street, for example, in 2 minutes. A fast trip in a Ferrari on Sunday morning would take longer. In addition, because drivers were penalised when they arrived late, they gave up rest stops and dashed into fast-food restaurants instead. And since the drivers were almost always late, the passengers were almost always angry. Drivers lacked control over a host of variables such as traffic and terrible shift arrangements, and drove during both morning and evening rush hours without enough time to go home in between shifts. At the end of a long day, many visited the local tavern. When they got home, they did not often socialise with family, but went to bed, only to get up at 4 a.m. to begin another gruelling day. They had health problems that needed attention, but obviously it was the job that had to be fixed to allow drivers some control of destiny and sense of empowerment (Syme 2004).

In addition to the social gradient in mortality across social classes for both males and females, it is evident that the gradient has become steeper over the period: that is, while life expectancy for all classes has increased, the rate of increase is much higher for class I than for class V, so that the gap between classes is greater.

Explanations for the gradient in health continue to be debated. Clearly it cannot be understood merely in terms of deprivation, or access to health services, or health literacy, for these differences between adjacent social classes are not substantial. The hypothesis put forward by Marmot (2004), Syme (2004), and others is that differences arise from factors such as self-esteem, status differences, self-direction in work, control over one's environment, social capital, and sense of social support—all variables that decline in strength as one descends the social ladder (Cockerham 2007, p. 94).

Social inequality and social exclusion

The Whitehall studies' finding of a social gradient in health status and life expectancy has been replicated around the world. Direct comparisons between countries are, however, made difficult by different measures of social class and **socio-economic status** (SES). Wilkinson and Pickett (2009) have developed comparisons for developed nations using per capita income as an indicator of SES, and a ratio of the per capita income of the top 20% to that of the bottom 20% as a measure of social inequality. Their findings can be summarised in two key graphs:

Further, they are able to show that health is related to the differences in income *within* societies, but not to differences *between* societies. It is inequality within a society, not that society's overall prosperity, which predicts the level of problems (Pickett & Wilkinson 2009).

Income is only a rough indicator of SES or deprivation, and more sensitive measures are now being developed. In Europe, social exclusion is increasingly used as an indicator of social inequality to reflect the complexity of the processes creating

Socio-economic status Represents how individuals and groups are 'placed' in a society, and how social and economic factors interact to affect health. These factors include social prestige, education, occupation, material resources, housing, and working conditions.

See Chapter 17 on social justice.

Figure 11.3 Health and social problems are worse in more unequal countries

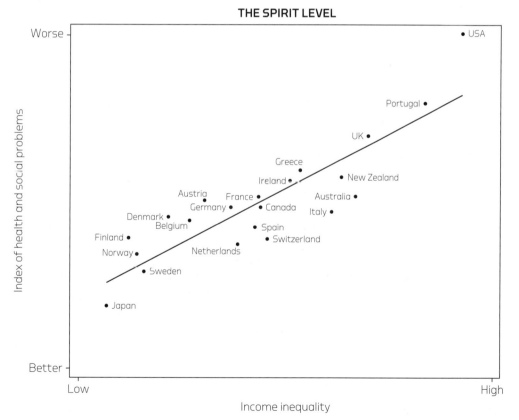

Source: From The Spirit Level by Richard Wilkinson & Kate Pickett, Allen & Lane. © Wilkinson and Pickett 2009

Figure 11.4 Life expectancy is longer in more equal rich countries

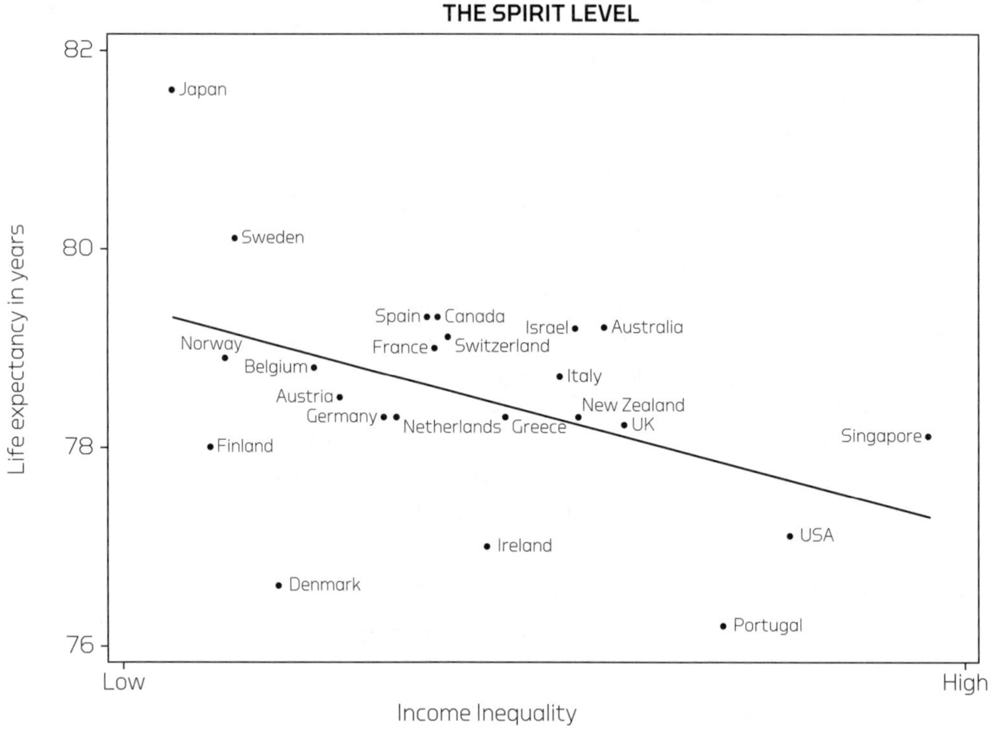

THE SPIRIT LEVEL

Source: From The Spirit Level by Richard Wilkinson & Kate Pickett, Allen & Lane. © Wilkinson and Pickett 2009

Social exclusion
A shorthand label for what can happen when individuals or areas suffer from a combination of linked problems such as unemployment, poor skills, low incomes, poor housing, high crime environments, bad health, and family breakdown.

Equity In healthcare can be defined as the absence of systematic disparities in health (or in the major social determinants of health) between social groups who have different levels of underlying social advantage/disadvantage.

inequality and provide a basis for addressing inequality. **Social exclusion** is a complex and multidimensional process. It involves the denial of resources, rights, goods, and services, and the inability to participate in normal relationships and activities available to the majority of people in a society, whether in economic, social, cultural, or political arenas. It affects both the quality of life of individuals and the **equity** and cohesion of society as a whole (Levitas et al. 2007). The Bristol Exclusion Matrix (Figure 11.5) provides an overview and summary.

Social exclusion is one of the most serious consequences of poverty and inequity. There are strong interconnections between the many social determinants of health, and the construct of social exclusion holds these multiple contributions together, demonstrating that social exclusion is an active process within societies. Being socially included means that people have the resources (skills and assets, including good health), opportunities, and capabilities they need to learn, work, engage, and have a voice (Social Inclusion Unit 2009, p. 3). Australia's **social inclusion** policy and strategy has been designed as a whole-of-government tool to be used in evaluating all policy initiatives in all sectors. The policy contains both aspirational and practical principles as follows:

Aspirational principles

- Reducing disadvantage
- Increasing social, civil and economic participation
- A greater voice, combined with greater responsibility

Figure 11.5 Bristol Exclusion Matrix

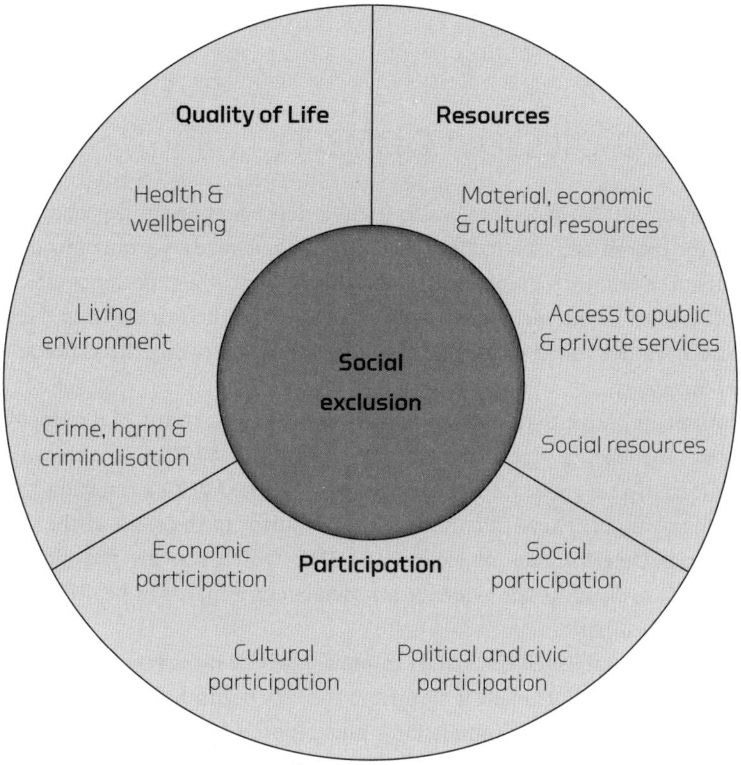

Source: Reproduced by permission from Professor Ruth Levitas and Dr Eldin Fahmy,
Copyright University of Bristol.

Principles of approach
- Building on individual and community strengths
- Building partnerships with key stakeholders
- Developing tailored services
- Giving a high priority to early intervention and prevention
- Building joined-up services and whole of government(s) solutions
- Using evidence and integrated data to inform policy
- Using locational approaches
- Planning for sustainability

Social Inclusion Unit 2009, p. 21

A primary aim of such policies is to remedy the mechanisms of social exclusion, identified principally as stereotyping, discrimination, and stigma.

A major influence upon social exclusion theory is the capabilities model devised by Sen (1984) and developed with Nussbaum (2001, 2005). This approach recognises the relationship between personal agency and social structure. Each nation has the responsibility, through its governance of social life, to ensure that individuals have the capacity to make choices about key aspects of their lives; each individual must take responsibility for their choices. A number of lists of capabilities exist, but

Social inclusion Used to describe strategies and policies designed to create a **socially inclusive society**, and also the experience of belonging to such a society.

Socially inclusive society One where all people feel valued, their differences are respected, and their basic needs are met, so they can live in dignity.

See Chapter 15 on deviance and stigmatisation.

Nussbaum's (see tutorial exercise) is indicative. The reforms called for in the *World health report 2008* (WHO 2008) and *Closing the Gap* (WHO CSDH 2008b) outline structural changes that are needed to nurture capabilities.

Health as a global concern

Wilkinson and Pickett (2009) show that health status is dependent on the degree of social inequality of a nation, not the overall average income. Obviously, income matters—some income is required to sustain life—but as the following graph, the Preston curve, shows, life expectancy effectively plateaus once a relatively low per capita income has been reached. From there, increasing the overall wealth of a nation may have less effect on health (as reflected in increasing life expectancy) than will reducing social inequality.

A major current initiative that aims at improving the health status of developing nations, in particular those at the leading edge of the Preston curve, is the WHO's Millennium Development Goals. These goals are strongly linked with the WHO's assertion that health is a human right. They are an immediate precursor to the work of the Commission on Social Determinants of Health (CSDH), which was given a global brief by the WHO to examine the evidence for social determinants of health in developing and developed nations.

See Chapter 17 on the WHO's Millennium Development Goals.

In 2005 the WHO established the CSDH to provide advice on ways of reducing the widening inequalities in health. The CSDH made it clear from the very beginning that health equity was to be the cornerstone of their work. The Commission's final report, *Closing the gap in a generation: Health equity through action on the social determinants of health*, was released in 2008 (WHO CSDH 2008) and contained three overarching recommendations:

- Improve daily living conditions.
- Tackle the inequitable distribution of power, money and resources.
- Measure and understand the problem and assess the impact of action.

The work of the Commission provides guidelines for practitioners and policymakers alike and provides the evidence for how action on these recommendations will improve health status for the most vulnerable members of our society. Of necessity, it does not commit itself to specific strategies for radical social reform (Green 2010; Lee 2010); rather, it enunciates principles and values to guide implementation in particular contexts. It is worth noting, however, that the CSDH implications for health system reform have been taken up in the *World health report 2008*, which asserts the central importance of primary care and critiques the structure and leadership of individualistic and medicalised health systems (WHO 2008).

See Chapter 19 on CSDH guidelines for reform.

Already the report has provided an important foundation for further national policy documents, among them *A healthier future for all Australians* (NHHRC 2009b,c) and *Fair society, healthy lives: The Marmot review* (Strategic Review of Health Inequalities in England post-2010 2010). Further major collections of evidence also continue to be published, such as *Equity, social determinants and public health programmes* (Blas & Kurup 2010). These reports reinforce Beauchamp's contention that 'the historic dream of public health...is a dream of social justice' (Beauchamp 1996, p. 105).

See Chapter 17 on social justice.

Figure 11.6 Preston curve

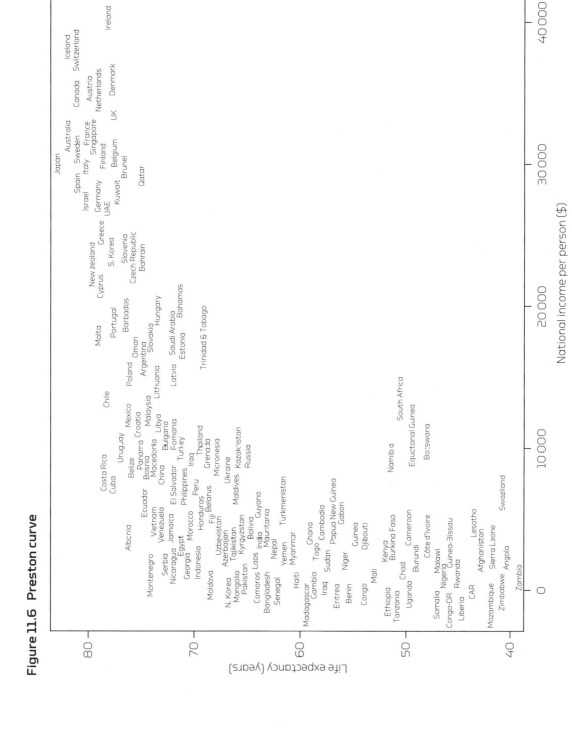

Source: From The Spirit Level by Richard Wilkinson & Kate Pickett, Allen & Lane. © Wilkinson and Pickett 2009

Getting the balance right

Because this chapter has been arguing the case for taking social determinants of health seriously, it may have conveyed an impression that we are playing down or even questioning the contribution of clinical science to a population's health. This is certainly not our intention. What we are arguing is that clinical advancements need to be seen in their social and global contexts, and that we need as societies to work out how the illness-management strategies of the clinical disciplines can best serve each nation's health. It is becoming abundantly clear that the largest proportion of national health budgets around the world is devoted to resolving or ameliorating health problems that could have been avoided, or reduced, or at the very least delayed in their onset. It is also clear that a significant proportion of these health budgets is spent on investigations and interventions that are, at best, of marginal benefit, at worst futile. But we seem unable to reorient our approach to health expenditure to accommodate the wider view, with the result that our expenditure on prevention and health education is still around 5% of the total budget.

Summary

The variation in health status between different societies and different groups within societies has always hinted that social and cultural factors contribute to illness, disability, and reduced life expectancy. The extent of this contribution has, however, not been clear, and some have suggested that differences are largely attributable to variations in the level and quality of healthcare services. Now that the primary causes of disability and death for most nations are found in so-called lifestyle illnesses—cancer, cardiovascular disease, diabetes—that are in turn linked with particular behaviours—smoking, alcohol abuse, obesity—and specific social contexts—unemployment, abusive relationships, social exclusion—it is becoming clear that social and cultural factors have a profound influence on health status both within and between nations.

Solid evidence from many epidemiological studies shows that health is shaped by social determinants, in particular social inequity and social exclusion, which produce a social gradient in health. As this evidence has emerged, so has a range of strategic responses. Most are strategies within the health system designed to address and enhance citizens' health knowledge and improve their agency to change unhealthy behaviours. A fundamental dilemma, however, is that action to address the social determinants of health also involves factors outside the control of the health system. Better health depends on changing settings and social structures that produce inequity and exclusion.

Healthcare reform thus involves not only a focus on preventive measures and primary healthcare, but also on social inclusion. Social justice is the key to building healthy societies that promote the well-being of the whole population.

Tutorial exercises

1   Return to the story of Samantha (Case Study 1.2). From the various contributions to her death that you identified then, list the social determinants. Consider where Samantha or her mother has agency, and where they are constrained by these determinants.

2   The suggestion has been made that some food companies are promoting some of their products in terms of their health benefits (high fibre, added vitamins, reduced fat...) while ignoring

dangerously high levels of sugar or sodium in those same products. Check this claim by a field trip to the supermarket during which you inspect the list of ingredients of some of these products. What strategies are needed to ensure that an accurate depiction of health benefits and risks is available to the public?

3   Go to the United Nations website <www.un.org/millenniumgoals> and look up the eight Millenium Development Goals. Choose one goal and examine any fact sheets that go with that goal. What has been achieved? What is still to be done? How might health workers ensure that this goal is met?

4   What are some of the main shifts in conceptualising and addressing social determinants that you see in comparing 2003's *The Solid Facts* with 2008's *Closing the Gap*?

5   What are some of the obstacles to implementing social inclusion strategies in Australia? In the light of this, what do you see as the benefits and risks of Australia's social inclusion policy?

6   Martha Nussbaum (2005) suggests that the core capabilities for living a good life are that each person should be able to
   a   live a life of normal length
   b   have bodily health
   c   maintain bodily integrity
   d   exercise the senses, imagination, and thought
   e   experience and express emotions
   f   develop practical reason (a conception of the good)
   g   affiliate with others
   h   have respect for other species
   i   play
   j   have appropriate control over their environment (political and material).
   Are there capabilities you would add to, or omit from, Nussbaum's list?

Further reading

Baum, F. (2008). *The new public health*, 3rd edn. Melbourne: Oxford University Press.

Blas, E., & Kurup, A. (eds) (2010). *Equity, social determinants and public health programmes.* Geneva: WHO Press.

Keleher, H., & MacDougall, C. (eds) (2009). *Understanding health: A determinants' approach*, 2nd edn. Melbourne: Oxford University Press.

Lin, V., Smith, J., & Fawkes, S. (2007). *Public health practice in Australia: The organised effort.* Sydney: Allen & Unwin.

Marmot, M. (2004). *Status syndrome: How your social standing directly affects your health and life expectancy.* London: Bloomsbury.

Marmot, M., & Wilkinson, R. (eds) (2006). *Social determinants of health*, 2nd edn. Oxford: Oxford University Press.

National Health and Hospitals Reform Commission (2009). *A healthier future for all Australians: Final report, May 2009.* Canberra: Commonwealth of Australia.

Wilkinson, R., & Pickett, K. (2009). *The spirit level: Why more equal societies almost always do better.* London: Allen-Lane (Penguin).

World Health Organization Commission on Social Determinants of Health (2008b). *Closing the gap in a generation: Health equity through action on the social determinants of health. Final Report of the Commission on Social Determinants of Health.* Geneva: WHO.

Websites

<http://aihw.gov.au/>

This is the website of the Australian Institute of Health and Welfare. It provides data on the health of Australians.

<www.marmotreview.org>

The 2010 Marmot Review *Fair Society, Healthy Lives* was an independent review into health inequalities in the UK. The site continues to report on many developments based on the approach advocated in the review, and provides links to other related European studies.

<www.equalitytrust.org.uk/resource/the-spirit-level>

The Equality Trust conducts a program of public and political education designed to improve the understanding of, and create action on, income inequality. It is non-partisan, and draws heavily on the research of Wilkinson, Pickett and colleagues.

<www.socialinclusion.gov.au/Pages/default.aspx>

This is the Australian Government website on social inclusion policy and strategy. It provides resources, regular reports from the Australian Social Inclusion Board, and research papers.

<www.un.org/millenniumgoals>

The UN Millennium Development Goals (MDG) website gives an overview of the global action plan implementing the millennium goals. It provides a wealth of resources and current information concerning a range of MDG initiatives.

<www.who.int/social_determinants/en>

This is the central global resource for data on the social determinants of health. The Commission's website contains a wealth of documents supporting the *Closing the Gap* report, and continues to be updated with fresh material on program developments and publications arising from the CSDH Report.

12 | Health as a social construct

Claire Henderson-Wilson

TOPICS COVERED

This chapter covers the following topics:
- social and cultural constructions of health, illness, and well-being
- social model of health
- health sociology
- social skeleton: health, illness, and structure agency model
- ecological models
- social ecological model

KEY TERMS

Biomedical model of health
Gender
Health sociology
Social class
Social construction of health

Social ecological model
Social model of health
Social Skeleton: health, illness and structure agency model

Introduction

The concept of health is...complex and dynamic. Its meanings are embedded in the unique individual, family, social and cultural contexts in which the term is used; as such, it is said to be socially and culturally *constructed*. (Taylor 2008a, p. 5)

Social construction of health Refers to a range of social forces that combine to create and modify the experience of health, such as social groups, social institutions, and the wider culture.

See the discussion of social and cultural determinants in Chapter 1.

As Taylor (2008a) suggests, different people ascribe different meanings to health, so for some people 'health' may mean being free from disease and for others it may mean maintaining balance between the mind, body, and spirit. This is referred to as the **social construction of health** as it involves a range of social forces (i.e. social groups, social institutions, and the wider culture) that combine to create and modify the experience of health (Brown 1995). Constructions of 'health', 'illness', and 'well-being' have moved beyond traditional biomedical interpretations that focused on an individual's medically defined pathology (Keleher & MacDougall 2009) to an awareness of how they are influenced by social and cultural contexts and determinants.

The first section of this chapter will define and discuss the social model of health, using relevant examples; it will explore how valuable this model is for understanding the social construction of health, illness, and well-being. The next section will discuss how health sociology can aid an understanding of health, illness, and well-being. Drawing on Germov's (2005) Social skeleton: Health, illness and structure agency model, the chapter will explore how social groups, social institutions, and the wider culture influence perceptions of health, illness, and well-being. Finally, it will discuss how ecological models can be used to explore social constructions of health, illness, and well-being, using Bronfenbrenner's social ecology model.

Social model of health

The social model locates people in social contexts and conceptualises the physical environment as socially organised, and understands ill health as a process of interaction between people and environments. (Broom 1991, p. 52)

Biomedical model of health Suggests that illness results from a malfunction of the body (i.e. germs or disease) and that each disease affects the body in a predictable way.

Social model of health Suggests that health is influenced by a dynamic set of social structures and aims to identify the factors within a society that inhibit the health of individuals.

For much of the 20th century, the 'biomedical model' dominated understanding of health, illness, and well-being. This model suggests that illness results from a malfunction of the body (i.e. germs or disease) and that each disease affects the body in a predictable way (Germov 2009). However, the quote from Broom above indicates that illness is much more than just a 'mono-causal model of disease' (Germov 2009, p. 10), and this is the main focus of this chapter, which will demonstrate how our constructs of health, illness, and well-being are shaped by social and cultural context.

By moving beyond the limitations of the **biomedical model of health**, which draws on biochemical explanations of health and illness, the **social model of health** can be useful in understanding how perceptions of health, illness, and well-being comprise a dynamic interaction of social structures (Germov 2005; Yuill 2010). The social model aims to identify the factors within a society that inhibit the health of individuals (Moon & Gillespie 1995). It acknowledges that infectious pathogens can affect health, but the focus is more on how these pathogens are not distributed randomly or shared equally among the population (Broom 1991). Therefore, the social model of health aims to address health inequities by directing attention towards the prevention of illness via social reforms that concentrate on living conditions (Jirojwong & Liamputtong 2009). Essentially, 'the social model gives equal priority to the prevention of illness along with the treatment of illness and aims to alleviate health inequalities' (Germov 2005, p. 17).

See also Chapters 1 & 17 for discussion of equity and social justice.

According to Yuill (2010), there are six key features of the social model of health:

1 Individual health is enabled or inhibited by social context.
2 The body is simultaneously social, psychological, and biological.
3 Health is cultural.
4 Biomedicine and medical science is something—but not everything.
5 Health is political.
6 Other voices matter.

Consideration of these features allows the social model of health to provide deeper understanding of health, illness, and well-being.

In terms of the first feature, perceptions of health and illness are often thought to be based on personal choices. For example, someone may choose to smoke cigarettes or eat foods high in saturated fat. Yuill (2010) contends that while personal choices can influence health, it is vital to consider the social context in which people find themselves and how this affects their ability to exercise control over their health. This is supported by Wilkinson and Marmot (2003), who argue that people who have more control over their lives tend to be healthier than those who do not. They cite examples of people who experience stress and a lack of control over their home and work life (i.e. social contexts) and how this can lead to poor mental and physical health and eventually premature death.

Second, Yuill (2010) proposes that bodies are made up of more than just biology and anatomy; they are based on relationships involving social, cultural, psychological, biological, and individual processes. For example, one of these processes concerns identity, whereby people develop a sense of identity through their pursuit of a certain body shape. When people experience chronic illness, their self-identity may be challenged or questioned. Martin and Peterson (2010, p. 580) support this contention and propose that when people experience illness, 'this implies a threat to the individual's inner and social being by the biological component of their own body'.

The third feature proposed by Yuill (2010) suggests that perceptions and assumptions of health and illness vary by culture. In Western cultures, people tend to see slenderness as equating to healthiness, particularly for women, whereas in other cultures larger women are seen as healthy (Parson 1990). Additionally, Blaxter (2004) points out that in countries like China, India, and some African nations, herbal therapies are often prescribed to people experiencing illness along with Western biomedical treatments. Furthermore, Germov (2005) states that Vietnamese people believe that emotional and physical illnesses are a result of the imbalance in the forces of *am* and *duong* (commonly translated as hot and cold). From these examples, it is clear that culture influences how people construct and perceive health and illness.

See Chapters 1 & 14 for more discussions on the impact of culture on health.

The fourth feature of the social model of health acknowledges that the biomedical model has merits that should not be ignored by social scientists. Germov (2005) agrees with this argument and states that the social model does not deny the requirement for medical intervention, and therefore it coexists with the biomedical model. Thus, the biomedical model focuses on treating

Stop and Think

» What social and cultural factors influence how you perceive health, illness, and well-being?

» How much influence do you think social contexts have on your health status?

illnesses with medical intervention but the social model focuses on social contexts that bring about illnesses in populations (i.e. social exclusion, bullying, and exposure to environmental pollution).

The fifth feature described by Yuill (2010, p. 13) proposes that 'health is not separate from other spheres of society'. In other words, an individual's health is influenced by the provision of health services and resources. This is supported by Perry and colleagues (2010), who conducted a study to examine the use and availability of health services by young people with type 1 diabetes by comparing those living in regional New South Wales with those using city and state capital services. They found that regional services had fewer resources and limited access to specialists compared to city and state capital services. The authors concluded that health service redistribution is required to ensure equity of access to services and resources for young people with type 1 diabetes living in regional Australia.

Last, Yuill (2010) proposes that in understanding perceptions of health and illness, the social model considers viewpoints beyond the medical profession. It can draw on the knowledge and perspectives of lay people, including those experiencing illness. For example, often people with chronic illness are believed to experience social constructions of illness that are considered more relevant and important than healthcare professionals' interpretations (Martin & Peterson 2010; Yuill 2010). By shifting the focus away from a healthcare/biomedical model towards the social model, understandings of health and illness can be viewed within a framework of individuals and society (Habibis 2009).

In summary, the social model allows for a comprehensive understanding of health, illness, and well-being by exploring the range of influential social and cultural contexts within an individual's environment. Some policy and practice responses to the social model of health in the Australian context will now be briefly discussed.

Social model of health: Policy and practice responses

The biomedical model is considered to dominate healthcare practice in many countries, including Australia, but over time it has become more inclusive of the range of social and cultural contexts influencing health and illness (Taylor 2008a). As Taylor writes: 'Public health proponents, for example, have questioned the effectiveness of biomedicine in improving the overall health of the Australian population and socially disadvantaged groups' (p. 28). This has resulted in a move towards adoption of a social model of healthcare, with a range of social and economic determinants being addressed at the level of health policy (Taylor 2008a). For example, the Victorian Department of Health (2010) recently published *Using policy to promote mental health and well-being: An introduction for policy makers*, which is a guide aimed at enabling policymakers in Victoria to consider, when developing or reviewing policy or programs, the range of social and environmental determinants of mental health. Additionally, many local governments within Victoria prepare Integrated Health Promotion Plans that place emphasis on addressing the social, economic, and cultural determinants impacting on the health, illness, and well-being of their communities.

In addition to the social model of health being recognised at a health policy level, it is also acknowledged by many health service providers. For example, Women's Health West (WHW) is the regional women's health service for the western metropolitan region of Victoria. This organisation provides a range of health services including health promotion, community development, research, training, and advocacy around women's health, safety, and well-being (Women's Health West 2008). WHW recognises that women's lives are shaped by political, economic, cultural, and social forces and 'as a result, WHW places great importance on identifying the structural factors that impact on women's health and well-being' (p. 2).

The shift from a biomedical to a social model of health has clearly been adopted by many health policy and healthcare providers within Australia, so it is worth considering how 'health sociology' has evolved to provide a perspective for understanding how health is socially constructed.

Health sociology

> Health sociology...provides a second opinion to the conventional medical view of illness derived from biological and psychological explanations, by exploring the social context of health and illness—the social, economic, cultural and political features of society that influence why some groups of people get sicker and die sooner than others. (Germov 2005, p. 5)

As the above quote suggests, '**health sociology**' encompasses multidimensional ways of thinking about social worlds and recognises that while illnesses are experienced by individuals, they are also influenced by a range of social determinants (Earle & Letherby 2008; Germov 2009). Aligned with the social model of health, health sociology is not necessarily focused on the individual but rather the social group to which they belong (Willis & Elmer 2007; White 2009; Weitz 2010).

Health sociology came to fruition during the 1970s and 1980s when many sociologists working in the area of health and illness began to question the biomedical model of health (Germov 2009; White 2009). They felt that only considering that people become ill because of the incursion of a germ overlooked the fact that living in social groups may also influence why people become ill (White 2009).

White (2009) asserts that when confronted by someone who is ill, sociologists do not think about why that person is ill but rather, what are the characteristics of the group to which they belong that leaves them at risk of becoming ill. Germov (2009, p. 4) agrees with White and states that 'health sociology focuses on the social patterns of health and illness, such as the different health statuses between women and men, the poor and the wealthy, or the Indigenous and non-Indigenous populations, and seeks social, rather than biological or psychological, explanations'. Some relevant examples will now be described to demonstrate how health sociology can inform understandings of health, illness, and well-being.

Health sociology
A discipline that recognises that health and illness are influenced by a range of social determinants and focuses on the social patterns of health and illness.

See also Chapter 5 on social factors in disease.

See also Chapter 1 for the varying health status of different groups of people.

Life expectancy

Life expectancy is significantly higher in developed and wealthy countries than in developing and poorer countries (Baum 2008; Germov 2009). Baum (2008) suggests that people in poor countries tend to earn lower incomes, are less likely to be educated, and have limited access to safe drinking water and sanitary conditions. Australia has a high life expectancy compared to other countries, with data indicating that a boy born during 2007–09 can expect to live 79.3 years, while a girl can expect to live 83.9 years (ABS 2009a). This long life expectancy could be attributed to the living and working conditions of Australia, such as access to a clean water supply, efficient sewage system, education, and employment. However, not all Australians experience long life expectancy, with data indicating that there is a gap in life expectancy for Indigenous Australians compared to non-Indigenous Australians: 12 years for males and 10 years for females (AIHW 2010a). This gap could be due to a range of social and cultural factors such as lower socio-economic status, unemployment, or lack of access to culturally appropriate health services (Baum 2008; Germov 2009).

Gender

Gender Socially and culturally constructed categories reflecting what it means to be 'masculine' and 'feminine' and associated expectations of roles and behaviours of men and women.

Gender is considered a vital element in the social construction of health, illness, and well-being, as it shapes exposure to health problems, accounts for differences in health-related behaviours, and influences how illness is experienced (Waldron 2005; Broom 2009). White (2009) suggests that women live longer than men (as indicated by the life expectancy example given previously), but they are also diagnosed with illness more than men. Several reasons account for why women experience illness more than men, such as complications related to reproduction, their social roles (working longer hours, being paid less, having a work/life imbalance), and the fact that they are reported to consult health practitioners more often than men (Broom 2009; White 2009). Temple-Smith and colleagues (2007) conducted a study, in Australia, to determine if there are any gender differences in seeking care for hepatitis C. They found that women were more likely than men to consult a general practitioner (GP) specifically for hepatitis C virus (HCV) related symptoms, consistent with previous research. However, they also found that women would seek the advice of a GP even when they had not experienced any HCV symptoms, suggesting that gender influences the health-seeking behaviours of individuals (Temple-Smith et al. 2007). Gender roles have also been found to influence rates of illness and mortality. Waldron (2005) argues that in some South Asian countries, boys receive better healthcare than girls, which contributes to a lower mortality rate for boys. This is largely due to a cultural preference for sons, which results in discrimination against girls in accessing healthcare and health-promoting resources (Reidpath 2004; Waldron 2005).

Income inequality

Social class The position of a person in a system of structured inequality; it is grounded in unequal distribution of income, wealth, status, and power.

Income inequality is reported to be one of the key indicators of **social class** inequality within populations (Germov 2009). Essentially, income inequality is the unequal distribution of income within a society, or in other words, the contrast between 'rich' and 'poor' (or high and low socio-economic status) (Atkinson & Leigh 2006). Societies with more equal income distributions have better health, but the unequal distribution of wealth within countries is believed to be increasing worldwide, and this may result in a range of health inequities (Wilkinson & Pickett 2006; Baum 2008). Cross-national research shows that the greater the degree of socio-economic inequality within a society, the steeper the gradient of health inequalities (Schrader 2004). The fact that class differences in health are smaller in Sweden than the UK and the USA has been attributed to Sweden's more even distribution of income (Schrader 2004). It is important to note that 'income distribution is related to health where it serves as a measure of the scale of social class differences in a society' (Wilkinson & Pickett 2006, p. 14). Wilkinson (1997a) has argued that income inequality in areas that are considered small has been influenced by the degree of residential separation of rich and poor people and that the health of people in disadvantaged neighbourhoods is poorer not because of the level of inequality within their neighbourhoods, but because they are perceived to be disadvantaged in relation to the wider society.

In summary, these examples demonstrate how social patterns of health and illness can be understood from a health sociological perspective. How the Social Skeleton model (Germov 2005) can be applied to understanding health, illness, and well-being will now be discussed.

Social Skeleton: Health, illness and structure-agency

Germov's (2005) **Social Skeleton: health, illness and structure agency model** (see Figure 12.1) represents the social structures individuals are part of and demonstrates how social groups, social institutions, and the wider culture influence perceptions of health, illness, and well-being. Germov (2005) contends that social structures are like the human skeleton; the various body parts (heart, lungs, muscles) need the skeletal frame to function and survive. Social structures include cultural customs and health, government, and education institutions that people experience in their lives and that influence their social interactions (Germov 2005).

The model allows us to see how our society is structured and to appreciate that the various components of the social skeleton are interconnected (refer to the two-way arrows). Germov (2005) suggests that a society's economy can influence its political system and culture. He also suggests that religion, via marriage and family, has influenced how personal relationships are structured.

> **Social Skeleton: health, illness and structure agency model** Represents the social structures individuals are part of and demonstrates how social groups, social institutions, and the wider culture influence perceptions of health, illness, and well-being.

Social institutions such as healthcare services, housing, education, welfare provision, and mass media are defined as 'formal structures within society that are set up to address identified social needs' (Germov 2005, p. 19). These social institutions are said to influence the formation of social groups. For example, different socio-economic classes evolve from the economic institutions in a society, and cultural attitudes and laws influence gender-based social roles (Germov 2005). Additionally, other social relationships can develop, for example, between patients and doctors, students and teachers, and employees and employers.

Another important component of the model is that of the 'structure/agency debate'. Germov (2005, 2009) suggests that this is a key debate in sociology that asks us to determine how much influence we have over our lives and whether we can blame society for some of the actions we take. It also suggests that we perceive structure and agency as interrelated and consider to what extent we shape society and simultaneously are shaped by society. In other words, 'structure and

Figure 12.1 Social Skeleton: Health, illness and structure agency model

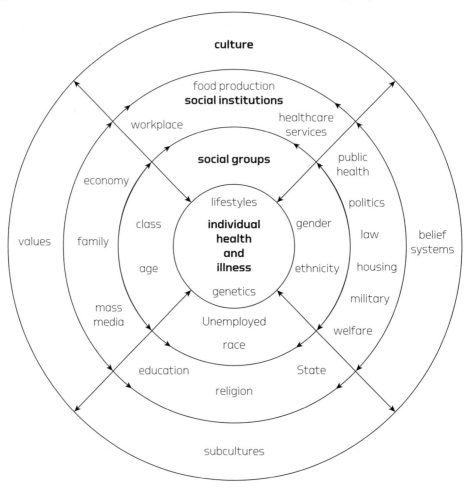

Source: Germov 2005, p. 19

Case Study 12.1   Social Skeleton: Health, illness and structure agency model

The following hypothetical example is provided to briefly demonstrate how key social structures, as represented in the Social Skeleton model, influence an individual's perceptions of health, illness, and well-being.

Katie is an 18-year-old university student living in an outer suburb of Melbourne. She is Anglo-Saxon and of a high socio-economic status. Belonging to these social groups, combined with her lifestyle, influences her perception of health. Katie considers herself to be a very healthy young woman as she consumes a balanced diet, exercises daily, does not smoke cigarettes or drink alcohol, and maintains positive relationships with friends and family members. Although Katie is responsible for controlling her health and lifestyle, a number of social institutions can be said to influence her life. The social relationships Katie shares with her parents would be considered to influence her perceptions of health and illness. For instance, Katie's dad Barry has always been a regular marathon runner and instilled the importance of regular exercise in his daughter from a young age. This no doubt has influenced how Katie perceives health but so too have the mass media. Often, television shows and magazines portray slenderness as equating to healthiness; this could be influencing Katie's perceptions of health. Furthermore, cultural attitudes towards women being seen as healthy if they are slender dominate Katie's society, including via the mass media, and this is another social structure that influences her perceptions of health, illness, and well-being.

Stop and Think

» If you think about the various parts of the Social Skeleton model, which social structures influence your perceptions of health, illness, and well-being the most?

» Thinking about the structure/agency debate, how much influence does society have over your health behaviours and actions?

Mythbuster

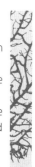

Consider whether you see the following as questionable. What does this tell you about your own values regarding the influence society has over health behaviours and actions?

- There are many who believe that an African male infected with HIV/AIDS can be cured of the infection by having sex with a virgin.
- In Pakistan, decisions about pregnancy and antenatal care are said to be usually made by older women. Often, this is the pregnant woman's mother-in-law, and the mother and father to be are distanced from the process.

These and other examples are reported on <http://en.wikipedia.org/wiki/Sociology_of_health_and_illness>

agency may be in tension, but they are interdependent—that is, one cannot exist without the other' (Germov 2005, p. 21).

In summary, Germov's (2005) Social Skeleton is a useful model for depicting a range of social structures influencing people's perceptions of health, illness, and well-being. However, ecological models are other useful tools for mapping the social, cultural, and other determinants impacting on people's health, illness, and well-being and they will be explored in the next section.

Ecological models

Human ecologists contend that an individual's health is part of a structure of relationships (contexts and determinants) and is altered by changes in that structure (McLaren & Hawe 2005). They are interested in the relationships between humans and the physical, natural, cultural, and social dimensions of their environment (Lawrence 2003). The notion that health is a result of connections between humans and the elements of their broader environments has gained prevalence since the mid-20th century (McMichael 2001). Following the development of the social model of health, a number of ecological models have been developed since the 1970s to show the relationship between humans and elements of their social, cultural, and broader environments that impact on health (Townsend & Mahoney 2004).

For example, Hancock and Perkins (1985) developed the Mandala of Health to demonstrate the links between humans, social and cultural environments, and the broader environment/ecosystem. The model displays human health in a broad context, with four critical factors influencing the health of an individual at the centre (Nicholson & Stephenson 2004). These four factors are human biology, personal behaviour, psychosocial environment, and immediate physical environment (Hancock & Perkins 1985). The Mandala sees health in its holistic sense, so the health of the individual at the centre is shown to have body, mind, and spirit dimensions. Hancock (1993) indicates that the Mandala has been widely used by educators and practitioners to map the determinants of health of individuals and populations.

Following this, Hancock (1993) developed two more ecological models. First, the Health-Environment-Economy model focuses on human development and is based on two key principles of public health first proposed in the 1980s—ecological sanity and social justice. It demonstrates the intersection between health, the environment, and the economy and indicates that 'the economy both underpins human health and the environment and, at the same time...the economy is—or should be—subservient to those broader imperatives. It also ensures that issues of human well-being and social equity are incorporated in the discussion of sustainable development' (Hancock 1993, p. 44). Second, the Community Ecosystem Model demonstrates that community health is found at the intersection of three circles: the community, the environment, and the economy. Hancock suggests that healthy community ecosystems should comprise six qualities within their environmental, economic, and community domains. They should be convivial, liveable, sustainable, viable, and adequately prosperous with equitable wealth distribution.

Social ecological model
A nested arrangement of interrelated structures comprising the microsystem, mesosystem, exosystem, and macrosystem, which have a trickle-down effect on an individual at the centre of the model.

Social ecological model

Urie Bronfenbrenner, a renowned human ecologist, argues that an individual's health and well-being is dependent on their interaction with the environment. He develops an ecological model to depict how various contexts and consequences impact on an individual's health and well-being. This model is now described in detail and a case study will be used to demonstrate the applicability of this model for understanding health as a social construct. Bronfenbrenner's **social ecological model** consists of a nested arrangement of interrelated structures comprising the microsystem, mesosystem, exosystem, and macrosystem, which have a trickle-down effect on an individual at the centre of the model (Bronfenbrenner 1979).

At the centre of the model is an individual and their particular characteristics such as gender, age, and health status (Bowes & Grace 2009). The first layer of the model, the microsystem, is the structure of activities, roles, and personal relationships (family members and peers) experienced by an individual that directly affects health and well-being (Bronfenbrenner 1979; Bowes & Grace 2009). The next layer is the mesosystem, which comprises the relationship between two or more settings (places where people can engage in face-to-face interaction) in the microsystem, such as the level of match between family and work (Bronfenbrenner 1979; Bowes & Grace 2009). A third layer of the model is the exosystem, which refers to one or more settings that do not directly involve the individual, but that affect the individual's health and well-being, such as extended family and community influences (Bronfenbrenner 1979; Bowes & Grace 2009). The macrosystem is the outer layer of the model and consists of cultural norms, values, and attitudes that are passed on through families and social and government institutions to shape an individual's health and well-being (Bowes & Grace 2009).

Traditionally, the social ecological model has been used to determine the range of factors impacting on an individual's development (Bronfenbrenner 1979). But it has also been useful for exploring the influence of family on an individual (Townsend & Mahoney 2004) and can be applied to a number of individuals and contexts. How the model can be used to map the factors affecting the health and well-being of inner-city high-rise residents is illustrated in the following case study.

Case Study 12.2   Adapted social ecological model

For her PhD, the author conducted an exploratory mixed-methods study that investigated the factors, including access to nature (i.e. parks, gardens, and/or bodies of water), impacting on inner-city high-rise residents' health and well-being (see Henderson-Wilson 2009, 2010). The study participants varied in age, gender, socio-economic status, housing tenure (owner-occupiers/private tenants and public housing tenants), city of residence, and degree of proximity to natural environments. Phase 1 of the study involved surveying 221 high-rise residents from inner Melbourne and Sydney to identify and measure relationships between access to nature, high-rise living, and health and well-being. Phase 2 involved interviewing 30 of the surveyed residents to gain a deeper understanding of their experiences with high-rise living, access to nature, sense of community, and sense of place. Analysis of the integrated findings (from Phases 1 and 2) revealed that numerous factors (including accessibility, choice and control, tenure, and community infrastructure) impact on residents' health and well-being, either directly or indirectly. Results of this study indicated that for disadvantaged populations (e.g. public housing tenants), the availability of a park, garden, and/or body of water can enhance residents' quality of life.

The social ecological model was applied to describe the range of factors affecting high-rise residents' access to nature, health, and well-being. The results of the study showed that a range of factors trickle down from the outer, macrosystem level to the high-rise resident at the centre of the model. The following section discusses the range of contexts and consequences at each level of the adapted social ecological model (see Figure 12.2).

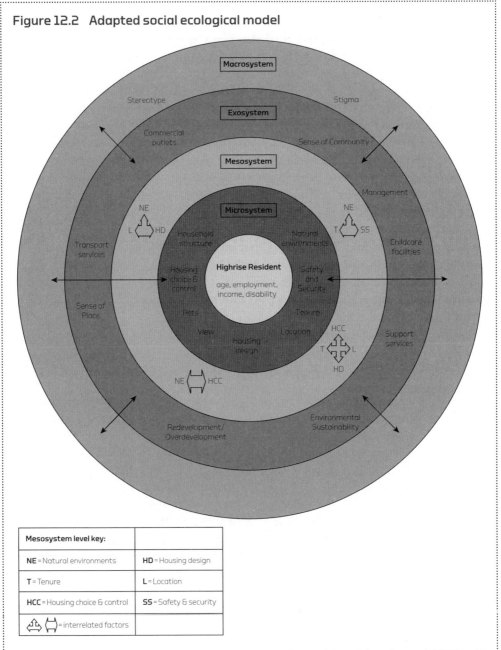

Figure 12.2   Adapted social ecological model

Mesosystem level key:	
NE = Natural environments	**HD** = Housing design
T = Tenure	**L** = Location
HCC = Housing choice & control	**SS** = Safety & security
= interrelated factors	

Source: Adapted from Santrock 2004, p. 40

Several demographic factors were found to impact on participants' health and well-being. These are displayed in the adapted model within the individual/high-rise resident level at the centre of the model as including:

- *Age*: being aged 55 years or more resulted in higher well-being. This could be due to the fact that residents at this age are more resilient to changing contexts.

- *Employment*: participating in paid work for 21 hours or more a week resulted in higher well-being. This is not surprising considering that residents who participate in meaningful occupation are likely to have enhanced well-being (Furnass 1996; Trewin 2001).
- *Income*: earning an income of more than $31,000 per annum resulted in higher well-being (linking to the findings on employment). It should be noted that at the time of data collection, 2004, less than half of the participants worked full-time (39.8%); the majority earned more than $15,000 per annum (64.7%), with about a quarter of them earning $90,000 or more (23.5%).
- *Disability*: findings indicated that participants who did not have a disability or medical condition had higher well-being.

At the microsystem level, that which is closest to the high-rise resident, a range of contexts and consequences was found to impact directly on the resident's health and well-being (Bronfenbrenner 1979; Bowes & Grace 2009). These factors are displayed in the first layer of the adapted model (refer to Figure 12.2) and include:

- *Household structure*: Findings indicated that participants who did not have children living with them had higher well-being.
- *Tenure*: Owning or privately renting an apartment resulted in higher well-being.
- *Location*: Satisfaction with housing location resulted in higher well-being. Factors found to influence residents' location satisfaction include access to natural environments, the availability of facilities, and efficient transport services.
- *Safety and security:* Vandalism and security were factors discouraging participants from public housing to access their nearby natural environments. In addition, safety and security within a participant's high-rise and neighbourhood impacted on their health and well-being.
- *Housing choice and control*: Choosing to live in an apartment resulted in higher well-being.
- *Pets:* Findings indicated that participants who do not own pets (majority) had significantly higher well-being. The main reason why residents do not own pets is because they do not feel apartments are suitable for housing them.
- *Natural environments*: Visiting available garden/s and park/s resulted in higher well-being.
- *Housing design*: Being very satisfied with an apartment's size resulted in higher well-being.

The mesosystem layer of the adapted model displays the relationship or congruence between two or more contexts and consequences of the microsystem layer (Bronfenbrenner 1979; Bowes & Grace 2009). A review of the findings indicated that the congruence between the following factors impacts on residents' health and well-being:

- *Natural environments and housing design*: The inclusion of natural elements (i.e. gardens and parks) within residents' development, or nearby, contributes to their accessibility, health, and well-being.
- *Natural environments and housing choice and control*: Good access to natural environments was a motivator for a number of residents to move into an apartment.
- *Natural environments and safety and security*: Residents' access to nature, and satisfaction with available nearby nature, was influenced by its safety and security.

The exosystem layer of the adapted model displays a range of contexts and consequences that, while not directly impacting on the high-rise resident at the centre of the model, affect the resident's health and well-being through a trickle-down effect (Bronfenbrenner 1979; Bowes & Grace 2009). These factors are displayed in the third layer of the model as including:

- *Sense of community*: Residents' sense of community ranged from strong to nonexistent and was influenced by body corporate/management bodies and access to nature.
- *Sense of place*: Residents' sense of place and connection to location varied from strong to nonexistent and, like the sense of community, was influenced by access to nature.
- *Childcare facilities, transport services, commercial outlets, and support services*: Safe and easy access to childcare facilities, transport services, commercial outlets, and support services influenced residents' health and well-being.
- *Management*: Body corporate/management bodies influenced residents' sense of community, sense of control, opportunities for accessing natural environments, and pet ownership.
- *Environmental sustainability*: Developments that were designed to be environmentally sustainable and gave residents the ability to practise environmentally sustainable behaviours enhanced residents' quality of life.
- *Redevelopment/overdevelopment*: The proposed redevelopment of public housing in Sydney was found to have a large impact on the well-being of the public housing tenants. In addition, overdevelopment of apartments was a concern for many residents because they felt it impinged on available open space.

The outer level of the adapted model, the macrosystem, consists of the attitudes and ideologies of the culture which trickle down to impact on the resident's health and well-being (Bronfenbrenner 1979; Santrock 2004; Bowes & Grace 2009). The factor contained within the macrosystem level is displayed as including:

- *Social exclusion*: Many residents experienced stigma and stereotyping, which may be components of social exclusion, i.e. derogatory comments relating to their living in high-rise developments.

As demonstrated, the social ecological model, like the Social Skeleton model, can be used to map the range of social, cultural, and other contexts and determinants impacting on an individual's health and well-being. In this example, the factors impacting on inner-city high-rise residents have been mapped. You may wish to use this model to map determinants impacting on a range of individuals.

Summary

The social model of health has moved beyond the limitations of the biomedical model to allow for an understanding that health is comprised of a dynamic interaction of social structures. Six key features of the social model of health proposed by Yuill (2010) include: 'individual health is enabled or inhibited by social context'; 'the body is simultaneously social, psychological and biological'; 'health is cultural'; 'biomedicine and medical science is something—but not everything'; 'health is political'; and 'other voices matter'.

Health sociology provides a useful perspective for understanding the social and cultural contexts influencing understandings of health, illness, and well-being. It is aligned with the social model of health and focuses on the social group to which people belong and the social patterns of health and illness. Examples of social patterning of health and illness include life expectancy, gender, and income inequality.

The Social Skeleton model can be used to depict a range of social structures influencing people's perceptions of health, illness, and well-being. In addition, ecological models can be useful aids for mapping the range of social and cultural contexts impacting on individuals' health and well-being, particularly the social ecological model.

🗓 Tutorial exercises

1 In small teams, debate which is the most effective model for mapping/depicting the range of social and cultural contexts influencing perceptions of health, illness, and well-being: the Social Skeleton: health, illness and structure agency model or the social ecological model? Why?

2 Now use the social ecological model to map/depict the range of social and cultural contexts influencing your health and well-being. How useful was the model in completing this exercise? Why? Discuss your responses with your team mates.

3 Reflecting on your responses to Question 2, which level contained the most contexts? What factors were located at the macrosystem level? What interrelationships were depicted at the mesosystem level? Were your responses similar to your team mates?

Further reading

Bowes, J., & Grace, R. (2009). *Children, families and communities: Contexts and consequences*, 3rd edn. Melbourne: Oxford University Press.

Bronfenbrenner, U. (1979). *The ecology of human development: Experiments by nature and design*. Cambridge, MA: Harvard University Press.

Broom, D. (2009). Gender and health. In J. Germov (ed.), *Second opinion: An introduction to health sociology*, 4th edn. Melbourne: Oxford University Press, 130–55.

Germov, J. (2009). Imagining health problems as social issues. In J. Germov (ed.), *Second opinion: An introduction to health sociology*, 4th edn. Melbourne: Oxford University Press, 3–24.

Habibis, D. (2009). The illness experience: Lay perspectives, disability, and chronic illness. In J. Germov (ed.), *Second opinion: An introduction to health sociology*, 4th edn. Melbourne: Oxford University Press, 288–306.

Taylor, S. (2008a). The concept of health. In S. Taylor, M. Foster, & J. Fleming (eds), *Healthcare practice in Australia*. Melbourne: Oxford University Press, 3–21.

White, K. (2009). *An introduction to the sociology of health and illness*, 2nd edn. London: Sage Publications.

Yuill, C. (2010). The social model of health. In C. Yuill, I. Crinson, & E. Duncan (eds), *Key concepts in health studies*. Thousand Oaks, CA: Sage Publications, 11–14.

Websites

<www.abs.gov.au>

This website provides the latest Australian statistics on everything from health through to housing. It is a useful resource for any health-related studies.

<www.aihw.gov.au>

Visit this website to access the latest 'Australia's Health': a comprehensive profile of the nation's health and welfare status.

<www.health.vic.gov.au>

This is the website for the Victorian Department of Health. Visit this website to obtain the latest health information relevant to Victoria.

<www.chs.unimelb.edu.au>

This is the website for the Centre for Health and Society at the University of Melbourne. Visit this website for links to research investigating the social construction of health.

<www.phac-aspc.gc.ca/ph-sp/determinants/index-eng.php>

This is the website for the Public Health Agency of Canada. Visit this website for information on social factors impacting on health.

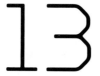

13

Health throughout the life course

Christopher Fox

TOPICS COVERED

This chapter covers the following topics:
- definitions of life course, life course determinants, and social gradient
- life course determinants and their effects on health
- life course determinants and the social gradient
- life course determinants and policy

KEY TERMS

Cohort
Human agency
Life and historical times
Life course perspective
Life event
Linked lives

Social gradient
Timing of lives
Trajectory
Transition
Turning point

Introduction

Life course determinants are considered to be a relatively new approach to exploring health. Although such determinants have been around for about 50 years, as a concept, policymakers, academics, and researchers rarely draw on the approach. Glen Elder is recognised as one of the early developers of the life course approach and continues to be its key proponent (Hutchison 2010). Elder is a sociologist and was working in the 1960s on data from three early longitudinal studies of children when he identified patterns in the analysis (Elder 1974). These cohorts appeared to have been affected in similar ways when it came to individual and family trajectories. The common factor for the participants was they were children of the 1930s Great Depression. Elder became fascinated with the influence of history, or past events, on family, education, and work roles of individuals and communities (Elder 1974).

The life course approach to health draws on several disciplines: psychology, sociology, anthropology, epidemiology, and social history to name a few (Elder 1994). As an approach, or theory, it has developed key ideas and concepts. In this chapter readers will be introduced to the life course approach and explore how it can be applied to understanding the determinants of the health of an individual or social group.

Defining the life course perspective

The life course refers to the course of our lives from birth to death. One way of viewing the life course is as a path or road—definitely not straight, but with corners, turns, and twists (Hutchison 2010). The life course can be influenced by intra-generational and inter-generational events (Blane 2006); in other words, events that occur within your generation that affect you, or events that occurred in your parents'—even your grandparents'—generation that affect you.

> **Stop and Think**
>
> Why not draw a map of the key events that have affected you? Start at birth and then draw in the events. The events may not have happened in a straight line. Some events may have happened to someone else but affected you. Other events may have occurred simultaneously. Now connect these events. The path you would have drawn is not likely to be straight and is likely to have arms off it—more like a street directory. This is one way to capture the winding road concept of life course determinants.

Life course perspective The cumulative effects of events from earlier life on later life.

The **life course perspective** is also concerned with the impact of one stage of life on another. In this situation, we even consider events that occur while still in the womb. 'Events' that may have occured while you were in the womb can have an impact on your life today, or even in your older age. Or decisions, or events, that occur now could impact on your later life. For example, Delisle (2002), in her review of the relationship between birth weight and coronary heart disease (CHD), reported on studies which found that babies born with a low birth weight had an increased chance of developing CHD at a later stage in life.

The life course perspective is also interested in the roles that culture and social structures, or institutions, have on an individual's life. Culture here not only refers to ethnicity, but also the cultural groups we belong to and the society in which we live. Culture can refer to non-biological aspects of life: the aspects of life that are learnt and/or are symbolic, like the unwritten rules of society, customs, and use of language (Willis 2004). Social structures or institutions can refer to organised institutions like the law or education, or phenomena like gender, race, age, and sexuality. For example, children who have limited exposure to books and reading in early childhood may experience reading difficulties in later childhood (Baydar et al. 1993).

See also Chapters 1 & 14 on language and culture.

So far we know that life course determinants are about the paths our lives take, that each life stage impacts on a later life stage, and that culture and social institutions also have an influence. These three elements form part of the definition of life course determinants. Blane (2006) suggests that most chronic diseases which result in death result from cumulative developmental stresses, with adulthood health being influenced by circumstances in earlier life. The life course approach to health can also be viewed as the intersecting of socio-historical and cultural factors, with personal biological development. Elder (1994, p. 5) states: 'The life course can be viewed as a multilevel phenomen[on], ranging from structured pathways through social institutions and organisations to the social trajectories of individuals and their developmental pathways'. Elder's definition is considered to be the original formulation of the idea. Yet theory, like language, is dynamic; it is ever developing. Elder's definition is still relevant: the life course perspective can be applied to areas beyond physical and emotional health. The life course perspective, in accordance with its multidisciplinary origins, has been applied to other areas in the human services: individuals, families, groups, and organisations. Hutchison (2005, p. 144) suggests the life course approach could be viewed

See Chapter 14 on language and culture.

> from the micro and macro advantage points. It has been studied from the perspective of the individual as *event history*, or the sequence of events, experiences, and transitions in a person's life from birth to death. It has also been studied from the perspective of the family, in terms of how family lives are synchronised across time. In addition, the life course has been studied as a property of cultures and social institutions that shape the pattern of individual and family lives. Some life course scholars have also conceptualised small groups, communities and formal organisations and social movements as having life courses marked by both continuity and change.

Hutchison's definition gives the approach broader perspective and a greater application beyond traditional ideas of health. In general, the life course is affected by historical, social, and cultural factors and the cumulative effects of circumstances and how these affect later events or outcomes. The life course approach can be applied to individuals, groups, communities, and organisations. In regard to health, the approach challenges the dominance of adult risk factors as causes of adult diseases.

Stop and Think

» The life course approach can be applied to more than individuals. Using your family as an example, how have earlier events affected later events in your family?

» You could also try the same exercise with an organisation (e.g. an AFL team).

Basic concepts
Cohorts

Cohort A group who share the same experiences, in the same time, in the same sequence.

Cohorts are groups of people who share the same time together in the same time period. A cohort could also be a group of people born in the same (historical) time, in the same culture, and who experience the same social changes in the same order (Hutchison 2005). For example, Elder's data analysis of people born in the USA during the Great Depression was the cohort he was studying when he noticed the effects of earlier life events on later life experiences (Elder 1974). Cohorts of people do not need to be born at the same time if we are talking about an organisation or group. In this instance, the cohort may be the people on a sporting team between 2008 and 2011. As a cohort on a sporting team, they share the same experiences in the same order with that team. A cohort could also be conceived as families who had their first child born in 1990. Cohorts can differ in size but face challenges in similar ways. For example, it is suggested that the baby boomer cohort faced the challenges of their demographic bubble by delaying marriage and childbirth, and having fewer children (Hutchison 2010).

See also Chapter 6 on health and ageing.

Stop and Think

» People generally think of themselves as belonging to a birth cohort (e.g. Gen X, Gen Y, Gen Z, baby boomers), but we can also belong to other cohorts. Make a list of cohorts to which you belong. What experiences, in what time-frame and in what sequence, help define these cohorts?

Transitions

Transition Moving from one life stage to another, or from one life event to another.

Transitions can be viewed as stage changes in life. Transitions are often culturally bound, yet at a macro level may be similar to other groups of transitions. Transitions can be thought of as markers in life as we transit from one state (childhood) to another (adolescence). Transitions can revolve around family life: birth, marriage, divorce, death (Hutchison 2005). Transitions are about changes, exits, and entrances. In the workplace, transitions may be marked by the change of managers in a job, or the start of a new group of graduates in an organisation.

Case Study 13.1   Micro transitions and macro transitions: Markers of adulthood

The markers of entry into adulthood have changed, yet have not changed, since Dickens was chronicling life in the mid-1800s. Although on a micro level there are profound differences between Dickensian England and Australia in the 2010s, there are similarities on a macro level. When reading Dickens, we learn about some of the markers of the transition from childhood to adulthood, and one thing that is substantially different is the cultural idea of adolescence.

Adolescence is marked as the transition from childhood to adulthood. Biologically, it is defined by the development of secondary sex characteristics. Socio-culturally, it is marked by different experiences in different times and cultures. Adolescence is often referred to as a liminal state—not quite one state (childhood); not quite the other (adult). In contemporary Anglo-Australian culture, adolescence is (culturally) defined as the teenage years, where we experiment with adult identities and behaviours. Adolescence for most Australians begins at 13 and ends around 19. If we were to use biological markers for adolescence, it would begin somewhere around 9 or 10 years for girls, and 11 to 13 years for boys; and end at around 17 years for girls and 20 years for boys.

One of the markers of entering into adulthood in Anglo-Australian society is finishing school and beginning employment. Another possibility is moving out of home (although 'Dependults'—young people remaining in the family home until well into their twenties—challenge this notion), or getting married.

If we take adolescence as being culturally defined as the liminal state between childhood and adulthood, then in Dickensian England this lasted around two to three years. Childhood ended, as chronicled by Dickens, at around the age of 12. Dickens writes of young people entering employment in their early teenage years. In some cases, young people moved out of home to take up service (in the case of girls) or an apprenticeship (in the case of boys). If the same markers of entry into adulthood were applied in Dickensian England, then adulthood would have begun around the age of 14. Society in mid-1800s England managed this transition by delaying the onset of adulthood until the young person had completed their service or apprenticeship and could function as an independent person.

So, on a micro level the transitions are quite different, yet on a macro level there are similarities. The markers of entry into adulthood are about independence in both cases. This is how transitions can be similar and different at the same time.

Case Study 13.2   Life transitions

One of the key issues with working with transitions is how we define them. One model is proposed by Bartley and colleagues (1997). Another possible way of looking at critical transition periods is to use Erik Erikson's Psychosocial Stages of Development (1968). Erikson argues that at critical times in our lives we need to resolve a conflict in order to progress positively through life. It is not so much the 'conflict' to be resolved that this model offers; rather the age range represents critical periods of transitions. Erikson's model, like that of Bartley and colleagues, covers the life span.

Bartley and colleagues (1997)

Transition from primary to secondary school

School examinations

Entry to the labour market

Leaving parental home

Transition to parenthood

Job insecurity, change, or loss

Onset of chronic illness

Exit from the labour market [retire]

Erikson's Stages of Psychosocial Development (1968)

Infants, 0 to 1 year = Hope: Trust vs. Mistrust

Toddlers, 2 to 3 years Will: Autonomy vs. Shame & Doubt

Preschool, 3 to 5 years = Purpose: Initiative vs. Guilt

Childhood, 6 to 11 years = Competence: Industry vs. Inferiority

Adolescents, 12 to 19 years = Fidelity: Identity vs. Role Confusion

Young Adults, 20 to 40 years = Love: Intimacy vs. Isolation

Middle Adulthood, 45 to 65 years = Care: Generativity vs. Stagnation

Seniors, 65 years onwards = Wisdom: Ego Integrity vs. Despair

Stop and Think

» Bartley and colleagues (1997) and Erikson (1968) provide two potential lists of key transition periods in life. What would you list as key transitions in life?

» What do you consider to be key transitions you have experienced in your life? It might be turning 13, or starting secondary school or university.

» Draw two columns on a page. On one side write the transitions you have experienced. In the other column, write down the effects these had on you at the time.

Trajectory A stable path towards a life destination.

Transitions and **trajectories** are two key concepts in understanding life course determinants (Elder 1985). Where transitions are transitory, or moments in time, trajectories are more stable and follow a path towards a 'life destination' (Wheaton & Gotlieb 1997). Trajectories can consist of a number of transitions (Elder 1985; Macmillan & Elliason 2004). They can influence and be influenced by other trajectories. A change in trajectory results in a new 'life destination' (Wheaton & Gotlieb 1997). Trajectories, or 'careers', are multidimensional and interdependent (Elder 1985). Elder classes work, life, marriage, and parenthood as trajectories one might face in one's life. As one can see, these trajectories are interdependent or interrelated. Macmillan and Elliason (2004, p. 2) define trajectories as the 'stable component of a direction toward a life destination [which] is given by the probability of occurrence'.

Life events

Life events can be defined as unexpected and sudden with an outcome markedly different from what was previously expected (Settersten & Mayer 1997; Wheaton & Gotlieb 1997). Life events require the individual to change and can result in experiences of great stress (Hutchison 2005). Some events in our lives are expected, for example, marriage after an extended period of dating. If one of these events happens out of normative sequence and this results in significant change—marriage at a younger age because of an unplanned pregnancy and so not completing university—then this is a life event. The change is unexpected, significant, and has consequences for our trajectory.

> **Life event** Abrupt and sudden change in life resulting in significant change in trajectory and stress.

Turning points

Turning points are classed as significant changes or change of direction in life (Rutter 1996) and result in crucially important moments in life (Wheaton & Gotlieb 1997). A turning point may not become apparent at the time, and to identify turning points we need a baseline that is stable over time. Turning points, unlike life events, may not be abrupt single events, unusual events, or anything dramatic (Wheaton & Gotlieb 1997). Rutter (1996) identifies three types of life events that can also be turning points:

> **Turning point** A crucial point in time that leads to significant change of direction.

1 An opportunity is closed off or opened up.
2 A change in the individual's personal environment (e.g. marriage) results in a change in social networks.
3 Changes in the individual's self-concept, beliefs, values, and views.

Trajectories are made up of transitions and life events. A change of trajectory results from a turning point in an individual's life. Turning points are not mere detours but result in a significant change of direction.

> **Stop and Think**
>
> » So far you thought about the cohorts you belong to and transitions you have experienced. Now consider what trajectories you have been on in your life. What life events have resulted in detours? When did these trajectories change? What turning points occurred for the change in trajectory?
>
> » Now what possible impacts will these phenomena have on your later life?

Elder's four themes of the life course

Elder (1994) posits four central themes in the life course approach. These overarching themes account for the interaction between the social and developmental trajectories. He argues that the link between our lives and historical events (times) accounts for some dynamic features of the life course, while the timing of events, the interdependence of our lives (with others), and our agency are all avenues that influence the paths we take (Elder 1994). Below is a summary of each of the four central themes.

Lives and historical times

Life and historical times A way of accounting for cohort effects and how they affect the individual now and in the future.

Elder's phrase **'life and historical times'** refers to the intersection of our lives with the (historical) events that occur around us, for example, a cohort affected by the Vietnam War. Different birth cohorts experience a different social world. Elder (1994) suggests that historical effects are cohort effects. Yet, these effects not only affect us at the point at which they occur but will affect our future and therefore indirectly affect the next generation. When applying a life course approach, we also need to consider how the historical event and its effects, and how we embody these effects, become part of our life course. For example, does the event result in a transition, a life event, or a turning point? Does the historical event effect a change in trajectories? For the people of Queensland in late 2010 and early 2011, who were hit by floods or cyclones, how will this historical event affect their lives and how will they embody the changes? What will be the outcome of these events on their health, in ten or 15 years' time? A life course approach can account for this question.

In exploring life and times, we also need to consider the individual's agency: what they contribute and how significant the event is to them and the subsequent change (Elder 1994). The impact of technological growth on young people is minimal and they have the skills to cope with a technological change in the workplace, whereas an older person might not have the skills and could therefore experience a greater impact of the change. In this example, the lack of skills in the older person will possibly lead to the introduction of new technology as having greater significance and therefore the subsequent change may also have greater impact.

Stop and Think

» In developing the map of your life course, ask yourself what significant historical events have occurred in your life? Are these events unique to you or your family? If so, maybe these are life events or turning points. Remember, we are talking about events that affect cohorts.

» Make a list of historical events and then describe how they affected your cohort.

The timing of lives

See also Chapter 6 on ageing.

Timing of lives An account for the age-graded perspective of social markers, roles, and events.

In developed nations, especially, there are parallels between chronological and social ageing (Elder 1994). In other words, the social events and transitions associated with marking periods of life are now prescribed for the individual according to their chronological age. Adulthood in Australia is marked by an 18th birthday party. The party is the social marker of the legal definition of adulthood. Social timing is the defining of values and beliefs of a role, alongside the incidence, duration, and sequence of roles (Elder 1994). So, a childbirth in a marriage at a 'planned stage' has minimal impact, yet parenthood in adolescence is costly. The importance of **timing of lives** is that the impact of an event is moderated by where the person is in their life stage. Elder (1994) cites his exploration of the service of men in the Second World War: men who entered service young with no family had minimal social disruption, while men in later life with families felt the full brunt of social disruption.

Case Study 13.3   Understanding age: How old are you?

Age is not universally defined. It is a dynamic concept. The author can recall working with a colleague, who was an anthropologist, on a survey. The author wanted to ask respondents the question, 'how old are you?' He was quickly informed that the question had different meaning to different people—how age is defined is culturally bound. He needed to ask, 'In what year were you born?' in order to calculate the age he needed for analysis.

Think of how in the past we have described our age. When we were children, we might have said, 'I am nearly 4', when in fact we had not long turned 3. Or during our late adolescence when we were trying to convince our parents we were old enough to make a decision, we might have said, 'I am nearly an adult', or believing that our physical maturity allowed us to look adult enough in order to purchase alcohol. And we hear older people say, 'I'm only 40.' All of these statements mark age differently. Earlier, we looked at the markers of childhood, adulthood, and adolescence. Now we can consider the different ways we can define age.

Chronological age is the age according to our birth year. This is how many of us think of age when we talk about it. If you were born in 1990, then in 2011 you will be 21 years old. Hutchison (2010) argues that chronological age is not the only aspect in the timing of our lives, but differences in roles and behaviours are also the result of biological, social, and psychological processes. For example, being able to drive is a widely recognised marker of adulthood in many societies. Permisson to engage in this adult behaviour is arbitrarily determined by law in various localities to occur at the age of 15, 16, 17, or 18, depending largely on social need and perception of the biological and psychological state of young people.

Biological age is when we use biological development as an indicator of age, for example, when a paediatrician uses the Tanner Stages of Puberty (Marshall & Tanner 1969, 1970) to define where a person is at in development. Biological age can also be defined according to our health and how well our organs function.

Psychological age is when age is defined according to the stages of psychological and cognitive development, for example, where an individual's cognitive or motor skills are in the developmental stages, or how well the individual copes with certain life crises (e.g. Erickson's Stages of Psychosocial Development).

Social age is the expected age-graded role and behaviours. For example, a society may have expectations of when it is okay for young people to begin romantic lives, or when it is appropriate for children to begin household chores. Social age is often defined by markers and events as recognition. Social age could also be defined by asking how old do you feel? Our perception of age is often based on social markers, or engagement with age-grade roles/behaviours.

Christopher Fox

Stop and Think

» Since age is dynamic and fluid and not easily defined, using the four examples of defining age above, write down how you fit into each category. Is there a difference in how you could perceive your age?

Linked lives

Linked lives The interdependence we have with others in our social networks and relationships and how these affect our life course.

Linked lives is Elder's (1994) recognition of the interdependence of our lives. We are all embedded in social relationships and networks. We are interdependent. We live in a family network with multiple social relationships. We study or work in a network with multiple social relationships. Sometimes our networks even overlap. The life course approach recognises that relationships and networks are structures of socialisation and management, and these relationships also provide us with necessary interaction. These relationships and networks influence our decisions, and therefore our transitions, life events, and turning points—if not directly, then in reaction to them, which is of equal importance. Our parents can influence us in our immediate world and can also affect us in our later life. For example, parental socio-economic level can have an impact on our infancy and childhood health and can also impact on health in later life.

Elder's (1974) work on the longitudinal data of the Great Depression children highlights the interdependence between parents and children over the life course. The parents expressed high levels of stress, depression, and marital discord which in turn affected their ability to care for and nurture their children. This too was to have an effect on the children's later lives. Linked lives are the interaction of our social worlds over the duration of our life (Elder 1994).

Stop and Think

» How is your life linked?

» Using a large piece of paper, draw the networks in which you are a member. What networks are interdependent? How are these networks part of the multiple trajectories along which you might be travelling?

» Consider the role these networks have in your life and what impact they might have in the future.

Mythbuster

Consider whether you see the following as questionable. What does this tell you about your own values?

A life course approach to addictions, whether smoking, gambling, or alcohol and other drugs, highlights the importance of past events and transitions in determining current experiences. Current health promotion campaigns to address addictions tend to focus on the individual to make a choice. To reorient our campaigns would mean greater interventions at earlier life stages. This is a costly exercise to govern and would lead to greater intrusions into people's lives, especially at the lower end of the social gradient.

Human agency

Human agency refers to our free will, or our ability to act independently of social constraints or structures (Abercrombie et al. 1994). In the life course approach, human agency is how we as actors in our social world make choices in relation to the world and events around us (Elder 1994). Elder believes that although we are influenced by the social structures around us, we can make decisions within and around the influences of the social structures. Human agency can account for some individual differences identified through the life course approach to exploring health issues.

Social structures, on the other hand, can be conceived of as key social institutions in society. These institutions can be constituted (e.g. school and education or the justice system) or can be more symbolic (e.g. gender, age, sexuality). Social theorists such as Durkheim and Marx argued that our lives are governed by social structures, while others, such as Weber and Habermas, suggested that life is about agency. There is a third school of thought which argues that our lives are influenced by our agency engaging with social structures (e.g. Bourdieu). For example, social structures can be used to account for successes in life. Children from high socio-economic groups are more likely to succeed at school; more likely to have professional jobs with higher salaries, therefore better superannuation savings, and resulting in a better quality of old age than someone of low socio-economic status (Blane 2006).

> **Human agency** Our ability to negotiate the social structures and a way to account for individual differences in the life course.
>
> See Chapters 1, 11 & 12 on the social determinants and construction of health.

> See also Chapter 1 on the social determinants of health.

Health effects and the life course

Hertzman (2000) sees life course effects as a gradient that increases in time and with age. These gradual effects provide one way for us to understand how life course events affect our health. According to Hertzman, there are three types of outcome effects to the life course approach when looking at health: latent effects, pathway effects, and cumulative effects. *Latent effects* are biologically or developmentally based and result in effects in later life, regardless of future experiences. They result from events occurring during foetal and infant development stages which program organ systems, for example, low birth weight and the increased likelihood of coronary heart disease (Delisle 2002). *Pathway effects* result from experiences which set us on particular trajectories that can later influence our health or well-being. Limited exposure to literacy in early childhood can lead to poor reading in early schooling (Baydar et al. 1993), in turn affecting educational outcomes and therefore later life experiences. Hertzman and Power (2004) suggest that children who are not prepared for school (emotionally, cognitively, and behaviourally) are more likely to experience 'education failure' and people with poor educational outcomes are less likely to engage in health-enhancing behaviours. *Cumulative effects* are a combination of latent and pathway effects (Hertzman 2000) and can refer to an accumulation of either disadvantage or advantage. Hertzman argues that these effects could be risks or protective factors. He cites the study by Power and colleagues (1999) of the effect of socio-economic class on adult health where low socio-economics status in early life may lead to cumulative effects on health outcomes in later adulthood. Cumulative effects are also affected by the social gradient.

Social gradient Life
expectancy is shorter
and most diseases are
more common further
down the social ladder.

See Chapter 5 on
chronic illness &
Chapter 11 on the social
gradient.

The social gradient and the life course

When we consider the effects thesis put forward by Hertzman (2000), we can also discuss the effects of the life course in terms of the social gradient. When we apply the **social gradient** to life course determinants and health, we note that the health of people is better towards the top of the gradient. Most diseases, especially chronic diseases, are concentrated at the bottom of the gradient and at earlier stages.

Case Study 13.4   The social gradient and mortality

As we have just seen, people at the lower end of the SES scale have on average poorer health for a longer time than do people at the upper end of the scale. These differences also affect not only when but also where people die.

The social gradient in health was first recognised through the relationship between age of death and social class: the lower people's SES, the lower their average age of death in comparison with higher SES groups. Further, people with lower SES have a higher average number of years of disability before their earlier deaths (Marmot 2010).

The most detailed studies of causes and place of death as a function of deprivation have been carried out in the UK (National Audit Office 2008; National End of Life Intelligence Network 2010). These show higher rates of death from cancer and respiratory diseases, and more deaths in hospital, in more deprived (lower SES) groups. The available Australian data is consistent with this. For example, male mortality in Victoria is lower than average in most rural areas and the western suburbs (Victorian Department of Human Services 1999; Draper et al. 2004). Tobacco- and alcohol-related diseases contribute more to deaths in lower SES groups, while accidents and suicide further reduce the average age of death for men in rural areas.

Surveys consistently show that the majority of people would prefer not to die in hospital but, as indicated above, people with lower SES are more likely to do so. The reasons for this are not yet clearly established, but it has been shown that a combination of informal care (from family and friends) with formal care in the community significantly increases the odds that a person will be able to die at home. A recent study in Western Australia found that people who accessed community-based specialist palliative care had a seven times higher chance of dying in their usual place of residence (McNamara & Rosenwax 2007). Studies in Australia and overseas show that many people die in hospital when there is no clinical reason for them to be there. Not only is this contrary to their wishes in many cases, but it also contributes to increased healthcare expenditure in the last days of life. Governments have recently endorsed Advance Care Planning (ACP) as a means by which people can document their wishes about end-of-life care, but evidence to date indicates that the options available may not be able to deliver on people's choices. The National Health and Hospitals Reform Commission even suggested that ACP could become a consumer tool for shaping end-of-life services—but these services are inextricably linked with health service provision in general.

The policy implication seems clear. Providing more community services that are more accessible—that is, shaped by local needs and demand—should both meet dying people's expressed wishes to die at home (or in a 'homelike' environment such as a residential aged care facility) and reduce demand on expensive acute hospital services. It is clear that in the coming decades Australia will need to accommodate a large increase of ageing and deaths. A health service focus on providing primary care services that allows not only ageing in place, but also dying in place, is imperative.

This case study is contributed by Bruce Rumbold

According to Blane (2006), dis/advantage accumulates cross-sectionally and longitudinally, with dis/advantage in one stage of life affecting other phases of life. To accommodate this idea of accumulation of positive or negative impacts, Blane uses three processes: social accumulation, social mobility, and social protection. *Social accumulation* is used to explain the continuity of parental socio-economic status to conditions throughout the life course (infancy, childhood, adolescence, adulthood) (Blane 2006). It also accounts for the intersection between biological programming and social conditions of life. Two possible disruptions to the cumulative role of social disadvantage are, first, when a person shifts social class and, second, when a socio-economic system evolves or changes. For example, in Australia we have moved from a production economy to a service economy. A similar effect is felt when economic events like the global financial crisis occur.

Social mobility accounts for the accumulation of health and social factors that can lead to better or poorer health in later stages of life (Blane 2006). Parental socio-economic status can influence whether their offspring move up the social ladder, down the social ladder, or remain in the same position. If a person moves up the social ladder (i.e. increases in status), they will add 'advantage' to their life course; they will have less advantage than those of already equal footing, but more advantage than those left behind. The corollary is also true. Downward mobility adds disadvantage, with the individual experiencing less advantage than those left behind and more advantage than those they have joined (Blane 2006).

Social protection also explores the interaction between health and life course events. Social protection moderates the experience of impact of new disadvantage (Blane 2006). New disadvantage has minimal impact on previous advantage—this is positive social protection. A new disadvantage, however, will have an increased impact on previous disadvantage. Blane (2006) explains the idea of social protection by using examples from the Analysis of General Household Survey in the UK (Bartley & Owen 1996). Working men with a restrictive chronic illness were more likely to be unemployed compared with men who reported good health. Blane argues that people of low socio-economic status with a chronic illness were more likely to experience disadvantage from the chronic illness, as it affects life choices like employment, whereas people of high socio-economic status are likely to be protected from further disadvantage.

Policy implications

Little has been undertaken in Australia in using life course determinants as a basis for developing social and economic policy. The UK Government made moves to include life course determinants in social and economic policy development in 1994 with the establishment of an interdepartmental working group (Dorozynski 1994; Bartley et al. 1997). One of the first acts of the working party was to set a research agenda which explored factors that accumulate over the life course (Bartley et al. 1997). The Queensland Government acknowledged the significance of life course determinants in health (Queensland Health 2001), yet this has not to date been explicitly articulated in policy development.

Bartley and colleagues (1997, p. 1194) recommend that policy development should focus on key transitional periods in life which could have material effects and psychosocial effects by 'preventing dramatic falls in living standards and by a wider effect on the degree to which citizens experience a sense of control over their lives'. Policy that builds resilience will strengthen individual and community health and well-being (Queensland Health n.d.). The Queensland Government suggested key transitional periods (e.g. birth, school, adolescence, changes in employment, and ageing). One of the problems with this idea is knowing how to define key transitional periods in life that can accommodate the differences in population—though it can be argued that we all experience some critical points in the life course.

See Case Study 13.2 for a discussion of critical periods in the life course.

Summary

Points in the life course are one of the social determinants of health and well-being. When we consider the causes of illness and disease we need to look beyond the individual and explore their history (and possibly that of their families and communities) to gain a better understanding of the effects their past has had on them. What we now know is that effects accumulate over the life course and when combined with the social gradient we see greater impact. The utility of life course determinants has also moved beyond health and can focus on other areas of well-being such as families (Hutchison 2005).

Although the early history of life course determinants focuses on foetal and early childhood development, researchers have acknowledged that events that happen at any time in our lives can have an impact (Lynch & Smith 2005). The challenge for us as health and well-being practitioners is to advocate for acknowledgment of life course determinants and to advocate for policy change that addresses these determinants in the policy response.

Tutorial exercises

1   Throughout this chapter you have undertaken a number of exercises. You now need to bring this information together and explore how your life course is affecting or could affect your health.

2   Many people confuse life course determinants with the life span approach to development. How are each of these terms defined? How can life span approaches be integrated into life course approaches?

3   What is the role of life course determinants in young women living with HIV in sub-Saharan Africa?

4   What policy action could we take to address the issues of life course determinants in the experiences of women living with HIV in sub-Saharan Africa?

5   Which critical periods in life would impact on domestic violence? How can we address this issue at those critical periods?

Further reading

Bartley, M., Blane, D., & Montgomery, S. (1997). Socioeconomic determinants of health: Health and the life course: Why safety nets matter. *British Medical Journal*, 314, 1194–95.

Blane, D. (2006). The life course, social gradient and health. In M. Marmot & R.G. Wilkinson (eds), *Social determinants of health*. Oxford: Oxford University Press, 64–80.

Elder, G.J. (1985). *Life course dynamics: Trajectories and transitions, 1968-1980*. Ithaca, NY: Cornell University Press.

Elder, G.J. (1994). Time, human agency, and social change: Perspectives on the life course. *Social Psychology Quarterly*, 57(1), 4–15.

Hertzman, C., & Power, C. (2004). Child development as a determinant of health across the life course. *Current Paediatrics*, 14(5), 438–43.

Hutchison, E. (2010). A life course perspective. In E. Hutchison (ed.), *Dimensions of human behavior: The changing life course*. London: Sage Publications, 3–38.

Liu, S., Jones, R.N., & Glymour, M.M. (2010). Implications of lifecourse epidemiology for research on determinants of adult disease. *Public Health Reviews*, 32. <www.publichealthreviews.eu/upload/pdf_files/8/Glymour_for_website.pdf>.

Mayer, K.U. (2009). New directions in life course research. *Annual Review of Sociology*, 35, 413–33.

Mortimer, J.T., & Shananhan, M.J. (2004). *Handbook of the life course*. New York: Springer.

Power, C., Manor, O., & Matthews, S. (1999). The duration and timing of exposure: Effects of socio-economic environment on adult health. *American Journal of Public Health*, 89(7), 1059–66.

World Health Organization Commission on Social Determinants of Health (2007). *A conceptual framework for action on the social determinants of health*. Geneva: WHO. <www.who.int/social_determinants/resources/csdh_framework_action_05_07.pdf>.

Websites

<www.who.int/social_determinants/en>

This is the website of the WHO's Commission on Social Determinants of Health. It is a good source of discussions on social determinants and provides crucial background papers and reports as well as examples of actions in relation to social determinants.

<www.longstudies.longviewuk.com/index.shtm>

The Society for Longitudinal and Life Course Studies is an international, multidisciplinary society. It aims to increase the visibility and influence of life course studies. The website has access to publications and links, including to the *Longitudinal and Life Course Studies: An International Journal*.

<http://aging.utoronto.ca>

The Institute for Life Course and Aging is based at the University of Toronto. It focuses on ageing research from a life course perspective.

<www.sfb186.uni-bremen.de/frames/main.htm>

The Special Collaborative Centre 186: Status Passages and Risks in the Life Course is a research centre based at the University of Bremen. The website provides a link to an extensive bibliography and links to other organisations.

<www.lebenslaufarchiv.uni-bremen.de/index.php?id=567&no_cache=1&L=>

The Archive for Life Course Research is an archive for qualitative social science research and is available for life course researchers.

<www.ucl.ac.uk/icls>

The International Centre for Life Course Studies in Society and Health is a UK-based centre with a focus on the UK birth cohort studies. The Centre is under the directorship of Mel Bartley and David Blane, two leading researchers in life course determinants.

<www.journal.longviewuk.com/index.php/llcs>

Longitudinal and Life Course Studies: An International Journal's website has archived copies of past issues.

<http://caepr.anu.edu.au/population/lectures2011.php>

The Centre for Aboriginal Economic Policy and Research at the Australian National University, 2011 Online Lecture Series is on 'Measures of Indigenous wellbeing and their determinants across the life course'. There are 14 lectures, with a transcript, a copy of the presentation, and an audio file.

Acknowledgment

The author would like to thank Dr Bruce Rumbold for his assistance in writing this chapter and for providing the text on which The Social Gradient and Ageing is based.

14 | Language, culture, and health

Rebecca Fanany

TOPICS COVERED

This chapter covers the following topics:

- what culture is and how it is related to language
- the effects language and culture may have on people's conceptualisation of health
- the nature and importance of cultural competence in health professionals
- the concept of illness behaviour and how it is shaped by culture

KEY TERMS

Cultural competency
Culture
Disease
Health

Illness
Illness behaviour
Sociolinguistics

Introduction

The language people speak and the culture they are part of play an important role in shaping their understanding of **health**. The terms and concepts they have available to talk about health and illness and what exactly these terms and concepts mean are determined by the language they speak (Reynaert & Gelman 2007). Similarly, a society's accepted norms about what it means to be healthy or sick, what kinds of symptoms indicate illness, and what is the right thing to do if someone is sick are all determined by culture (Heggenhougan & Shore 1986). These things are not universal. That is, while each person's understanding of health and illness is an integral part of their way of thinking, people from different cultural backgrounds may have a very different idea of what health and illness mean.

It is very important for health professionals to understand that conceptualisations of health in different parts of the world differ as these views underlie many aspects of health behaviour and may be significant in working with patients or clients from a variety of backgrounds. We must be aware of our own culture and language-based conceptualisation of health and recognise that it affects our perceptions just as much as our patients' or clients' affects theirs. This chapter gives an overview of the ways in which the language and cultural background of individuals can affect their understanding of health. The need for cultural competence among health professionals is also discussed along with a consideration of **illness behaviour** and culturally determined expressions of disease.

Culture

Culture is a system of shared meaning, representations, and practices that make up our social life. These principles are known and understood in more or less the same way by all members of a given society and are characteristic of that society (Danesi & Perron 1999). Most people never think about the culture they are part of and how it affects their ideas and understanding. We begin to absorb the principles of our culture from birth, and eventually they become the basis for our worldview. We do not need to think about our own culture but we use it as the basis for making decisions about everything we experience.

Culture is reflected in language and is also shaped by it. This is a reciprocal relationship where language acts as the means to express culture, while the demands of culture also contribute to the development of terms to express them (Kramsch 1998). To a great extent language provides a structure for our thoughts and ideas, and culture supplies a set of norms within which we express ourselves such that these two elements make up our cognitive framework. Our cognitive framework gives structure to the way we perceive the world and allows us to interpret and understand our surroundings and experiences. This extends to health; we should not assume that people from different cultures will conceptualise health and illness in the same way.

Any culture has clearly identifiable characteristics that give it a unique identity. We often speak about the national character of various countries or invoke (frequently negative) stereotypes about some group. In many cases, the elements that contribute

Health There is no definite meaning of health. Its meaning can be different depending on individuals, social groups, and cultures and can differ at different times. In general, it means not just the absence of illness or disease but a total sense of well-being.

Illness behaviour The socially acceptable way to act when sick.

Culture A system of shared ideas, attitudes, and practices that defines the social system of its members.

See also Chapter 1 on the ways in which we conceptualise health.

See Chapter 15 on deviance and difference.

to these set ideas represent observable but superficial characteristics of the culture in question as seen through the lens of our own culture. Going beyond the superficial, a more objective understanding of other cultures may be useful as a guide to behaviour and perception, although it cannot guarantee any particular reaction from members of the culture. Every society is composed of individuals who may share knowledge and understanding that derive from a shared background but who may also use this common understanding differently according to their particular personalities. It is important to remember that every culture is really composed of subcultures, groups, or individuals whose perceptions may be significantly different from the accepted social norms (Danesi & Perron 1999).

Language and culture cannot really be separated because, as noted, language gives us the means to express the understandings culture gives us. People who are native speakers of the same language, even if they come from different countries, often share understandings of culture. If we think about native speakers of English, who may come from Australia, the USA, or the UK, we realise that the culture of these three countries is quite different but the common language, English, means that these cultures are necessarily more similar than the culture of any one of them would be to people from a non-English-speaking country, simply because the means of expressing culture is the same.

Language

The languages of the world are divided into families that share general characteristics of grammar, lexicon, origin, and so forth. Within linguistic families, individual languages are different, and each has unique aspects. The structures available in a given language are related to how speakers perceive and categorise events and, by extension, how they think about their experience (Crystal 1997).

The Sapir-Whorf hypothesis describes this situation and is taken as an important tenet of the field of **sociolinguistics**, the area of study that relates to the social uses of language. The hypothesis states that differences in languages affect the way speakers think. This is called linguistic relativity (Dirven & Verspoor 2004). Linguistic relativity suggests that while every language can express anything its speakers might wish to say, each language has a unique set of words and structures that are the means by which speakers convey their ideas (Crystal 1997). Because the linguistic material available to discuss a particular issue, health for example, differs, it is likely that speakers of different language will also have different conceptualisations of this issue, and these conceptualisations will be more different for languages that are further apart.

Sociolinguistics The study of language in the social/cultural context.

For instance, the Indonesian language has a single word, *sakit*, that is used to mean both 'sick' and 'in pain'. Indonesian is very dependent on context and position, and speakers have to interpret the meaning of each utterance based on the social situation in which it occurs. In English, by contrast, we distinguish between being sick and being in pain and, in fact, have a number of different terms to further distinguish what exactly is wrong. We might wish to indicate that a pain is an ache or soreness or is stabbing. Indonesian has none of these distinctions. This does not mean that Indonesian speakers do not experience the same physical manifestations of pain that English speakers do, only that their conceptualisation of health does not require that the concept of being in pain be further specified.

The result of these differences in language, which are underpinned by the nature of the culture that uses the language, may be difficulty in understanding or even communication breakdown between healthcare professionals and their clients and patients. We normally expect health issues to be expressed in the way we are familiar with and rely heavily on culturally determined phrases and terms that are part of our cognitive framework (see Reynaert & Gelman 2007). When we work with speakers of other languages (even if they are speaking our language), we often find that they conceptualise their own health problems in ways that are unexpected and unfamiliar because we each tend to use our first language and culture as a template or model for what we say. This is an important issue for healthcare professionals and will be discussed further under the heading 'Cultural competency'.

Another important aspect of sociolinguistics that may affect us as healthcare professionals is the difference between our manner of discussing health and disease and that of the general public (see e.g. Keller & Carroll 1994; Chang & Fortier 1998). Health professionals generally spend many years completing their training, and part of this training is learning the ways of the profession. We can think of each health profession as a subculture that has its own conventions, ways of using language, and means of talking about clients or patients and their conditions. Being able to fit into this subculture is a part of successfully carrying out our duties. The general public who are not trained in our field have a completely different way of talking about health and disease. If we are members of the same culture, we understand what lay people mean when they talk about their health in this way, but it is often imprecise compared to our professional usage. It is easy to forget that lay people may not understand our own way of speaking or may be uncomfortable with it.

The use of medical language is often viewed by patients as a problem for them in understanding what their condition is and what they are supposed to do. Research has shown that patients feel much more comfortable using ordinary language to discuss their health, while doctors, in particular, tend to use the technical language that they use with their colleagues (Castro et al. 2007). It is often nurses who have to mediate by translating medical terminology and phrasing into more ordinary terms patients feel comfortable with (Hadlow & Pitts 1991; Bourhis et al. 2002). It is worth noting that patients and clients often react to non-verbal communicative cues as well as to language. What is considered the usual conversational manner differs considerably from culture to culture, and common hand gestures, making eye contact, smiling, and a whole range of other mannerisms contribute to how comfortable a patient or client feels with a healthcare professional and, indirectly, how much they might gain from the conversation (Larsen & Smith 1981; Harrigan et al. 1985; Griffith et al. 2003).

Language and culture in health

We understand that there are many universal aspects of human experience anywhere in the world and that people everywhere from every culture have the same potential for health and disease. We also understand that the state of health of different populations in different places may vary significantly because of a whole range of factors, including language and culture issues. This extends to what are viewed as signs of health and signs of illness (Kleinman et al. 1978).

The human condition includes a multitude of minor problems and pains that most people have suffered at one time or another. We have all had a headache which we might have treated ourselves with an over-the-counter pain medication. Or we might have done nothing, knowing that the headache would go away itself and did not represent a major problem. Most of us have an idea of what kind of symptoms are more serious and warrant a visit to the doctor for further treatment. The set of symptoms that may be ignored and those that should not are part of our cultural understanding and are often understood quite consistently by members of the same population.

This shared understanding derives from the culture and language shared by the group but also develops from a shared environment with specific characteristics in which the population in question lives. For example, drinking water in many Western countries is fluoridated, and toothpastes and other dental products often contain fluoride as well. Dentistry is highly developed, and awareness of dental hygiene is high among much of the public. For this reason, while still an important public health concern, dental health has improved greatly in Western societies over the course of the 20th century. Tooth loss due to decay or disease, especially among the young, is much less common than it once was, and most people expect to retain all or most of their teeth into adulthood. In other parts of the world, however, there is no treatment of drinking water and fluoride is generally not added to toothpastes and dental products. Dentistry may be less advanced than in the West, and there are generally fewer dentists. More importantly, the public in these areas tend to be much less accepting and trusting of dentistry and may accept much higher levels of pain, disability, and tooth loss than would be tolerated by most people in the West. Tooth loss and dental pain, in many parts of the world, are considered a normal part of life and if people do seek dental treatment it is often too late to save the teeth in question. The idea that there is a great deal the individual can do to prevent dental problems is not well understood, and many people make little effort to protect their own teeth (see WHO 2005c).

This difference in understanding is based on the cultural norms of each population. We often encounter a conflict between expectations when people emigrate from one country to another. In Australia, where oral health is one of the national health priorities, dental health among refugees is a particular concern. Because of the nature of the cultures these individuals come from combined with the effects of the social disruption there that caused them to become refugees, many suffer from serious dental and oral health problems. These can be treated more readily in Australia than in their countries of origin, but in many cases their condition is far advanced, and it is no longer possible to save teeth. This may have the effect of further strengthening the idea among this population that dentists cannot really help, and tooth loss is inevitable. Deeply held cultural understandings are often extremely difficult to change because we are not aware of their subjective (at the societal level) nature and often do not or cannot consider another perspective. For this reason, it may not be possible for the first generation of immigrants to learn the health perspective of their new country, but their children who grow up with them generally absorb the views of the society they live in more readily (Davidson et al. 2006; Finney Lamb et al. 2009).

It is important to understand that people are rarely aware that their actions represent a cultural norm that relates to their background and upbringing. We generally feel that we are behaving in the 'right' way because we are doing something that comes naturally in the social context in which we find ourselves. This subjective perception of appropriateness applies to language use as well. People talk about health in the ways they have observed among family members, friends, and other social groups. For the lay person (someone who is not trained in a health field), as mentioned above, it is more natural to use the imprecise terms common in society to refer to health conditions than to use more technical terms even if they are known. For example, we often read that someone has died 'following a long illness' (often used euphemistically to refer to death from cancer), that someone needs 'an operation' (where the professional might speak of surgery or a procedure or an appendectomy), and so forth.

While it is important to understand the cultural and linguistic factors that may affect perceptions about health, we should also be aware that at best they provide a set of guidelines. It is probably never the case that every member of a given culture or language group shares the exact same attitude and perceptions about health and illness. Similarly, we should not expect that every member of a cultural or language group will use their culture's approach to health as a basis for their own actions, and members of particular groups may act very differently from what we expect. This extends to members of our own culture as well as to individuals from cultural backgrounds we are less familiar with. Overall, then, we should be cautious about making generalisations about expected health behaviour based on cultural and language background but we should be aware of differences in perception due to diverse backgrounds and train ourselves to be sensitive to their existence.

Stop and Think

We all have ideas about health that come from our cultural and language background, including what we learn from the media and from other people.

» What kinds of things does the average Australian believe about health?

» To what extent do lay people's ideas about health correspond to the evidence used by health professionals as the basis for their work?

Indigenous health in Australia and New Zealand

The Aboriginal and Torres Strait Islander populations in Australia and the Maori population in New Zealand provide important examples of how the health of specific population subgroups that possess specific linguistic and cultural characteristics can differ from that of members of the majority culture. In Australia, Indigenous people suffer a greater burden of disease than the general public, tend to have less access to healthcare, and experience higher rates of hospitalisation for a range of diseases and conditions. As a group, they also have more disability and a lower life expectancy than the rest of the population, as well as more emotional and mental illness. Levels of behaviours that tend to be detrimental to health have also been observed to be higher among Indigenous peoples (AIHW 2011). This discrepancy in health outcomes and experience between the Indigenous and non-Indigenous populations is often referred to as a gap that must be addressed through policy, service provision, and change in social attitudes. To address this, the Australian Government has introduced the Closing the Gap Strategy which addresses a range of health concerns affecting the Indigenous population, including basic health, education, and employment as well as social inclusion (Australian Government 2009).

See the discussion of social inequality and exclusion in Chapter 11.

Like Australian Indigenous populations, the indigenous Maori of New Zealand have specific health concerns and issues that differ from those of the non-Maori population. Over the last 50 years, life expectancy for Maori individuals in New Zealand has increased significantly, bringing the discrepancy to 8.6 years for men and 7.9 years for women (Ministry of Maori Development 2009a). Like the Indigenous population in Australia, the Maori population in New Zealand is affected by higher rates of some diseases, especially diabetes, than the general public. Although this group tends to be more physically active than the non-Maori, obesity remains a problem as do rates of smoking, which tend to be higher than for non-Maori despite dropping significantly since the late 1990s (Ministry of Health 2010).

The experience of the indigenous peoples of Australia and New Zealand with respect to health is characteristic of indigenous populations around the world for whom dramatic change in social structures and the living environment has occurred rapidly in the context of colonisation and integration into modern nation states. A range of social inequalities and socio-economic factors associated with globalisation, migration, loss of language and culture, and disconnection from the land have been implicated as the basis for current health discrepancies (King et al. 2009). Another important element of social change that has affected indigenous populations is the shift from the use of traditional languages to the majority language of the nation in which they are located (Gracey & King 2009). As discussed above, our understanding of health is embedded in language which, in turn, develops in such a way as to facilitate cultural conceptualisations, including ideas about health. It has been observed, for example, that indigenous conceptualisations of health, as expressed through traditional languages and cultures, tend to be more holistic and more centred on well-being. Recovering from illness may entail consultation with the wider community and participation in collective practices (King et al. 2009). The importance of the traditional community in indigenous health cannot be underestimated; it has been observed that many indigenous peoples define their personal identity in the context of the group (Durie 2005; Durie et al. 2009). This identity, as a member of a particular culture with its own language, practices, and worldview, is central to the emotional health of the individual and will also contribute to how people perceive illness in themselves as well as in others. It is generally agreed that, in considering the social determinants that affect the health experience of all people, a range of cultural factors in the special case of Indigenous health in Australia—loss of language and connection to the land, environmental deprivation, and spiritual, emotional, and mental disconnectedness—must also be taken into account (Mowbray 2007; Nettleton et al. 2007). The communal aspect of health is significant as well, and recognition of this conceptualisation is part of the rationale for the Australian Government's social inclusion agenda for Indigenous populations (Australian Government 2011). A similar approach has been taken in New Zealand to encourage greater participation by the Maori community in larger social issues and governance with the aim of further closing the gap between indigenous and non-indigenous health and welfare (Ministry of Maori Development 2009b).

Cultural competency

As health professionals, we are required to provide appropriate care to patients and clients that best meets their needs and represents best practice. This means that we have to be aware of the ways in which language and cultural background may affect people's perceptions and understandings about health and take these into account in our work. This is increasingly important as societies around the world become more multicultural; Australia is no exception to this. Our population is made up of people from many different backgrounds, and its diversity is continuing to increase (Department of Foreign Affairs and Trade 2008). For this reason, it is especially important that we are aware of cultural differences and how they may affect health and that we develop cultural competency in working with people from different backgrounds.

Cultural competency
The ability to work effectively with people from different cultural and language backgrounds.

Cultural competency for the healthcare professional means the ability to work appropriately with people from different cultures and who speak different languages. A culturally competent healthcare system is one that acknowledges the importance of cultural practices and the relationship between cultures in achieving health outcomes (Betancourt et al. 2003). Individually, we must be aware of our own cultural outlook and how it colours our understanding of health, but also that the people we work with may have a very different set of perceptions based on different assumptions. In the healthcare system, cultural competency is one way of eliminating some of the inequities in health that are observable in modern society. We know that a number of social factors, such as income (socio-economic status), education, and structural/institutional issues, can have an impact on health, but cultural factors can as well. Cultural competency allows us to address the effects of the social environment that are shaped by culture and language.

It is important to understand why cultural competency has become so important in healthcare and the training of its professionals. There are two main reasons for this. The first is that individuals from different cultural backgrounds may describe their symptoms quite differently according to their own understanding of illness. They may also have limited ability in English (or whatever the language of interaction is in a given situation). Their decisions about when to seek care may vary, and their expectations for treatment and beliefs about their condition may affect their adherence to health advice (Berger 1998; Betancourt et al. 2005). The second is that a great deal of research has shown that communication between health professionals and patients or clients is closely related to patient/client satisfaction, adherence to advice, and health outcomes. In other words, poorer health outcomes may result when sociocultural differences between health professionals and patients/clients are not acknowledged and addressed (Stewart et al. 1999; Williams & Rucker 2000; Institute of Medicine 2001; Smedley et al. 2002).

See Chapter 1 under the heading 'Health, illness, well-being, and culture'.

In Australia, the National Health and Medical Research Council (NHMRC) has produced a set of guidelines about cultural competency for healthcare professionals. Cultural competency is especially important in the Australian context because our population is very diverse, and, like many other countries, we must address a number of health inequities between different population subgroups. The Australian model for cultural competency addresses four dimensions of the healthcare system as a whole: systemic (how the whole national healthcare system is structured); organisational (how the various agencies at different levels of government are structured); professional (relating to the various health professions whose work contributes to the well-being of the population); and individual (how each person in the healthcare system does his or her job). According to the NHMRC (2005, p. 4), a culturally competent healthcare system is one that

> acknowledges the benefits that diversity brings to Australian society; helps health
> providers and consumers achieve the best, most appropriate care and services;
> enables self-determination and ensures a commitment to reciprocity for culturally
> and linguistically diverse consumers and their communities; and holds governments,
> health organizations, and managers accountable for meeting the needs of all
> members of the communities they serve.

This emphasis on cultural competency is based on the fact that different Australian population subgroups have a very different experience of health. For example, statistics collected by the Australian Government show that certain communities have higher than average rates of diabetes (immigrant groups from southern Europe, the South Pacific Island states, North Africa, the Middle East, and Asia). The population that emigrated to Australia from the UK and Ireland has higher than average rates of breast cancer and lung cancer, while rates of skin cancer for the population born overseas are less than half those of the population born in Australia (AIHW 2004, 2005).

Stop and Think

It is important that health professionals be aware of cultural differences that might affect the health of the patients or clients.

» Why do you think this is viewed as the responsibility of those who provide healthcare instead of part of the responsibility of the patient/client?

Illness behaviour and culture

The idea that each culture has a 'sick role', a set of behaviours and attitudes that are accepted by members of the culture as the appropriate way for a sick person to behave, is long established in the field of health sociology (see e.g. Parsons 1951). Continuing research in this area has shown that the cultural perspective of health professionals as well as their patients and clients is an important influence on illness behaviour. It is now accepted that the way people behave when they are sick derives from a complex interaction between their particular biological determinants, the nature of their symptoms, the social context in which illness occurs, the characteristics of the healthcare system of which they are part, and learnt responses to illness that are rooted in their language and culture (Mechanic 1995; Kirmayer & Sartorius 2007).

A learnt response to illness comes from all the observations of the behaviour of people around them that an individual absorbs from birth. Young children come to understand what is expected of a sick person, what kind of illness means a person is sick enough not to participate in normal activities, what symptoms require professional assistance, and how various diseases are viewed in the context of their own family, culture, and social group. These culturally determined lay understandings of health often differ dramatically from the evidence-based, best practice approaches of health professionals. For example, evidence indicates that early ambulation is an important factor in recovery after certain kinds of surgery (Oldmeadow et al. 2006; Izumi et al. 2010). However, lay conceptualisations of health in many cultures suggest that a person who has undergone a serious operation should not move around too much, especially if they are in pain. These opposite interpretations may lead to disagreement and conflict between patients and their family members and health professionals.

Illness behaviour has been shown to influence several important dimensions of health, particularly in relation to when and how an individual might seek treatment. First, culturally influenced illness behaviour may affect who is vulnerable to illness (Hartog & Hartog 1983). In this, it is important to distinguish between **illness** and **disease**. *Disease* refers to a clinical condition that is acknowledged to be abnormal and detrimental to a person's health. By contrast, *illness* is the state of being sick or having something wrong as perceived by the individual in question. Many people who have a disease do not feel that they have an illness, but it is also the case that many people who feel that they have an illness do not have a detectable disease. Different cultures

Illness A condition adversely affecting health as perceived by the individual in question.

Disease A condition adversely affecting health that has measurable (clinical) symptoms.

See also Chapter 1 on illness, health, and well-being.

allow, in the sense of deeming it socially acceptable, for certain people to suffer from illness as part of their social role. Second, culturally influenced illness behaviour can determine who decides to become a patient (Hartog & Hartog 1983). That is, some cultures do not recognise certain symptoms or problems as evidence of a health concern, and individuals who experience these symptoms may not be willing to seek treatment. This is often the case in mental illness but may apply to physical symptoms as well (see e.g. Roy et al. 2005; Canino & Alegria 2008). And third, culturally influenced illness behaviour may dictate how a person behaves once they are a patient (Hartog & Hartog 1983), including to what extent they are likely to follow health advice given to them by professionals or what the meaning of illness is in their culture (Bhui & Dinos 2008). For example, for individuals from a low socio-economic background whose earnings allow for few savings, it may be impossible to take on the role of patient and hence deprive the family of necessary income. In socio-cultural contexts like this, there may exist deeply ingrained behaviours and rationales that encourage people to ignore symptoms and continue to work until it is physically impossible to ignore pain or other problems.

Culture-bound syndromes

Culture-bound syndromes are usually said to be locally defined patterns of discrete behaviour (Littlewood & Lipsedge 1985). That is, they are illnesses that occur only in specific communities and are identified by a set of symptoms that derives from the culture of the society that experiences them. For a long time, culture-bound syndromes were seen as exotic, occurring generally in cultures that were viewed by Westerners as less developed, more traditional, and lacking the institutions of modernity (Hughes 1996; Bhugra & Jacob 1997). Culture-bound syndromes depend on the recognition of symptoms reported by the person who is affected that often cannot be confirmed clinically. That is, the symptoms of these conditions typically do not have physiological effects that can be measured by Western tests. For this reason, culture-bound syndromes are usually psychiatric or psychological conditions, as opposed to strictly medical ones.

Case Study 14.1   Being sick in Indonesia

Illness behaviour in Indonesia is very different from Australia or other English-speaking societies. As we have seen, how people act when they are sick and how their condition is perceived are determined by a combination of factors that derive from the language, culture, and shared environment of the people in question. We should also understand that every country has a number of cultures. Indonesia, for example, is very diverse with more than 300 ethnic and language groups. Nonetheless, there are also aspects of culture that are shared by many people in the country. Illness behaviour is one of these.

In Indonesia, illness behaviour is related to how serious a particular health condition is viewed. Some health issues are seen as serious by definition. These include broken bones, fevers, pain of any kind, and recovery from childbirth. Whether a condition is viewed as serious is not always related to how the individual feels but instead is based on how others react to any visible signs and symptoms. It is perhaps for this reason that broken bones or injuries are always considered serious. In Australia, for example, a person with a broken arm would be expected to go about most of their usual activities. The injury would certainly not prevent them from leaving the house or going to work (assuming they were physically able to do their job with one hand).

In Indonesia, when a person is viewed as having a serious health condition, even if this is only a headache, they are expected to lie in bed. Other family members will normally wait on them, bringing them food, helping them walk to the bathroom, and so forth. A sick person is not supposed to watch television, read, or do anything around the house and will not be allowed by family to go outside. If someone is sick, they must rest, and the appropriate illness behaviour will be enforced by others. Needless to say, the sick individual also understands this sick role and tends to adopt the culturally appropriate behaviour. From a Western point of view, Indonesians frequently take to their bed for what we perceive as no reason at all. However, the social need to do so is part of their culture and represents correct behaviour in the context of their shared expectations and experience.

Indonesia does not have a tradition of diagnosis and did not develop techniques for examining and understanding how the body works beyond what is visible to the eye. Traditional medicine relies on what we would call magic, herbal remedies, and basic technical skills such as bone-setting. In the modern era, Western, allopathic medicine forms the basis of the nation's healthcare system, but diagnosis remains much less important than in the West, and many people are more familiar with traditional conceptualisations of health and disease than with the evidence-based understandings of health professionals with modern training. For this reason, the determination of what constitutes a serious illness to the average Indonesian is based on a different set of considerations from those a modern doctor would use. For example, it is common to see people on the street or in the market with coughs so severe it is difficult for them to breathe. A cough is rarely considered enough to require illness behaviour on the part of the sufferer, however, even though to a health professional it might be a sign of serious illness or represent a threat to public health. Similarly, diseases like diabetes, which is very common in Indonesia, that do not have pronounced symptoms very seldom change people's behaviour (including diet), even when they have received a medical diagnosis.

When working with patients or clients from another culture, it is important to recognise that their understandings of disease and what they consider to be appropriate illness behaviour may be very different from what we consider to be usual. It is important to approach these differences without making judgments and without criticism. This is where communication between the healthcare professional and their patient or client becomes central in providing the best care that also meets the needs of all involved.

Although culture-bound syndromes have been viewed largely as occurring in non-Western populations, Western societies do, in fact, experience these illnesses. For example, it has been suggested that the type A behaviour pattern that has received as great deal of attention in the media since the 1970s is a culture-bound condition. People suffering from this condition say that they feel chronically pressed for time, extremely frustrated when they cannot achieve what they expect to, aggressive, overly ambitious, and impatient (Hughes 1996). The type A behaviour pattern has been thought to lead to greater incidence of heart disease, but the evidence supporting this is inconclusive (Matthews & Haynes 1986; Ragland & Brand 1988). Similarly, bulimia nervosa has also been observed to be a Western culture-bound syndrome (Littlewood 1996).

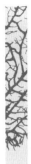

Mythbuster

Emotional response is not universal. While all human beings have the same range of emotions, the events or perceptions that trigger a particular emotion are culturally determined, as is the way in which that emotion is expressed. For this reason, we have to be very careful in interpreting the emotional reaction of people from another culture. Even the experience of war, which might be expected to be universally traumatising regardless of culture, has been observed to produce different reactions in different populations. In fact, post-traumatic stress disorder, the expected response to severe emotional trauma in the West, is increasingly viewed as being culture-bound or determined by the specific cultural understandings of the population affected by it.

There are indications that Western health problems that are culturally defined in terms of their nature and symptoms are spreading around the world. One cause of this may be the dominance of Western health paradigms in health fields and the fact that a large part of research and study in these areas comes from Western societies. Another contributing factor may be the globalisation of healthcare through the activities of multinational companies that may seek to create and maintain global markets for their products (Watters 2010). Examples of Western patterns of illness being transferred to societies where they did not previously occur include depression in Japan (Vickery 2010) and anorexia nervosa (with the Western characteristics of the condition) in Hong Kong (Lee & Lee 1996).

The existence of culture-bound syndromes emphasises the important role that culture plays in people's conceptualisation of health. The fact that a set of subjectively constructed symptoms can be generally understood to indicate the presence of a particular condition that is recognised by members of specific linguistic/cultural groups shows that the nature of health and illness is not necessarily universal but depends to a significant extent on how people think about themselves and their physical and emotional reactions. It is important to understand that perceived health conditions are real to those involved, even when they do not have observable clinical signs, and contribute greatly to how people evaluate their own well-being. As health professionals it is important that we are aware of the degree to which culturally formed conceptualisations of health affect individuals and try to understand how others understand the experience of being ill.

Summary

Language and culture shape our understanding of what it means to be healthy or sick. Language provides the means of expressing perceptions about health and disease, while culture is a shared set of understandings that direct behaviour, attitudes, and views. Language and culture are related, and this relationship is studied in the field of sociolinguistics, which is concerned with the social uses of language.

While knowledge of culture may provide guidelines for how members of that culture may understand their own health, generalisations of this kind are not absolute, and there may be a great deal of variation among members of a group. Nonetheless, it is important to be aware of cultural differences in how people understand health and disease. Cultural competency is the ability to work effectively with people from different language and culture backgrounds. Australia is becoming more diverse, and health professionals have to be increasingly aware of and sensitive to cultural differences. Understanding the specific health needs and experience of Indigenous populations is an important aspect of cultural competency.

Cultural differences are often observed in the context of illness behaviour. These culturally determined behaviours relating to health are often at odds with evidence-based best practice that would be recommended by health professionals, but are often very deeply ingrained. As health professionals, we must be aware of potential differences, be prepared to understand how a patient or client feels, and approach our work with that individual without making judgments or criticisms.

Tutorial exercises

1 Based on your own experience, what aspects of language use or social interaction that are considered usual and appropriate in Australia might be misunderstood by people from a different cultural background?

2 Does the behaviour of health professionals ever contribute to communication problems with patients or clients from another cultural or linguistic background? Explain.

3 What kind of illness behaviour is expected where you come from? Explain and discuss.

Further reading

MacLachlan, M. (2006). *Culture and health: A critical perspective towards global health*. Chicester, UK: John Wiley & Sons.

Ritter, L.A., & Hoffman, N.A. (2010). *Multicultural health*. Sudbury, MA: Jones & Bartlett.

Singer, M., & Baer, H. (2007). *Introducing medical anthropology: A discipline in action*. Lanham, MD: AltaMira Press.

Websites

<www.nhmrc.gov.au/publications/synopses/hp25syn.htm>

The National Health and Medical Research Council offers a set of guidelines as well as other information on cultural competency.

<www.cyf.vic.gov.au/indigenous-initiatives/archive/practice-guides/aboriginal-cultural competence-framework>

The Department of Human Services of Victoria has developed an Aboriginal cultural competency framework and matrix for working with the Indigenous community.

<www.indigenous.gov.au/About/Pages/closing_gap.aspx>

Close the Gap offers a variety of resources related to narrowing the disparity between Indigenous and non-Indigenous health in Australia.

<www.health.vic.gov.au/cald>

The Department of Health of Victoria offers information and advice on working with individuals from culturally and linguistically diverse (CALD) communities.

15 Deviance, difference, and stigma as social determinants of health

Pranee Liamputtong and
Somsri Kitisriworapan

TOPICS COVERED

This chapter covers the following topics:
- definitions of deviance, difference, stigma, and discrimination
- impact of deviance and stigma on health
- stigma and HIV/AIDS
- what has been done to combat HIV-related stigma

KEY TERMS

Deviance
Difference
Discrimination
HIV/AIDS
Labelling theory

Moral career
Social exclusion
Social norms
Stigma
Stigmatisation

Introduction

Sciologist Emile Durkheim (1895/1982) suggested that deviance is a universal feature of all societies because it implies the values and norms of a culture. Moral interpretation exists in all societies, and some qualities and conduct are perceived as more desirable than others, so deviance is always present in every society. By identifying what is deviant, societies identify what is not. This in turn creates shared standards within a society (Clinard & Meier 2008, p. 10).

Often, the notion that some people are different in an unacceptable way leads to stigma, which refers to certain traits and behaviours that are devalued by others. The word 'stigma' is derived from an ancient Greek word meaning 'mark'. Marks were impressed on slaves as a way to identify their position in the social structure, which was one of inferiority (Whitehead et al. 2001a; Sherman 2007). Although deviance, difference, and stigma are socially constructed concepts, they are often thought of as somehow intrinsic, and so have a negative impact on the life and well-being of the individuals and groups who are so labelled. As such, they form an important component of the **social determinants** of health.

This chapter will bring readers through several important issues relevant to deviance, difference, and stigma. The chapter will first introduce these notions, then discuss the impact they have on the health and well-being of those who are stigmatised. It also discusses stigma and HIV/AIDS and what has been done to combat HIV-related stigma as a case study.

> **Social determinants**
> A number of factors, including social, cultural, economic, and political, which can impact on the health of individuals.
>
> See the discussion of the social determinants of health in Chapter 1.

Deviance and difference

Deviance constitutes a universal aspect of our everyday social life (Roach Anleu 2006, 2009). Indeed, the ideas of conformity, rule observation, and correct conduct can only be comprehended because of the existence of deviance. Even a simple question like 'Why did you do it?' could suggest that the person has violated some social rule. Questions like this usually elicit unease or awkwardness and may eventually discourage individuals from violating those particular rules. As such, it is a form of informal social control that stops people from engaging in deviant behaviour (Roach Anleu 2006, 2009).

At the simplest level, Clinard and Meier (2008, p. 8) suggest, deviance marks out those who are **different**. Deviant people behave differently, and hence they are different from us. However, the concept of deviance goes beyond a simple examination of differences between individuals and their behaviour. Often, when we refer to the notion of deviance, we tend to think about some things we devalue or evaluate negatively (Clinard & Meier 2008). A common definition of deviance refers to 'behaviour which violates social norms' (Roach Anleu 2006, p. 420). Deviance symbolises nonconfomity to a norm or set of norms that is approved or observed by the majority of people in a particular society or culture (Scambler 2003). Deviant behaviour signifies behaviour which, 'once it has become public knowledge, is routinely subject to sanctions—to punishment, correction or treatment' (Scambler 2003, p. 192).

Social norms are rules or standards that guide or constrain individuals' actions or behaviour (Stuber et al. 2008; Roach Anleu 2009). A norm is a social rule

> **Deviance** Behaviour that transgresses social expectations and is likely to attract sanctions from other members of the society.

> **Difference** Used when an individual possesses characteristics that are dissimilar to or behaves differently from the majority of people within a society.
>
> **Social norms** Rules or standards that guide or constrain individuals' actions or behaviour.

indicating what individuals ought to or ought not say, think, or do in a given situation (Blake & Davis 1964). Transgressions of norms usually elicit negative responses or sanctions from others in the society. These responses or sanctions put pressure on people to conform to social norms (Clinard & Meier 2008). Relevant to the concept of normatic deviance is social control—the use of strategies that attempt to compel comformity, or at least to deal with or deflect deviant behaviour (Roach Anleu 2006, 2009).

Although norms are shaped, encouraged, and sustained by the social and situational contexts within the society (Becker 1963a; Clinard & Meier 2008), most concepts of deviance are created by some segments of society who strive to harden their positions about what is proper and improper and what is right and wrong into norms (Clinard & Meier 2008). They tend to be those who have more power because of their social status (Roach Anleu 2009). When these groups sense threats to their interests from particular conditions or acts, they might try to advance those interests by convincing others of the authority of their concern (Clinard & Meier 2008). These processes have shaped criteria for many forms of deviance, for example, drink driving, consumption of illegal drugs, abortion, prostitution, and homosexuality.

See also Chapter 1 on gender, ethnicity, and social class.

Stop and Think

Emma, who is in her late thirties, has a great career path. She does not have any children, and has recently got a divorce. Because of a promotion, she moved to Melbourne. As she meets new colleagues and friends, Emma starts to feel that she is somehow being treated differently. In a number of conversations with them, it becomes clear to her that some of her new network regard her 'family situation' as unusual. Emma begins to feel that she is excluded from social gatherings where couples with children are welcomed. This makes Emma think that she is in some sense deviant. *But is she?* (adapted from Clinard & Meier 2008, p. 2).

Stop and Think

Consider the case of Emma presented above. Nowadays, more couples choose not to have children and divorce is common. There are no absolute standards which dictate that adults should have children or that one should not be divorced. But Emma feels uncomfortable around her social network because she is excluded from social occasions, and this is due to her social status as childless and a divorcee. But why would her colleagues and new friends see her as deviant? Clinard and Meier (2008, p. 7) contend that an answer might be that 'the norms of their groups suggest that couples and parents are statuses that are valued'. Emma might be feeling deviant because her new social network groups who have partners and children think that this is the way things *should* be in our society.

» What is your view about this theory? Is there any other theory that you can use to explain this case?

Concepts of deviance ebb and flow over time and can change in different situations (Roach Anleu 2006; Clinard & Meier 2008). For example, in most Western societies there is no longer much moral disapproval of premarital sexual intercourse, so it is no longer seen as deviant behaviour. Masturbation has also been increasingly accepted. Some may even perceive the practice as an essential part of 'normal sexual development' (Janus & Janus 1993, p. 106; Clinard & Meier 2008, p. 297). Homosexuality was once seen as an extremely deviant and morally wrong behaviour. However, it is now more tolerated by many people, and also seen merely as an example of difference (Roach Anleu 2006, p. 3).

Looking through the daily newspapers in Australia reveals that the kinds of deviance seen as requiring social control nowadays tend to include abortion, domestic violence, bottle-feeding practices, homelessness, drug trafficking, juvenile delinquency, sex work, environmental pollution, and tobacco consumption. These activities have always gone on in Australian society, but they have not always been labelled as deviant (Roach Anleu 2006). Cohen (1974) uses the term 'elasticity of evil' as the title of his book to suggest that activities and behaviour which are interpreted as deviance are always evolving. Hence, what is deviant at one point of time or situation might not be perceived as such in another (Roach Anleu 2006).

As we have suggested, some particular groups in society have more power to elicit, change, and sustain specific concepts of deviance. There are constant movements to abandon the perception of practices such as personal drug consumption, public drunkenness, and prostitution as 'deviant'. There have also been some attempts to make some activities sanctioned by law as deviant and hence criminal. A good example of this is the prevailing categorising of cigarette smoking as deviant, which has occurred in a number of nations including Australia and the USA. Up to the 1970s, cigarette smoking was an acceptable behaviour; nowadays, it is viewed as deviant. This can be seen through the 'no smoking' signs that appear in numerous public places, including restaurants, planes, and in Australia, all Commonwealth Government offices and buildings. Smoking is forbidden by law in these locations. There are penalties if this statute is violated (Roach Anleu 2006).

What is deviant in one culture, however, may be normal or acceptable in another. For example, in many Western societies, smoking marijuana is deviant but consuming alcohol is not. In some Middle Eastern cultures the reverse is true (Scambler 2003). Belching loudly when eating is acceptable in Japanese or Chinese culture (it is a form of food appreciation), but this is seen as rude by most people in Australia. Traditional practices regarding painful initiation ceremonies, arranged marriages, or the confinement of women during childbirth and menstruation, for instance, may seem highly deviant, if not barbaric, to Australian and other Western societies, but these practices are normal in some cultures and form an important part of their ways of life (Roach Anleu 2006).

Case Study 15.1   Breast and bottle-feeding: Moral and deviant mothers

Notions of deviance always elicit a strong moral stance. Even everyday conduct can have this moral tone. The argument on whether mothers should breastfeed or bottle-feed babies embodies a moral attitude of this kind. Murphy's (1999) study of first-time mothers in England and Liamputtong and Kitisriworapan's research with working mothers in Thailand (see Liamputtong & Kitisriworapan 2011) reveal that whether the mothers intend to breastfeed or bottle-feed, they face tremendous challenges from those who disagree with them. Clinard and Meier (2008, p. 2) put it succinctly, that 'not even the time-honoured institution of motherhood is immune from allegations of deviance'.

The dominant idea that 'breast is best' is pervasive in literature on infant feeding patterns and in policy and health promotion material which attempt to educate women about their infant feeding practices. Within the lay population, this idea is also promulgated. Due to the societal perception of the superiority of breastfeeding, mothers' intention not to breastfeed their babies may tarnish the 'moral status' of motherhood. By choosing to bottle-feed, a mother is subjected to the accusation that she is a 'bad' mother who 'places her own needs, preferences or conveniences above her baby's welfare'. On the contrary, the 'good mother' is 'deemed to be one who prioritises her child's needs, even (or perhaps especially) where this entails personal inconvenience or distress' (Murphy 1999, pp. 187–8), such as trying to breastfeed in the face of many obstacles.

Motherhood is 'often represented as the ultimate expression of womanhood while breast-feeding is represented as the ultimate experience of motherhood' (Nadesan & Sotirin 1998, p. 221). Because of this, the decision to bottle-feed 'leaves women open to the charge of being a poor mother, in short, of maternal deviance' (Murphy 1999, p. 188). The intention to formula-feed threatens women's claims to qualities such as selflessness, wisdom, responsibility, and far-sightedness, all of which are widely seen as evidence of being a 'good mother' (Murphy 1999, p. 188).

The discourses on motherhood have created this moral image of breastfeeding (Guttman & Zimmerman 2000). In Earle's study (2000, p. 327) with women in Coventry, England, women perceived breastfeeding as natural. A woman who did not breastfeed was perceived as a 'horrible mother' (Liamputtong 2006).

Deviance, according to Murphy (1999, p. 189), 'involves a charge that public morality is being violated' and in the case of infant feeding, mothers break the rules of infant feeding. But more than that, as Murphy (1999, p. 188) theorises, 'the moral mother is not simply one who follows the rules. Rather, she is one who follows the rules *knowingly*'. Hence, simply breaking the rules does not make the mother deviant. Rather, 'her deviance rests upon a judgement that she has broken the rules *knowingly*' (McHugh 1970, p. 188, original emphasis). In the case of infant feeding, mothers who choose not to breastfeed their infants despite knowing very well the likely impact on their infant's health are potentially subjected to the charge of deviance, or being stigmatised as 'immoral mothers'.

However, there appear to be some possibilities for women who intend to bottle-feed to 'challenge or resist the interpretation of their behaviour as morally sanctionable' (Murphy 1999, pp. 189–90). To do so, women who intend to bottle-feed must prove that, while it breaks the rule, it is nonetheless justified. When the decision to formula-feed her baby is questioned, a mother must justify that her intention is 'non-conventional'; that is, 'she could not have done otherwise' (Murphy 1999, p. 190). As she has no other choice, her intention is justified and therefore should not be sanctioned. When breastfeeding is socially valued in societies, women choosing not to breastfeed may use socially and culturally acceptable grounds for their actions, such as the need to work in a paid job or having insufficient milk. This will help them to escape being seen as 'bad mothers'.

Stigma, stigmatisation, and discrimination

Closely related to deviance is the concept of **stigma**. The foundation of stigma lies in 'differences'. These differences can be in physical appearance, personality, age, gender, sexuality, illness, disability, and specific behaviour which evoke discontent, abhorence, panic, or sympathy from others (Mason et al. 2001).

Stigma, according to Goffman (1963, p. 3) is a 'devaluation' process that links with stereotyping and prejudice. It is used by individuals to interpret specific traits of others as 'discreditable or unworthy' and this results in the person stigmatised becoming 'discounted' or 'tainted' (Thomas 2006, p. 3175). Those who are stigmatised will then be 'disqualified from full social acceptance' (Goffman 1963, preface). Following Goffman's theory of stigma as an attribute, Jones and colleagues (1984) used 'mark' to indicate stigma, which would eventually lead to the definition of someone as 'flawed' or 'spoiled' (Yang et al. 2007, p. 1525). On the basis of a social position which dictates that some individuals are 'tainted' and 'less than', stigma is a mark that separates people from one another (Pescosolido et al. 2008, p. 431).

According to Mason and colleagues (2001, p. 4), the main element of the stigmatising strategy is to create the 'them and us' principle (see also Foucault 1973). Its aim is to lay a foundation which could separate individuals who are perceived as 'good and in favour' from those who are 'bad and out of favour' within a given social norm (Foucault 1973). Once this principle is initiated, **stigmatisation** and **social exclusion** are permitted. This process is then established and confirmed by the prejudiced position that accentuates the difference between 'them' and 'us'. As Sontag (1991) suggests, HIV/AIDS symbolises 'sinful' and 'evil'. Hence, people living with HIV/AIDS tend to be perceived as discredited individuals who have immoral characters. As a consequence, they are socially conditioned as not 'one of us' (Mason et al. 2001, p. 4). Often, this leads to **discrimination** against the discredited persons.

Goffman (1963) suggests that there are three kinds of stigmatising conditions. The first is 'tribal identities', which include such characteristics as gender, race, religion, and nationality. Second is the 'blemishes of individual character', which may include having mental illness, having a history of addiction or imprisonment, and living with HIV/AIDS. Third is 'abominations of the body' which include such bodily conditions as deformities and physical disabilities (LeBel 2008, p. 411). Based on Goffman's stigmatising conditions, there are many individuals who would be stigmatised because of their social and health status in many societies. More recently, Falk (2001) proposes two types of stigmatising states which are based on the 'cause' of stigma. First, 'existential stigma' occurs when an individual does not create stigma or has very little control over it. These include being old, having a certain race and ethnicity, and having a mental illness. Second, 'achieved stigma', which happens when an individual has acquired a stigma because of their own action and behaviour and/or because they have personally cultivated it. These may include such actions as becoming a refugee, immigrant, prisoner, homeless, or living with HIV/AIDS (LeBel 2008).

Similar to the concept of deviance presented above, stigma theorists have focused more on the position of social norms in the process of constructing stigma (Stuber et al. 2008, p. 422). Goffman (1963), for instance, contends that because deviations from social rules are inescapable,

Stigma An attribute or characteristic that separates people from one another. It is used by individuals to interpret specific attributes of others as 'discreditable or unworthy' and this results in the stigmatised person becoming devalued.

Stigmatisation The process of stigmatising a person.

Social exclusion The exclusion of individuals from social networks and resources because of their different and stigmatised status.

Discrimination The idea that someone is of less value and should be excluded from social networks and the benefits of society.

stigmatisation is a common characteristic of any society. Others suggest that stigmatisation is a characteristic of all socio-cultural groups and that it is employed to elicit conformity with the social standings of society so that law and order can be enforced. From this perspective, stigmatisation is the result of deviating from social rules that attempt to make the deviant individual conform. It is also used to illustrate to other group members the behaviours that are not condoned, and the effects that will be felt by those who engage in such actions. However, it can only be used in these ways to enforce conformity around voluntary behaviours, for example, illicit drug consumption and cigarette smoking (Stuber et al. 2008). Stigma has also now been defined by scholars in terms of a person's social identity, and their unique social contexts has been more emphasised. According to Crocker and colleagues (1998), the central feature of social stigma is that stigmatised persons have, or are believed to have, some characteristics that are associated with a devalued social identity in a particular social situation.

How does stigma occur? Goffman (1963) contends that stigma is a process grounded within the 'construction of social identity' (Yang et al. 2007, p. 1527). Stigma eventuates through what Goffman (1963, p. 32) refers to as a **'moral career'**: when a stigmatised individual initially makes sense of their social position in society and later acquires a set idea of what it would be like to have a specific stigma. The person will then pass from 'normal' to a 'discreditable' status, and through social interaction, they will eventually obtain a 'discredited' status. In Goffman's term, when an individual's new identity is 'assumed through interaction (i.e., "re-identifying") with socially constructed categories', stigma will occur (Yang et al. 2007, p. 1527). A good example is the case of mental illness. A person with mental illness (a non-visible stigma) passes from a 'normal' status to a 'discredited' one. Their 'discredited' status is gained when they disclose the mental illness condition to others.

Stigma also occurs through the process of 'labelling'. Scheff (1966) posits a **labelling theory** and applies it to the case of mental illness. He suggests that when an individual living with mental illness is given a deviant label, it will eventually lead them to change their self-perception and lose social opportunity (Yang et al. 2007). Scheff argues that individuals learn about the stereotypes of mental illness through the process of socialisation and daily reinforcement. Because of its highly discrediting status, once the stereotype is fully formed, the person's 'patient' role will appear as a 'master status' (Markowitz 2005). Consistent reactions from others, particularly the application of social exclusion, will prevent the person from reclaiming their former ('normal') social functions (Yang et al. 2007).

Moral career A process when a stigmatised individual initially makes sense of their social position within the society and later acquires a set idea of what it would be like to hold a specific characteristic.

Labelling theory The process of labelling a person with stigma, which through the process of social interaction will eventually lead the person to change their self-perception and lose social opportunity.

The impact of deviance and stigma on health

For the stigmatized, stigma compounds suffering. (Yang et al. 2007, p. 1528)

The greatest suffering inflicted by stigma in modern times can be seen in what is now called 'ethnic cleansing'. The mass killing of harmless people occurs simply because they are of different race, ethnicity, religion, or culture, or merely because they are different. This is proof of what humans can do to others if the reactions to stigma are not taken seriously (Whitehead et al. 2001b).

Health and illness conditions that tend to produce stigma are those connected with negative characteristics, those that have uncertain or unknown causes and limited treatment, and those that produce intense reactions such as fear and disgust (Sontag 1991; LeBel 2008). Historically, leprosy and tuberculosis were met with revulsion and later on we witnessed the same emotional responses towards cancer, mental illness, and, more recently, HIV/AIDS (Sontag 1991; LeBel 2008) (see later section on stigma and HIV/AIDS). Currently, we still see numerous health-related issues which have attracted stigma: abortion, infertility, being overweight, obesity, bottle-feeding, and cigarette smoking. Those who belong to stigmatised classifications (or the deviants as we outlined earlier), such as poor people, homeless people, gays and lesbians, refugees, indigenous people, and ethnic minority groups, are also likely to have to deal with the negative repercussions of stigma-related health issues (Pescosolido et al. 2008).

The effect of stigma on the stigmatised individuals can differ in its manifestation and magnitude (Link & Phelan 2001; Mason et al. 2001; Corrigan et al. 2003a,b). Often, stigma generates negative credibilities, in other words stereotypes. It then gives legitimacy to the negative credibilities; this is referred to as prejudice. This prejudice then leads to a wish to shun individuals who possess stigmatised status; this is discrimination (Pescosolido et al. 2008, p. 431; see also Link & Phelan 2001; Williams et al. 2008). Any form of discrimination and prejudice may lead to social exclusion as it functions to disconnect stigmatised persons from society and prohibits them from having societal benefits such as access to education, housing, social support, and healthcare (Mason et al. 2001; LeBel 2008).

Individually, the effects of stigma and social exclusion can be very destructive. They can result in isolation, low self-esteem, depression, self-harm, poor academic achievement and social relationships, and poor physical and mental health (Mason et al. 2001; Major & O'Brien 2005; Yang et al. 2007). For stigmatised individuals with major health problems, the stigma they carry can 'intensify the sense that life is uncertain, dangerous, and hazardous' (Yang et al. 2007, p. 1528). Therefore, it is clear that stigma and discrimination are harmful to the quality of life of stigmatised persons (Pescosolido et al. 2008).

Importantly, an emphasis on the association between a person's behaviour and health has created a 'new morality' (Becker 1993, p. 4). 'Being ill' is reinterpreted as 'being guilty'. For example, people with obesity are stigmatised because they let themselves go and smokers are stigmatised because they 'have no willpower' to stop (Bayer 2008, p. 468). Guilt is used as a prompter, and it might be successful in certain situations. However, guilt itself has tremendous ability to produce adverse physical and emotional effects on health (Becker 1993). It may be worth noting that the idea that health conditions, poverty, non-standard lifestyles, and so forth have long been considered a failure of will and evidence of lack of moral fibre. The reconstruction of alcoholism as a disease, for example, was an attempt to shift the focus from a moral problem to a physiological one.

The impact of stigma on the public health of the stigmatised individuals and groups is huge. Herek (2002, p. 604) states bluntly that 'stigma and discrimination are the enemies of public health'. The fact that stigma has a damaging effect on people's health has led public health officials and advocates to notice the powerfully negative results of stigmatisation for public health. In the area of HIV/AIDS, for example, it is now clear that the stigmatisation of certain groups such as commercial sex workers, injecting drug users, and gay men would only make them more susceptible to HIV infection and push them out of reach of those who attempt to help them to modify the behaviours that put them and others at risk (Stuber et al. 2008).

Within healthcare settings, Whitehead and colleagues (2001b, p. 29) contend that perceptions of difference may 'become professionalised'. Within a medical framework, it may be acceptable to treat someone differently because they are seen, in some ways, to be too 'dis-ordered'. For example, because of the lack of an interpreter, healthcare providers might be reluctant or refuse to provide care to individuals living with mental illness who are from ethnic minorities. This is simply because healthcare providers think that these people cannot or do not speak English and would not understand what they are told. This means that these individuals could be excluded from healthcare services to which others in the society have access. This is what we have referred to as 'social exclusion', which can have a negative impact on the lives of many marginalised people.

Stop and Think

» An injecting drug user who has no history of HIV infection is not allowed to donate blood at a local blood donation event. What do you think may explain this?

» A new mother who has been living in her local residence for a number of years is told not to bring her newborn baby to a play group in her local area because the baby has a visible physical malformation. What impact will this have on her and her newborn?

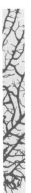

Mythbuster

Consider whether you see the following as questionable. What does this tell you about our societal values?

• A nurse refuses to provide care to a female patient who lives with HIV/AIDS because of her own ideas about the cause of HIV/AIDS. She believes that the woman acquired the disease through promiscuity, which she does not approve of.
• A mother of an autistic boy has difficulty placing him in the local school because the school thinks he would not be able to learn or fit in with others, and his condition may lead to discrimination against him.
• An overweight young woman who works at a local business office is told to lose a substantial amount of weight or she will be sacked from her work, even though such an action is illegal.

Stigma, discrimination, and HIV/AIDS

HIV/AIDS Human Immunodeficiency Virus (HIV) and Acquired Immunodeficiency Syndrome (AIDS) emerged as a major public health issue in 1981 in North America. It is a highly stigmatised illness because it is seen to be associated with individuals who engage in deviant sexual behaviour or anti-social behaviour of other kinds.

Globally and locally, the **HIV/AIDS** epidemic has offered the circumstance for a powerful argument that connects stigmatisation and public health (Bayer & Stuber 2006). From the onset of the epidemic, HIV/AIDS has been seen not only as a medical condition, but also as a stigmatised state (Herek & Glunt 1993; Letteney & LaPorte 2004). Scambler (2003, p. 199), states clearly that HIV/AIDS 'has been both medicalized as "disease" and moralized as "stigma"'. HIV/AIDS was first recognised in 1981 and since then it has provoked forceful reactions from others (Scambler 2003). HIV/AIDS uniquely combined 'sex, drugs, death and contagion' (Scambler 2003, p. 199). This unique combination made HIV/AIDS a powerfully stigmatising disease. It is also prevalent among those who are already members of stigmatised groups, initially gay men, and later injecting drug users (Parker & Aggleton 2003; Scambler 2003). Globally, in countries where HIV/AIDS is predominantly heterosexually transmitted, stigmatisation and discrimination are also pervasive. Those who are from marginalised groups such as poor people, women, mothers, sex workers, and injecting drug users heavily bear the brunt of the impact of HIV/AIDS. Some have suggested that the stigmatisation and discrimination of these people have violated human rights. Mann and Tarantola (1998, pp. 4–5) put it succinctly: 'Those who—before the arrival of HIV/AIDS—were societally marginalized, stigmatized or discriminated against, were found gradually and increasingly to bear the brunt of the HIV/AIDS epidemic. Human rights violations are now recognized to be primordial root causes of vulnerability to the epidemic.'

See also Chapter 17 on social justice and human rights.

Despite the fact that society now has better understanding of the causes and impacts of HIV/AIDS, the burden of prejudice continues to exist (Carlisle 2001; Liamputtong et al. 2009; Vlassoff & Ali 2011). Goffman (1963, p. 70) warns that 'familiarity need not reduce contempt'. Research continues to reveal the ways in which society neglects the need for healthcare for those living with HIV/AIDS (Carlisle 2001; Deng et al. 2007; Anderson et al. 2008).

It is suggested that HIV and AIDS have particular traits which initiate a high level of stigma (Parker & Aggleton 2003). As stigma is socially constructed and is attributable to cultural, social, historical, and situational factors, stigmatised individuals can be beset by feelings of shame and guilt. As discussed earlier, a major consequence of stigmatisation is discrimination and it occurs when an individual 'is treated unfairly and unjustly' because of the perception that the individual has deviated from a norm observed by others (Deng et al. 2007, p. 1561). As such, the HIV/AIDS stigma is perceived as 'an individual's deviance from socially accepted standards of normality' and these can include such deviance as 'immorality', 'promiscuity', 'perversion', 'contagiousness', and 'death'. Hence, people living with HIV/AIDS (PLWHA) are socially constructed as the 'other' who are 'disgracefully different from and threatening to the general public' (Zhou 2007, p. 2856).

The HIV/AIDS stigma continues to manifest inequalities in class, race, and gender (Parker & Aggleton 2003; Reidpath & Chan 2005; Simbayi et al. 2007). Those who are seen to be associated with sexual promiscuity, homosexuality, and drug use are particularly vulnerable to stigma. Women are more vulnerable to the stigma associated with HIV/AIDS as a sexually transmitted disease (Lawless et al. 1996; Cullinane 2007; Ndinda et al. 2007). In African and Asian countries, women living with HIV/AIDS are frequently referred to as 'vectors', 'diseased', and 'prostitutes', but these terms are seldom used about infected men (Ndinda et al. 2007, p. 93). Clearly, discrimination against PLWHA is not simply about HIV/AIDS as a disease. Rather, it intersects with other social prejudices and these include homophobia, racism, and sexism (Parker & Aggleton 2003). Hence, when women living with HIV/AIDS feel stigma, it is not 'only their internalization of the AIDS stigma, but also an effect of their interactions with others or actual experiences with public attitudes through which AIDS-related social standards are manifested' (Zhou 2007, p. 2856).

Often, stigma is multidimensional. There are three broad types of HIV/AIDS-related stigma. First is self-stigma which occurs through 'self blame and self-deprecation' in those living with HIV/AIDS. Second is perceived stigma, which is related to a person's fear that if they disclose their HIV positive status, they may be stigmatised. Third is enacted stigma, which occurs when individuals are actually discriminated against because of their HIV status—actual or perceived (Thomas 2006, p. 3175).

Stigma may be manifested in actions such as gossip, verbal abuse, and distancing from people living with HIV/AIDS. It ranges from subtle actions to 'extreme degradation, rejection and abandonment' (Thomas 2006, p. 3175). These manifestations may change over time (Thomas 2006).

Case Study 15.2   Stigma and Thai women living with HIV/AIDS

There is currently a high prevalence of HIV and AIDS among Thai women. Despite the fact that Thailand has a progressive national approach to dealing with HIV and AIDS, the stigma of HIV/AIDS and the fear of the infection remains. Liamputtong and colleagues (2009) suggest that stigma and discrimination towards PLWHA in Thailand, as experienced by the women in their study, still exists, although it was not as marked as others found earlier. Thai people, even family members of the women in their study, still have fears about HIV and AIDS. This fear is created by the AIDS campaigns in the nation (Lyttleton 2000). Although the initial mass media campaigns in Thailand acted as an 'effective buffer against high rates of transmission' (Lyttleton 2000, p. 224), the aggressive campaigns have also created fear of AIDS among Thai people and a continuing sense of the stigma that people attach to HIV and AIDS. Although there is more local acceptance in some parts of Thailand, such as in the north and in rural areas because of the common presence of HIV/AIDS (Lyttleton 2004; VanLandingham et al. 2005), PLWHA are still rejected by their family, close kin, and particularly others in the community (Lyttleton 2004; Maneesriwongul et al. 2004; Sringernyuang et al. 2005; Apinundecha et al. 2007). The advancement of HIV treatments such as antiretroviral vaccine (ARV) has prolonged the lives of many PLWHA as well as reduced AIDS to a manageable chronic condition (Lyttleton et al. 2007). This has, however, also increased the disclosure of HIV/AIDS and many PLWHA are now subjected to stigma and discrimination in the community (Apinundecha et al. 2007).

Often, ignorance, a lack of accurate information about HIV and AIDS, and misunderstanding about HIV transmission are the common sources of HIV/AIDS stigma (Apinundecha et al. 2007; Zhou 2007; Vlassoff & Ali 2011).

However, as Parker and Aggleton (2003, p. 17) warn, it is crucial to recognise that stigma occurs 'within specific contexts of culture and power'. They also suggest that 'discrimination is characterized by cross-cultural diversity and complexity' (p. 14). Hence, socio-cultural beliefs, values, and morals within local contexts have played a major role in constructing stigma and discrimination (Zhou 2007). Stigma also changes over time. What was stigmatised in older times may not be seen as carrying too much of a stigma now. The HIV/AIDS stigma may also appear far more transparent to some groups of people, but not so to others (Reidpath & Chan 2005; LeBel 2008). Some individuals or groups are more likely to be perceived by society as 'innocent victims of HIV' (Sontag 1991), for example, infants who have contracted HIV through maternal transmission or infected blood. The label of 'innocence' is applied because they are perceived as 'blameless' (Katz 1981). On the contrary, those who have contracted HIV/AIDS through homosexual activities and drug use tend to carry an extra stigma because of their own 'deviant behavior' (LeBel 2008, p. 411).

What has been done to manage stigma

According to LeBel (2008), in order to entirely reshape public perceptions and reactions towards stigmatised people, there is a need for more organised and structural attempts that include both policy and legal action. The results of these attempts may produce a long-term effect on our anti-stigma efforts (see Link et al. 2002; Parker & Aggleton 2003; Puhl & Brownell 2003; Heijnders & Van Der Miej 2006). It has been suggested that through contact with the stigmatised persons and educational campaigns, the stigmatising attitudes of the public could be improved. It has been shown that when the general public have a direct interaction with individuals from stigmatised groups, public attitudes towards the stigmatised have improved (Corrigan & Penn 1999; Brown et al. 2003). Similarly, involving stigmatised individuals as speakers in educational sessions to educate the general public is effective in promoting favourable perceptions and responses of the target audiences as these people can give more accurate information and debunk many misconceptions about them (see Corrigan et al. 2002; Couture & Penn 2003).

Additionally, LeBel (2008) suggests that protest and advocacy can work effectively as a strategy to reduce stigma. Collective tactics such as 'social activism' have proved to be valuable. Thus far, we have witnessed these collective tactics among several stigmatised groups including gays/lesbians, individuals with physical disabilities, people living with mental illness, and other stigmatised groups, and they have been successful in changing official policies and laws. It is argued that this strategy is the most powerful and long-lasting way of reducing and eradicating prejudice and discrimination (Major et al. 2000; see also Sayce 2000; Corrigan & Lundin 2001; Parker & Aggleton 2003; Shih 2004).

The motive and ability to resist or deny the label of deviance among stigmatised groups is an interesting aspect of stigma-related reduction and eradication. In Foucault's term (1981), these people would employ 'reverse discourse' as a way to resist the label of deviance and hence avoid being stigmatised. This discourse allows individuals and groups to 'present a positive affirmation of their identity and perspectives rather than a deviance designation' (Roach Anleu 2006, p. 422). Collectively, the stigmatised groups can generate a strategy that can be used to reject the standard social values and norms (Anspach 1979). In the HIV/AIDS area, according to Taylor (2001, pp. 795-6), there have been many strategies that individuals and groups have used to combat and abolish stigma. Gay men have adopted such symbols as the pink triangle, which is a symbol that the Nazis used in the Holocaust to mark out homosexuals before slaughtering them, to counteract their stigmatisation (Gilmore & Somerville 1994). Two UK voluntary organisations, 'Gay Men Fighting AIDS' and 'ACT UP' (AIDS Coalition to Unleash Power) are good examples of political activation which make use of power as a response to combat stigma. See also Case Study 15.3 below about a stance that Thai women living with HIV/AIDS adopt as a way to resist the stigmatisation of their condition.

Case Study 15.3   AIDS support group and women living with HIV/AIDS in Thailand

Because of stigma and discrimination, many people living with HIV/AIDS attempt to find strategies to deal with or fight against it. A study by Liamputtong and colleagues (2009) revealed that joining AIDS support groups was a strategy used by some Thai women to counteract the stigma of their conditions and lives. As Lyttleton and colleagues (2007, S49) contend, PLWHA support groups act as 'a panacea for stigma and alienation', hence it is not too surprising to see many women in this study joining and participating in group activities regardless of their physical condition.

Support groups offered women more knowledge about the illness and how to deal with it better. As Foucault (1980) theorises, with more knowledge, individuals feel that they have more power to deal with their situations. Support groups also provided women with a sense of belonging. The Thai women got to know more about others who were in the same situation as themselves. Joining the group made them realise that they were not alone in the lonely world of living with HIV and AIDS. With more knowledge and an increased sense of belonging from being part of the support groups, the women attained greater emotional strength to deal with their health condition and the stigma associated with it. Joining support groups created collective power for all women, and this collective power allowed the women to defend their conditions and see their situations in a more positive light.

The most powerful way to fight against stigma and discrimination against HIV and AIDS occurs when the communities are able to mobilise themselves to do so (Parker & Aggleton 2003). Several studies have clearly demonstrated empowerment and social mobilisation in response to HIV and AIDS in various societies (see Daniel & Parker 1993; Altman 1994; Epstein 1996; Parker 1996; Liamputtong et al. 2009). Parker and Aggleton (2003) advocate that it is time for us to begin thinking more seriously about using new models for advocacy and social change in our response to HIV/AIDS-related stigma and discrimination, and building community strength is one of these models. The development of AIDS support groups in Thailand as presented by Liamputtong and colleagues (2009) and elsewhere is a good example of community strength.

Summary

Deviance is a common characteristic of all societies because it signifies the values and norms of a culture. It is based on the idea that some individuals are unacceptably different and this often leads to stigma. Although deviance and stigma are socially constructed, they can impact on the lived experiences of many individuals and groups, particularly those who are already vulnerable to ill health such as individuals with mental health concerns or living with HIV/AIDS. In order to eradicate deviance and stigma, the authors agree with Scambler (2003, p. 201) who contends that there should no longer be any sanction to 'mark' some individuals as deviant and stigmatised and then treat them as 'outsiders'. Instead of treating difference as a basis for discrimination and rejection, it should be credited as 'a source of celebration'. As primary deliverers of healthcare, health professionals are in the best position to embark on local and global dialogue, which can influence the creation of new policies and laws that would make the experiences of stigmatised individuals and groups more positive. This will inevitably enhance their health and well-being and make the lives of marginalised and vulnerable people better in many ways.

Tutorial exercises

1   Watch the Australian film *The Black Balloon* (Film Finance Corporation Australia Limited 2007) which portrays the lives of the parents and a brother of an autistic child. It is accessible in most university libraries and DVD shops. How can the film help you make sense of the concepts that are included in this chapter, particularly in terms of difference, deviance, and stigma?

2   Gay and bisexual men and injecting drug users have been labelled 'guilty HIV/AIDS carriers' by the media (Scambler 2003). What is your opinion of this accusation? How has this label come about? What can we explain about this accusation?

3   Cigarette smoking used to be a norm in society, but recently it has been seen as 'deviant behaviour'. As a result, there have been many bans on smoking in offices and public places such as restaurants. What are the main reasons for this change in societal norms? What arguments have people put in place to make the behaviour deviant? Is there any benefit in making cigarette smoking a deviant behaviour?

Further reading

Bayer, R. (2008). Stigma and the ethics of public health: Not can we but should we. *Social Science & Medicine*, 67, 463–72.

Becker, H.S. (1963b). *Outsiders: Studies in the sociology of deviance*. New York: Free Press.

Falk, G. (2001). *Stigma: How we treat outsiders*. Amherst, NY: Prometheus Books.

Goffman, E. (1990). *Stigma: Notes on the management of spoiled identity*. Harmondsworth: Penguin.

Liamputtong, P., Haritavorn, N., & Kiatying-Angsulee, N. (2009). HIV and AIDS, stigma and AIDS support groups: Perspectives from women living with HIV and AIDS in central Thailand. *Social Science and Medicine*, special issue on Women, Motherhood and AIDS Care in Resource Poor Settings, 69(6), 862–8.

Link, B.G., & Phelan, J.C. (2001). Conceptualizing stigma. *Annual Review of Sociology*, 27, 363–85.

Mason, T., Carlisle, C., Watkins, C., & Whitehead, E. (eds) (2001). *Stigma and social exclusion in healthcare*. London: Routledge.

Roach Anleu, S.L. (2006). *Deviance, conformity and control*, 4th edn. Sydney: Pearson Education Australia.

Scambler, G. (2009). Health-related stigma. *Sociology of Health and Illness*, 31(3), 441–55.

Stuber, J., Galea, S., & Link, B.G. (2008). Smoking and the emergence of a stigmatized social status. *Social Science and Medicine*, 67, 420–30.

Yang, L.H., Kleinman, A., Link, B.G., Phelan, J.C., Lee, S., & Good, B. (2007). Culture and stigma: Adding moral experience to stigma theory. *Social Science and Medicine*, 64, 1524–35.

Websites

<http://community-2.webtv.nct/stigmanet/LINKSAntiStigma>

This website is maintained by the National Stigma Clearinghouse and provides information on anti-stigma programs, resources, and research.

<www.sdsmt.edu/online-courses/is/soc00/Deviance.htm>

This website includes a collection of different sites that discuss issues relevant to deviance and criminology.

<www.avert.org/hiv-aids-stigma.htm>

The website provides good discussions on the impact of stigma and discrimination on people living with HIV/AIDS.

This is a good website that provides information on news, research, and other material. It aims to provide information about how to combat and eradicate HIV/AIDS-related stigma.

<http://nortonbooks.typepad.com/everydaysociology/2010/03/rethinking-nudity-and-deviance.htm>

This is an interesting blog that discusses deviance in the context of cosmetic surgery, which has been a popular trend among celebrities and movie stars and many others.

<www.positivedeviance.org>

This website explores the notion of positive deviance, which is an interesting concept that readers might like to explore further.

16 | **Health and the media**

Linda Portsmouth

TOPICS COVERED

This chapter covers the following topics:
- impact of the mass media on public health
- utilising the mass media to promote public health
- developing media materials to communicate health messages

KEY TERMS

Entertainment-education
Health literacy
Marketing
Mass media

Media advocacy
Public health communication
Semiotics
Social marketing

Introduction

The mass media constitute one of the social determinants of health. They are one of the many features of a society that impacts on people's knowledge, attitudes, and beliefs about health—and thus on their health behaviours. The mass media that people are exposed to, and interact with, have a measurable impact on their health choices and outcomes. Many people gain much of their understanding of health from what they see and hear on television, the internet, radio, and in newspapers and magazines.

The mass media are pervasive and persuasive, reaching population-wide with health information in a way that promotes and normalises the health concepts portrayed. The mass media play a part in the socialisation of children and adolescents—influencing them as to what to expect and what is expected of them in their society.

This chapter will discuss the impact of the mass media on health and how they can be used to promote health. News and current affairs, entertainment, the internet—and the advertising that pays for most of it—often contain messages of significance to public health. Public health professionals seek to explore the impact of the mass media—aiming to describe, quantify, and counter any negative influence on population health. We also study the effective techniques used by media professionals and learn to work in partnership with media professionals. This enables public health professionals to successfully communicate health messages via the mass media in a way that promotes population health. We seek to influence news and current affairs content to increase people's awareness of health issues, often advocating for a change in policy or legislation. We seek to influence existing entertainment and develop entertainment-education media. We have also successfully developed social marketing campaigns that include the use of advertising (among other activities) to promote health.

The chapter will also outline the process by which successful media materials and campaigns can be developed. Working closely with members of population groups at risk allows us to develop concepts, messages, and media materials that will communicate most effectively with that particular group—and thus have a greater impact on their health.

The mass media

Media means 'middle' in Latin and the media lie in the middle of the communication process—between the people who send messages and the people who receive them (O'Shaugnessy & Stadler 2008). The media are the means by which we 'transmit information and entertainment across time and space', with the **mass media** enabling mass communication to a large audience (p. 3). The mass media require technology and electricity to produce—and some mass media also require technology and electricity to consume at the other end. The mass media are one of society's ways of communicating with its members.

The mass media can be contrasted with 'limited-reach' media—which communicate with individuals or smaller groups of people within a limited geographical area. Limited-reach media include items such as pamphlets, DVDs, posters, T-shirts, drink bottles, stickers, and fridge magnets. Mass media can also be contrasted with 'folk media' or 'popular media'—the traditional media that humans used to communicate long before we could read and write. People everywhere enjoy music, song, theatre, puppetry, and dance as a form of entertaining communication. Public health

Mass media The means by which messages are communicated throughout a society, transmitting the same message to large numbers of people over a large geographical area at the same time, e.g. television, cinema, radio, the internet, newspapers, and magazines.

professionals use folk media when these are the best way to communicate their health message; they might be the most culturally appropriate form of communication for the health issue and the target group. It may also be that the target group has low literacy levels and/or limited access to those mass media that require technology and electricity. The traditional dividing line between mass media and both limited-reach and folk media has become blurred over the last 15 years as limited-reach media such as pamphlets are now routinely put up on websites and gain frequent hits as people search for health information using their web browsers. Videos of folk media performances can now be seen on YouTube by people all over the world. Some may argue that social network services on the internet are limited-reach media as people need to sign up to access other members—but how many hundreds of millions of members are needed before Facebook can be considered a mass media tool in its own right?

The mass media constitute a powerful, far-reaching social influence—particularly with the impact of globalisation of media and the internet over the past couple of decades. Never before, in the history of the planet, have such a large proportion of the population been exposed to the same messages at the same time. O'Shaughnessy and Stadler (2008, p. 34) argue that the media 'show us what the world is like; they make sense of the world for us' as they represent, interpret, and evaluate the world, noting that many media products 'do not show or present the real world; they construct and re-present reality' (p. 35). The authors also acknowledge that the media are 'not the only social forces to make sense of the world for us, nor do they have total control over how we see and think about the world' (p. 35), noting the influence of, for example, family, religion, and education.

Mass media impact on health

Seeking health information via the mass media

When people look for health information, the media sources they seek out and trust are influenced by their level of health literacy, educational level, age, gender, ability to access the digital media, culture, and religion. **Health literacy** is 'the wide range of skills and competencies that people develop to seek out, comprehend, evaluate and use health information and concepts to make informed choices, reduce health risks, and increase quality of life' (Zarcadoolas et al. 2006, p. 5). Health literacy is related to, but not the same as, the ability to read and write. People can have high educational levels and yet not have highly developed health literacy—and vice versa. In an Australian study, Dart (2008) found that the internet is considered an important source of health information for most people, noting that people from lower socio-economic backgrounds had less access. He also noted well-developed health literacy skills—most people did not fully trust the internet, as they were aware that the credibility of websites varies.

Health literacy The individual's ability to successfully seek out, identify, interpret, and act on health information so as to protect and improve their health.

Mass media representation of health

The knowledge, attitudes, beliefs, and behaviours of many people are influenced by the health messages they are exposed to via the mass media. The health issues reported in the newspaper, explored on a television current affairs program, shared by celebrities on the front cover of a magazine displayed at the supermarket checkout, and experienced by characters on television dramas or in movies enters the public consciousness. People are stimulated to think about the particular health issue and, if they have no firsthand experience of the issue, will tend to think of it in the way it is presented by the media.

It is important to consider how the mass media can impact on the health of some of society's most vulnerable members: children and adolescents. Strasburger and colleagues (2009) discuss, for example, extensive research which concluded that aggression is a behaviour that children can learn from witnessing media violence and that while media violence is not the major cause of violence, it is a 'socially significant…part of a complex web of cultural and environmental factors that teach and reinforce aggression as a way of solving problems' (p. 193). Strasburger and colleagues also review the literature regarding children and adolescents' frequent exposure to sexual material via the mass media. They argue that most of this material is either suggestive or explicit, with few messages about safer sex and sexual responsibility. The authors note that several studies reveal that the media are an important source of information about sex for teenagers. Strasburger and colleagues also discuss several studies which conclude that teenagers who are exposed to a lot of media are more likely to

Stop and Think

Karl is 18. He is planning to go out to a nightclub with a group of his friends. He wants to have fun and would like to meet an attractive young woman and start a relationship. He is a bit shy and worries that he will say the wrong thing and not look or act 'cool'. In movies, he has noticed that the main male characters often seem to be having a drink while romantic things happen to them. A TV ad he has found amusing shows sporty guys having a great time together drinking beer and getting the attention of beautiful women by offering them a drink. Karl decides that he will have a few drinks to relax him and help him have a laugh with his mates.

» What could be the adverse health outcomes of his night out?

» How do you think his attitudes and behaviours are influenced by the media?

Jasmine is 13. She loves to access social networking media and has her own Twitter and Facebook accounts. Her parents have never accessed these media and so do not know how it works or who she is in contact with. She met a new friend in a chat room two months ago. He is a 14-year-old boy who lives a couple of suburbs away. They have been getting closer and closer and he has started to ask her about her body and if she has ever had sex. She has not told her parents about this boy because she thinks they would stop her talking to him if they knew that he had asked her to meet him in the local park next weekend.

» What could be the adverse health outcomes of this social media contact?

» How do you think Jasmine's attitudes and behaviours are influenced by the nature of the media she is using?

overestimate the number of their peers who are engaged in sexual activity, and feel pressure from the media to begin having sex; this increases the likelihood of earlier sexual activity.

The relationship between the mass media and mental health is another important example of mass media impact. In a review of two decades of research, Klin and Lemish (2008) conclude that the mass media have perpetuated misconceptions and stigma about people with mental illness due to 'inaccuracies, exaggeration, or misinformation' (p. 434). They argue that the mass media tend to portray people with mental illness as male, violent, and unpredictable. They note that through news coverage, entertainment, and advertising the mass media have shaped community attitudes towards people with mental illness and this has formed a barrier to such people seeking assistance. There is also a clear link between the mass media and suicide. Stack (2003) discusses the 'copycat effect'—that suicides reported in the media trigger people to emulate what they have seen reported. News reporting of real suicides (4.03 times) and suicides of celebrities (14.3 times) are more likely to trigger suicides than fictional suicides in the entertainment media (Stack 2003). Sudak and Sudak (2005) point to more suicides resulting from media reports that 'romanticize or dramatise the description of suicidal deaths' (p. 495). An Australian study supports these findings, reporting that 39% of media items resulted in increased male suicide and 31% resulted in increased female suicide (Pirkis et al. 2006). The effect noted by the researchers was more likely if there were several media reports, it was reported on television, and the suicides were completed rather than just attempted. Recommendations for media reporting were made by all of the above authors and a later study found more positive or neutral reporting of mental illness in the Australian news media (Henson et al. 2009). Media reporting of major disasters and terrorist attacks has also been implicated as a contributor to mental health problems such as post-traumatic stress disorder in children (Pfefferbaum et al. 2002; Saylor et al. 2003).

Marketing was defined by Kotler and colleagues (2009, p. 7) as 'an activity, set of institutions and processes for creating, communicating, delivering and exchanging offerings that have value for customers, clients, partners, and society at

Marketing The strategies used by commercial or non-profit enterprises—including the use of persuasive communications such as advertising—that aim to change attitudes so that the consumer feels positive towards, and decides to buy or use, the advertised product or service.

Stop and Think

Public health professionals are concerned when the product or service being marketed has a negative impact on health. Tobacco advertising is an important example. Tobacco was advertised in Australia—and still is in many places in the world—despite clear evidence that it damages health. How did the tobacco companies advertise their product? Australians only see tobacco advertising when they travel—or if the tobacco product is promoted by being placed into media they access such as movies at the cinema. Exploration of tobacco advertising gives an interesting insight into how advertising is crafted to be so persuasive to people. Link to these two websites to see some tobacco advertising posters—but do not be too influenced by them!

<http://wellmedicated.com/lists/40-gorgeous-vintage-tobacco-advertisements>

<www.tobaccofreekids.org/ad_gallery>

large'. Marketing is often thought of as just selling and advertising, but Kotler and colleagues (p. 5) describe these as 'the tip of the marketing iceberg'. Marketing discovers and meets the customer's needs, building an ongoing relationship that leads to profit. Marketers aim to provide the right product, at the right price, in the right place, at the right time—and advertising is one method used to promote this to customers. Advertising has an enormous impact on purchasing behaviours—or companies would not have advertising budgets worth millions of dollars.

Semiotics The study of the meaning of signs and symbols (e.g. images and colours) within a particular culture and how they communicate specific information and influence the interpretation of messages.

Semiotics is the study of sign systems and the meanings (feelings, beliefs, or ideas) that people within a culture attach to them (O'Shaughnessy & Stadler 2008). Signs and symbols include language, colours, objects, facial expressions, clothing, and hairstyles. Note the images and words that were used in the advertisements in the above two internet links. What were the advertisers promising when they placed the words and images alongside the cigarettes they were trying to sell? Analyse the semiotics. The people in the images are attractive and many of them are having a wonderful time with other attractive people. They are shown enjoying a golden and wealthy, carefree and relaxing, or highly romantic lifestyle. They are having fun or are quietly satisfied by their success. There are celebrities or trusted community members (e.g. doctors) promoting tobacco. The Virginia Slims ads promise a voice and freedom for women. The Marlboro ads connect their tobacco with a rugged outdoors cowboy lifestyle for men. Many of the ads suggest sexual success. Advertising often presents stereotypes of what is generally agreed in society as what we should aspire to be, do, or have in order to be successful. Stereotypes enable customers to quickly see that desirable people are connected to this product—thus the product must be desirable too. Tobacco advertising offers us a wonderful life if we smoke cigarettes.

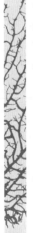

Mythbuster

Consider why you see the following as questionable. What does this tell you about our societal values?

- Tobacco companies, who are unable to advertise their product in Australia, are pouring millions of dollars into advertising in developing countries. Some of the advertising communicates the message—by use of stereotypes and images—that smoking is a thing done by people in rich countries and that if you smoke, you will appear more like them. The companies also use the full range of marketing techniques—such as giving away free cigarettes to young people at music concerts they sponsor. As the number of smokers in richer countries declines, the number in poorer countries is increasing.

- When people search for health information on the internet, some companies pay for advertising so that the link to their product appears at the top of the list of hits. Links to credible health information from reputable health organisations can be lower on the list than information pages put together by community members who do not know much about the health issue they are writing about.

- Some companies use the social media to market their products, particularly to children and young people. Marketers, for example, are able to enter chat rooms, posing as a child or teenager, and start off discussion about the product or service they are employed to promote.

Case Study 16.1   Television food advertising and children

The levels of childhood obesity are increasing globally with overweight and obese children more likely to become overweight adults who are at higher risk of health problems such as cardiovascular disease, diabetes, and some cancers (WHO 2010b). Using BMI measurements, it has been estimated that between 1985 and 1995 the proportion of Australian children who were overweight increased by between 60% and 70% and the proportion of Australian children who were obese more than tripled (Magarey et al. 2001; Booth et al. 2003). The most current Australian statistics, from the 2007 Australian National Children's Nutrition and Physical Activity Survey, indicated that 16.7% of children are overweight with a further 5.7% being obese (Commonwealth of Australia 2008).

Public health professionals have looked for the reason for this rise in childhood obesity. While there is a genetic predisposition to obesity (Wardle et al. 2008), this does not explain the rapid increase over the past two decades. The 2007 Australian National Children's Nutrition and Physical Activity Survey (Commonwealth of Australia 2008) revealed that 26.2% of children did not meet the recommended 60 minutes of moderate to vigorous physical activity per day and 66.6% of children exceeded the recommended two hours of screen time per day. There is a link between the amount of television watched and childhood obesity (Wake et al. 2003; Salmon et al. 2006). Public health professionals wondered if the time spent watching television rather than participating in physical activity has contributed to the development of obesity. The link between physical activity levels and obesity has been explored and it is now thought that the obesity causes the lack of physical activity rather than the other way around (Metcalf et al. 2010).

The Australian National Children's Nutrition and Physical Activity Survey (Commonwealth of Australia 2008) also discovered that Australian children's diets are higher in saturated fat, sugar, and salt—and lower in fruit and vegetables—than recommended by the Australian National Dietary Guidelines. Several Australian and international studies have demonstrated that children's television viewing is associated with a higher consumption of fatty foods, soft drinks, and sweet and salty snacks, and a lower consumption of fruit and vegetables (Woodward et al. 1997; Coon et al. 2001; Coon & Tucker 2002; Lowry et al. 2002; Boynton-Jarrell et al. 2003; Giammattei et al. 2003; Zuppa et al. 2003). Children from families that routinely watch TV during meal-times have been found to consume fewer fruits and vegetables and more fast foods than children whose families do not (Coon et al. 2001).

Australian children have been estimated to watch an average of 23 hours of television per week (just over three hours per day) (Woodward et al. 1997; Story 2003) with an average of eight food ads per hour, and thus are estimated to be exposed to over 10,000 food advertisements every year (Story 2003). Almost 80% of these food ads are for non-core foods and approximately 50% are for fast foods, chocolate, and confectionary (Zuppa et al. 2003; Neville et al. 2005; Chapman et al. 2006). Children of all ages who watch more television have consistently been found to desire more advertised products than children who watch less television (Robinson 2001). Children ask for and eat the foods that they see advertised (Hitchings & Moynihan 1998) and eat more of them after seeing television advertisements—particularly obese children (Halford et al. 2007). Giveaways (such as toys) and messages promoting taste or fun were the most used marketing strategies to Australian children, with the most frequently used features being cartoons and scenes of people eating the food within a social setting (Hill & Radimer 1997). Goris et al. (2010) attribute 10–28% of Australia's childhood obesity to television food advertising.

There has been an international call for the banning of television food advertising to children (WHO 2010b)—and this has already occurred in several countries. The Australian Television Communications and Media Authority has produced the Children's Television Standards 2009 which list standards that advertising to children is required to adhere to: <www.acma.gov.au/webwr/aba/contentreg/codes/television/documents/childrens_tv_standards_2009.pdf>. These standards stipulate that such advertising requirements as popular characters cannot be used to promote foods during children's viewing times, pressure cannot be put on children to ask parents to purchase, children who have the food cannot be shown as superior, and those who buy the food cannot be implied to be more generous. Chapman and others (2006) and Kelly and Chau (2007) have, however, reported frequent breaches of these standards.

Australian parents are concerned about the amount of advertising their children are exposed to and support tighter restrictions on television food advertising (Morley et al. 2008). Advocacy groups (see the media advocacy section below) are lobbying for the Australian Government to ban advertising of unhealthy food to children but this has not yet occurred. Some influential advocacy and information-sharing groups include the Public Health Association of Australia, who have written a policy document, <www.phaa.net.au>; the Australian Council on Children and the Media, <www.youngmedia.org.au>; Coalition on Food Advertising to Children, <www.cancercouncil.com.au/cfac>; and The Parent's Jury, <www.parentsjury.org.au>.

Utilising the mass media for health promotion

Health communication is the 'study and use of communication strategies to inform and influence individual and community decisions that enhance health' (National Cancer Institute 2002, p. 2). **Public health communication** can be seen as a subset of health communication and 'focuses more on the health of communities and populations', being 'inherently interventionist, seeking to promote and protect health through change at all levels of influence' (Bernhardt 2004, p. 2052). The major mass media communication strategies used in public health communication are discussed in the sections below: social marketing, media advocacy, and entertainment-education. Public health communication aims to change knowledge, attitudes, beliefs, and, ultimately, behaviours. The term 'behaviour change communication' is often used, particularly in developing countries, to refer to those communication programs aiming for behaviour change. In developed countries, 'social marketing' is more commonly used to refer to such programs.

Social marketing

The most commonly cited definition for **social marketing** is that of Andreasen (1995, p. 7), who explains it as 'the application of commercial marketing technologies to the analysis, planning, execution, and evaluation of programmes designed to influence the voluntary behaviour of target audiences in order to improve their personal welfare and that of society'. Social marketers can be seen as 'selling' health and social development. The advertising on television, radio, and in newspapers—urging the community to quit smoking, drive within the speed limit, watch their waistline or increase their physical activity levels—are very visible examples of this conceptualisation of social marketing.

Social marketing campaigns have successfully influenced population-wide changes in knowledge, attitudes, beliefs, and behaviours of relevance to public health. Campaigns have targeted a range of public health issues; see the list of websites at the end of this chapter to explore some current Australian campaign messages, materials, and evaluations. Social marketing is suitable for communicating simple messages about public health issues that affect a large proportion of the general population. There is a mass media campaign aiming to increase people's physical activity levels to 30 minutes a day, for example, but readers would not see a mass media campaign that promoted safer injecting techniques by injecting drug users (that very important public health message is best communicated in a trusted face-to-face setting). Messages and images that may offend sections of the community are usually avoided. While there are occasional safe sex campaigns in the mass media, for example, the messages and materials are not as explicit as the limited-reach media developed for specific target groups. Most of the links at the end of the chapter relate to physical health, but note the last link to the innovative Western Australian 'Act, Belong, Commit', which is the first population-wide attempt to promote mental health.

Social marketing campaigns are most effective if the mass media campaign is coordinated with limited-reach media and activities within the community that support and extend the reach of the 'brand' and the message (Donovan & Henley 2010). A current, successful, and comprehensive Australian social marketing strategy is the 'Go for 2 & 5®' campaign promoting increased consumption of fruit and vegetables (see Case Study 16.2).

Donovan and Henley (2010, p. 1) take a wider view of social marketing, arguing that it is 'the one discipline to embody, within one framework, most of the principles, concepts and tools necessary for the development and implementation of effective social change campaigns'. They believe that Andreasen's definition needs to be extended to include involuntary behaviours because we now know that behaviours are influenced by environment and are thus not entirely under an individual's control. Social marketing, they state, also needs to target policymakers in order to create supportive environments. They also propose that social marketing needs to enable individuals to reach their potential by seeking to change social structures and influence the social determinants of health. Donovan and Henley would thus argue that both media advocacy and entertainment-education—discussed in the following sections—are actually social marketing activities.

Case Study 16.2   The 'Go for 2 & 5®' Campaign

<www.gofor2and5.com.au>

<www.crunchandsip.com.au>

The 'Go for 2 & 5®' Campaign is a national multi-media campaign successfully using the mass media (television, radio, newspaper, magazines, and the internet). This campaign developed paid advertising, gained publicity via public relations events, and launched excellent websites.

There has also been the development of many limited-reach media (e.g. cookbooks, pamphlets, posters, billboards, signs on taxis), point-of-sale marketing (e.g. signs on supermarket trolleys, cooking demonstrations) and school-based activities (such as 'Crunch & Sip®', a program in which schools take a formal break every day for children to drink water and eat fruit or vegetables).

Australians do not eat the recommended amount of fruit and vegetables for good health and the prevention of many chronic diseases such as cardiovascular disease and some cancers. The 'Go for 2 & 5®' campaign, as summarised by Pollard et al. (2008a, 2009a), was first run by the Department of Health in Western Australia for the three years from March 2002 to June 2005. Research revealed that people knew fruit and vegetables were 'good for them' but they did not know the recommended level of intake and thought that they were already eating enough. Research also uncovered that people did not believe they had enough time or the skills to prepare vegetables. The campaign aimed to increase Western Australian adults' knowledge about the required number of serves, inform them as to what constitutes a serve, increase their perceived need to eat more (especially vegetables), and persuade them that vegetables were easy to prepare and eat. The main target group was the family meal preparer and grocery shopper. All of the campaign materials were strongly branded with the registered, colourful, memorable logo and attention-grabbing vegetable characters based on the celebrities who provided their voices. Explore the 'Go for 2 & 5®' website above to see many current campaign materials. The first message was: 'It is easy to get an extra serving of vegies into your day.' In 2003, a question was added to encourage honest self-assessment: 'How many servings of vegies did you really eat today?'

Pollard and colleagues (2008a, 2009a) also detailed how telephone surveys tracked the responses of thousands of Western Australian adults over time—before, during, and after the campaign. These surveys discovered that 90% of adults in the Perth metropolitan area were aware of the campaign—mainly via the television advertising. The surveys revealed that the campaign successfully increased awareness of the recommended servings and improved attitudes towards eating more fruit and vegetables, and that consumption rose as a result. From 2002 to 2005 there was an increase from 1.6 to 1.8 serves of fruit, and vegetable intake rose from 2.6 to 3.2. The proportion of the adult population who reported eating the recommended two or more serves of fruit a day and five or more serves of veg rose from 7% in 2001 to 13.4% in 2005. Pollard and colleagues (2009b) noted the direct link between increasing knowledge and behaviour change—people who knew what a correct serving size was were more likely to eat more fruit and vegetables. Other Australian states without the campaign did not show this increase and had consumption levels similar to Western Australia before the campaign (Pollard et al. 2008a). These increases were so impressive that the campaign has been implemented by all other Australian states and territories.

This success was not just due to the visible campaign. 'Go for 2 & 5®' also demonstrated the successful impact of taking the wider view of social marketing discussed by Donovan and Henley (2010). Partnerships were developed between government organisations, non-government organisations, and industry in order to increase the availability of affordable, high-quality fruit and vegetables and to increase opportunities for the consumption of fruit and vegetables within different community settings (Pollard et al. 2008b). The authors listed some achievements that targeted the environmental and social determinants of fruit and vegetable consumption.

> Examples included the development of nutrition policies for schools and childcare centres; award schemes that rewarded the food industry; promotion of the correct storage, handling, and preparation of fruit and vegetables; and supporting welfare agencies in the provision of fruit and vegetables.

Media advocacy

'Advocate' comes from the Latin word meaning 'to be called to stand beside' (Stafford et al. 2009) and advocacy is 'the pursuit of influencing outcomes—including public policy and resource allocation decisions within political, economic, and social systems and institutions—that directly affect people's lives' (Cohen 2001, p. 7). Chapman (2004a, p. 361) states that **media advocacy** aims to 'develop and shape...news stories in ways that build support for public policies and ultimately influence those who have the power to change or preserve laws, enact policies, and fund interventions that can influence whole populations'. While some advocacy is more behind-the-scenes, such as meetings with politicians or policymakers, media advocacy involves public health professionals carefully planning and telling their 'story' so that it is reported in the mass media in a way that can bring about the changes in society that they desire.

Media advocacy Aims to stimulate public support—and obtain the attention and sympathy of policymakers and legislators—to gain changes in law and policy which impact on public health.

Gaining this kind of publicity for a health issue can be cost-free—as compared to the high cost of a large social marketing campaign, for example—but it is less within the control of public health professionals. Journalists and news editors decide what will be reported—as well as how, when, and where it will be reported. News is also a 'perishable commodity'—it will only be reported for a short time before it is 'yesterday's news' (Howard & Mathews 2006, p. 27).

Public health professionals working in media advocacy need to develop good working relationships with journalists. They need to know what journalists consider 'newsworthy' as this will affect how health messages need to be 'framed' so as to gain maximum media interest. Newsworthy issues, according to Howard and Mathews (2006), are those that are considered important; interesting (e.g. unusual, entertaining, human interest, emotional); timely (e.g. current, new); close to people (e.g. local issues); or prominent (i.e. famous). Public health professionals are more likely to have their message communicated if they can provide memorable stories that will connect with people's emotions. They need, for example, to give local statistics; introduce local members of the target group who are willing to be photographed or filmed and tell their story; give a new angle to the issue such as recent and compelling evidence; suggest powerful images that can be photographed or filmed; and involve celebrities or high-profile spokespeople.

Public health professionals working for large organisations will usually have a public relations or media department to assist them—while those who work for small community-based organisations will need to develop some media relations skills. After careful planning, the issue in question needs to be brought to the attention of journalists. Large organisations have the skills and resources to hold press conferences; this works well when the issue is of interest to journalists and you can be sure they will attend. Many health organisations fax or email media releases (short written pieces summing up the main points about the issue) in order to interest the journalist, to contact them or attend an event. Journalists are often also open to clear, concise emails or clear telephone messages, particularly if they have worked with the public health professionals before. The events can be initiated in order to show that many and/or prominent people feel strongly about the issues. A media release, for example, can invite journalists to a protest, a public meeting, the presentation of a petition to a politician, or the launch of an intervention that is being attended by a politician or a concerned celebrity. Another effective, no-cost strategy is to write a letter to the editor of the newspaper. This way—should the letter be well written and topical enough to be chosen—a public health viewpoint can be put onto the public agenda quickly using a few words in an email. Once media interest is shown in their issue, public health professionals need to plan for newspaper, television, or radio interviews. They need to find and train articulate and credible spokespeople—while being aware that some interviews about urgent issues can happen with little warning!

Stafford and colleagues (2009), in the reading list at the end of this chapter, is an excellent and easily accessible 'how to' guide for public health professionals. This manual describes how public health professionals can plan and implement media advocacy strategies—including how to write media releases and letters to the editor, how to prepare for interviews, and how to influence journalists and politicians.

Case Study 16.3   Anti-tobacco media advocacy

Australia has implemented a highly successful social marketing campaign encouraging people to quit smoking: <www.quitnow.info.au>. It supports cessation activities and is an international leader in the use of media advocacy to create supportive environments that encourage people not to start smoking and assist smokers to quit.

Chapman and Wakefield (2001, p. 274), in their exploration of 30 years of tobacco control in Australia, cited tobacco company documents that stated that 'Australia has one of the best organised, best financed, most politically savvy and well-connected anti-smoking movements in the world. They are aggressive and have been able to use the levers of power very effectively to propose and pass draconian legislation...Australia is a seed-bed for anti-smoking programs around the world'. Chapman and Wakefield went on to chronicle the achievements gained by tobacco control advocacy since 1970: harm reduction via reduction in the tar and nicotine levels in cigarettes; 'civil disobedience' as activists 'graffitied' tobacco advertising billboards with anti-tobacco messages; banning of tobacco advertising and sponsorship; tobacco taxes; replacement of tobacco sponsorship of sport and arts by using some of the tobacco tax income; warnings printed on cigarette packs; banning of the small packs popular with children; banning of smokeless tobacco; and the banning of smoking in transport, workplaces, and domestic environments.

Smoking rates in Australia have fallen from their peak levels of 72% for adult males in 1945 and 31% for females in 1983 (Chapman & Wakefield 2001) to some of the lowest in the world: 18% for males and 15.2% in females aged 14 years or over—as estimated from the 2007 National Drug Strategy Survey (AIHW 2010a). This survey also revealed that more than half the Australian population have never smoked and approximately a quarter of people are ex-smokers. Statistical projections released in 2006 estimated that if current trends continue, smoking will disappear in Australia by 2028 (Daube & Walker 2008).

Chapman and Wakefield (2001, p. 278) noted that media advocacy 'challenges radio and television audiences and newspaper readerships—including the politicians at whom it is often ultimately directed—to locate themselves in a moral debate'. They argued that casting the tobacco industry as 'pariahs' who require heavy regulation has been an essential part of this process—giving the examples of how advocates 'framed' tobacco as a series of 'newsworthy' issues such as advertising seducing vulnerable children, and the hidden and dangerous chemical additives in tobacco which should be revealed. Advocacy's role was to successfully frame the public health issue so it gained the support of the public and politicians—and to communicate problems which require solutions that politicians are usually responsible for finding (Chapman & Wakefield 2001).

The media advocacy in Australia was first undertaken by the advocacy group Australian Council on Smoking and Health (ACOSH), which was formed in 1967 out of frustration with the government response to calls for tobacco control (Daube & Walker 2008). ACOSH worked in partnership with government health departments and non-government organisations such as the Heart Foundation, Cancer Council, and the Australian Medical Association. Daube and Walker described ACOSH's attention-getting media strategies which reduced the credibility of the tobacco industry, increased the sympathy of the media, and eventually gained the required legislation. These strategies included buying shares in tobacco companies so they could attend AGMs and ask questions; holding a press conference releasing a report on the number of body parts removed each year due to smoking; a 'death cards' campaign where doctors sent postcards to politicians when their patients' deaths were smoking-related; a report for each MP showing the impact of smoking in their electorate; and presenting statistics in forms that could be easily understood and reported on—such as bookies' odds.

It is interesting to note that, after exploring the concepts of deviance and stigma in Chapter 15, 'smoking, smokers and the tobacco industry are today routinely depicted in everyday discourse and media representations in a variety of overwhelmingly negative ways' (Chapman & Freeman 2008, p. 25). Mass media advocacy and social marketing, according to Chapman and Freeman, have been so successful in 'denormalising' smoking behaviour that this national 'culture change' may be impacting on the mental and social health of people who smoke. Smoking is now seen as dirty and smelly and smokers are now publically framed as selfish, undesirable, undereducated, lower class, or addicts, who are a drain on health services and should not be employed (Chapman & Freeman 2008). A 2007 Western Australian survey revealed that smokers now feel like 'social pariahs' and reported that they receive 'disdainful looks' and 'social verbal bashing' when they smoke in public—with many stating that they would consider quitting so that they could 'rejoin society' (Carter 2008, p. 28). This situation presents an ethical dilemma. Public health professionals used effective media strategies that aimed to reduce the population level of smoking—placing the overall population health 'good' above the mental and social health of the minority of people who smoke. Public health would normally seek to promote the health of all population groups—so this is a rare case where public health is culpable of a negative impact on the mental and social health of a particular group in society.

Entertainment-education

The terms **entertainment-education** and *edu-tainment* have been used interchangeably in the past. De Fossard (2008) notes that a clear difference between the two is becoming widely accepted and described the key difference. Edu-tainment is education made entertaining, by the use of a story for example, so that learners are emotionally engaged in the educational experience.

Entertainment-education
A mass media 'vehicle' which is designed to entertain a wide general audience while changing societal attitudes and norms. It models and normalises behaviour change that promotes health and social development.

Entertainment-education is an entertainment experience that is sought out and appreciated by a general audience who are emotionally involved with characters they identify with. Within this entertainment experience, the 'behavior change messages are woven and modeled gradually, naturally and subtly' (De Fossard 2008, p. 19). Entertainment-education connects with people in a unique way, becomes a part of the social fabric of their lives, and thus a social influence on their health.

Most interestingly, Singhal and Rogers (2004) point out that the first recognisable entertainment-education intervention was in Australia with a radio series called 'The Lawsons' in 1944—which encouraged farmers to adopt new agricultural innovations. However, they also note that for a long period the most common form of entertainment-education was donor-supported television and radio soap opera in developing countries which communicated health messages to audiences without much mass media exposure. According to Barker (2005), one soap opera was based on the successful formula pioneered by Miguel Sabido in the late 1970s and early 1980s, who made an enormous impact on family planning in Mexico using serial television dramas (telenovelas). The 'Sabido Methodology' results in a serial drama that captures people's attention and emotions over several months or years. This allows the audience to increasingly identify with the main characters as they change their behaviour slowly, in a realistic way, in a realistic social context—with various subplots enabling the introduction of different issues in a believable way through different characters (Barker 2005). Techniques used to keep the audiences thinking and wondering about the storylines include mystery, suspense, dilemmas, and 'cliffhangers' at the end of episodes (Singhal & Rogers 2004). Piotrow and De Fossard (2004) point out that when communicating health risks that are routine or longer-term, well-written drama scripts can make the health issue appear more important, urgent, or dangerous. They mention examples such as contraceptive pills being thrown into the fire, highlighting that they need to be taken daily, and a fruit seller who contaminates his fruit due to poor personal hygiene, resulting in a stampede of people to the latrine. Singhal and Rogers (2004) note that evaluation of this type of entertainment-education reveals that it is memorable—people can recall health messages years later—and it has resulted in millions of people changing their health behaviours.

Entertainment-education is now widely applied and many forms of entertainment media are utilised. Some entertainment-education reaches a local audience—particularly when folk media such as theatre is used. Other media, such as comics and fotonovelas (stories told by the use of photos with brief dialogue in 'bubble text'), are reaching an increasingly wider audience due to dissemination via the internet. The scope of mass media entertainment-education ranges from the placement of a few lines of dialogue into an existing mass media program (e.g. the Harvard Alcohol Project; see Case Study 16.4) to an ongoing multi-media TV, radio, internet, and print program spanning several countries over several years (e.g. Soul City; see Case Study 16.5).

Case Study 16.4   The Harvard Alcohol Project, USA

The Harvard Alcohol Project (Winsten 1994; Winsten & DeJong 2001) is the first, biggest, and most famous example of public health working with the existing commercial mass media to successfully promote a health message to an entire population. This project was launched across the USA in 1988 and ran until 1992. It demonstrated how a new concept and new behaviour could be introduced and disseminated via entertainment programming to a whole society—and actually shift social norms (i.e. what is considered normal behaviour).

All of the major Hollywood studios and the ABC, CBS, and NBC television networks worked with the Center for Health Communication at Harvard School of Public Health to promote the idea of the 'designated driver'. The designated driver is the one in the group who does not drink alcohol because they are driving—and getting everyone else home safely. It was intended, according to Winsten (1994), to give the non-drinker's role 'social legitimacy' and to encourage people to plan for their transport if they intended to drink. The author outlined how he met with more than 250 television producers and writers who agreed to insert drink-driving prevention messages, including mention of designated drivers, into scripts of top-rated television programs, such as 'Cheers', 'L.A. Law', and 'The Cosby Show'. The characters of the shows acted as role models for safer behaviours. Over four years, more than 160 prime-time television programs, with audiences of up to 45 million, incorporated the health message. At the same time, the networks also agreed to air frequent Public Service Announcements promoting the designated driver concept; a number of prominent individuals and organisations endorsed the message and the campaign was widely reported in the news media (Winsten 1994; Winsten & DeJong 2001).

The term 'designated driver' became a household phrase in the USA, appearing in the 1991 edition of Webster's College Dictionary (Winsten 1994). Research revealed that, by 1998, 62% of adults who were frequent drinkers had been designated drivers or had been driven home by one (Center for Health Communication 2011). The Center for Health Communication reported that a 30% reduction in alcohol-related traffic fatalities was gained over the six years following the launch of the campaign—compared with a reduction of 0% in the three years preceding the campaign. This was equated to 50,000 lives saved by the end of 1998.

Case Study 16.5   Soul City, South Africa

<www.soulcity.org.za>

'Soul City: Institute for Health and Development Communication' is a highly successful mass media entertainment-education program. It is a highly recognised and trusted source of health information in South Africa and was the first to address national health priorities with an ongoing nationwide multi-media strategy.

Soul City was established in 1992 by two medical doctors, Garth Japhet and Shereen Usdin, who wanted to prevent the serious health and social issues they saw impacting on the lives of their patients. Dr Japhet had been writing a newspaper column but realised that he was only reaching people who were literate (UNAIDS 2005). He then discovered that educational programs on South African television might reach an audience of 500,000 while 'prime-time' television drama would reach an audience of more than 7 million (UNAIDS 2005). Drs Japhet and Usdin brought together government, donors, and business to develop prime-time, health-promoting mass media that is entertaining and well made (Singhal & Rogers 2003; UNAIDS 2005).

Singhal and Rogers (2003), UNAIDS (2005), and Usdin and colleagues (2004) describe the media materials produced by Soul City and how success is ensured by undertaking extensive research with audience groups to develop realistic scripts that resonate powerfully with their audience. Each year Soul City produces a 13-part one-hour television drama on the most popular television channel; 60 episodes of 15-minute prime-time radio drama (with different characters and storylines to the television series) in nine languages covering all regional stations on a daily basis; and three nationally distributed 36-page booklets which are designed around the television characters and serialised in 11 major newspapers. Soul City also has relationships with newspaper journalists who regularly publish features based in Soul City activities. In 2000, for children aged 8 to 10, they began 'Soul Buddyz', which also includes a television series, radio series, and print materials.

Soul City reaches millions of people in South Africa and in the neighbouring countries of Botswana, Zimbabwe, Lesotho, Swaziland, Namibia, and Zambia. The most recent evaluation available from Soul City (Health and Development Africa 2007) is of Series 7, which broadcast in 2005 and 2006. Research revealed that 87% of the total adult population of South Africa was exposed to at least one Soul City program component in 2006—with wide reach across rural and urban areas and all educational levels—particularly among black Africans; 76% of women and 69% of men watched Soul City on television in 2006—with 60% of those watching nine or more episodes. This series had a measurable impact on the HIV issues it raised including increased HIV testing, increased condom use, and an increased willingness to accept and assist people living with HIV/AIDS. Soul City has been identified by the World Health Organization as an example of best practice in the use of mass media to communicate about HIV/AIDS (UNAIDS 2005).

Soul City has also had an influence on knowledge, attitudes, and behaviours relating to many other health and social issues. Usdin and colleagues (2004) detail the famous example of the impact that 1999's Series 4 had on community practices relating to domestic violence. In one episode, people in a neighbourhood gather around a house where a husband was beating his wife, loudly banging cooking pots and pans to show their disapproval. This newly suggested practice of pot beating—or making other loud banging noises—was reported to occur in response to domestic violence in several locations after this episode was broadcast. This series also resulted in communities organising several protest marches to highlight violence against women. An evaluation of this series reported that it stimulated public discussion of domestic violence; increased recognition of the abuse of women; increased knowledge and use of a telephone hotline; and many viewers subsequently did something to stop domestic violence in their lives or in the lives of others. Interviews with viewers revealed that some women had invited their husbands to watch episodes so that they could recognise their perpetration of domestic violence—and that some men who saw it recognised for the first time that their violence against their wives was wrong.

Developing media materials to communicate health messages

The National Cancer Institute (2002) in the USA has developed a useful way of conceptualising the process of developing health communication media materials. Media materials are most successfully developed when public health and media professionals follow the four stages described below. This process can be used for the development of mass media, limited-reach media, and folk media materials. The process is a cycle because, after evaluating the health communication program they have undertaken, public health professionals are better informed as they plan for future communications.

Figure 16.1 The stages in the health communication process

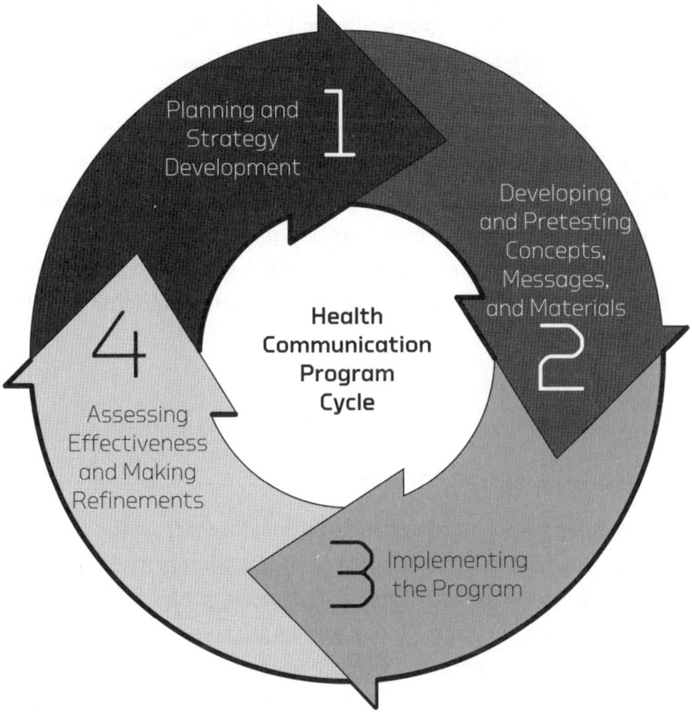

Planning and Strategy Development 1

Developing and Pretesting Concepts, Messages, and Materials 2

Health Communication Program Cycle

4 Assessing Effectiveness and Making Refinements

3 Implementing the Program

Source: NCI 2002, p. 11

Stage 1: Planning and strategy development

Adequate time spent at this vital stage will ensure a greater chance of success at later stages, and for the health communication program's overall objectives. Some people want to rush into developing their media materials as the first stage of their intervention; these people need to be held back and made to wait.

Public health professionals first need to assess the health issue and identify all parts of a possible solution. It could be that communication to the community via media materials is not the best plan of action—or that it is an excellent idea but needs to happen concurrently with communication with policymakers about changes in policy or with healthcare providers about changes in health services. It could be that the communication needs to be accompanied by changes to physical infrastructure or the social environment. It can be impossible for individuals to decide to change their behaviours if the things they need to do this are not available. We cannot, for example, produce a social marketing campaign encouraging women to go for breast screening if they are unable to access affordable, acceptable screening services close to where they live. It is difficult for people living in remote and rural areas of Australia to 'Go for 2 & 5' when the local shops do not stock affordable, high-quality fresh fruit and vegetables.

Public health professionals need to find out as much as possible about their intended audience. The target group may be of a different culture, language, religion, gender, age, and educational level than the public health professionals. Research will often reveal that the target group is made up of different audiences that require different media and messages. Surveys, interviews, or focus groups can be used to ask members of the target group such questions as: What do you know about this issue? What are you doing now? What have you tried before? What happened then? What do you think about it? What do you believe has caused it or is making it worse? What would help you to change? What is stopping you from changing? What would be the benefit—or the cost—of change to you? Do you think it is worth changing? What media do you pay attention to? What media do you believe? What media would you trust communicating about this health issue? Where are you and what are you doing when you access this media? The answers to these sorts of questions are invaluable in developing communication objectives and planning for the communication program. If these questions were not asked, public health professionals would develop media materials that made sense to them—not to a target group with a different understanding and lived experience of the particular health issue.

Stage 2: Developing and pretesting concepts, messages, and materials

The first thing public health professionals need to do in this stage is to review existing media materials and discover if there are any that meet their needs. If the decision is made that new materials need to be developed, it is useful to work with experienced media professionals who have expertise in research to ensure the concepts, messages, and materials are going to be the most effective for that particular target group. The concepts and messages need to be put together (in terms of words, images, colours, and sounds) in a way that is understandable, believable, convincing, and culturally appropriate. All of the information discovered in Stage 1 needs to be considered as this will shape the concept and the message. It is good practice to involve members of the target group in developing the concepts, messages, and materials. It is essential to then test the materials with different members of the target group to check that they are having the intended effects.

Stage 3: Implementing the program

The concepts, messages, and materials implemented are as varied as the health issue and the target group. Mass media approaches can be expensive and may not be the correct approach for the issue and target group. Mass media campaigns have been found to work best when an appropriate range of limited-reach media and person-to-person approaches also form part of the plan of action. Public health professionals can discover the kinds of messages and media that have worked for other people in similar projects—but must always be most influenced by what their target group tells them. Members of the target group are the experts on what will work for them, and it might not be what the public health professionals expect to be doing. Public health professionals may find that directly involving the target group in the program implementation (e.g. peer outreach and support) may enhance the impact of the media materials produced.

Stage 4: Assessing effectiveness and making refinements

Public health professionals need to ask such questions as: How appropriate was the message for the target audience? How effective were the media channels? How well did the message reach the target audience? What changes resulted? To what extent were the goals achieved? Were the benefits worth the cost? Evaluating the health communication program is not something that can be left until the end. Stage 1 activities include putting plans in place for evaluation. The program, methods, and media materials need to be evaluated while they are being developed and used. Surveys, interviews, and focus groups can assist in gaining the required information, but information can also be collected while the program is running. The people delivering the program can record useful information while they work (e.g. number of calls to the telephone information and support line or hits on the website after advertising appears in print, television, or radio).

Summary

The mass media constitute a powerful social determinant of health. Many people gain much of their understanding of health from messages in the mass media. This influences their health knowledge, attitudes, beliefs, and behaviours.

The mass media can have a negative impact on health. Media representation and reporting of violence, sexuality, body image, mental health, and suicide, for example, have been implicated in poor health outcomes. The marketing of products and services detrimental to health (such as tobacco) are of public health concern. Public health professionals need to recognise and study these negative impacts—and then act to counter them.

Once the mass media impacts on health are understood, the public health professional can use this knowledge to work in partnership with media professionals to utilise the mass media to promote health. Social marketing, media advocacy, and entertainment-education are the forms this activity usually takes—and all have demonstrated a strong, positive impact on public health.

Public health professionals need to carefully plan, implement, and evaluate health communication programs. It is vital, at all stages of the health communication process, to work closely with members of the media audience (target group) in order to successfully develop media materials to communicate appropriate health messages.

Tutorial exercises

1   Watch the American documentary *Super Size Me*, which won the Academy Award for best documentary in 2004. It is accessible in most university libraries and video shops. This film documents one man's decision to consume McDonald's food and drink for every meal for 30 days—with the resulting negative impact on his physical and mental health. What role do you think fast food marketing plays in the 'obesity epidemic'? Note how the documentary was made. What choices did the filmmakers make (in terms of words, vision, sound, music, and graphics) in order to make the film more persuasive?

2   Watch a commercial television station during a timeslot for children's programs. Note the advertisements for food and drink. Choose one of them and record it if possible to bring to

class. What messages are being communicated by the advertisement? What stereotypes, images, sounds, music, and colours were brought together to make the advertisement more persuasive to children? Do you think the advertisement adheres to the Australian Children's Television Standards?

3 Find an internet site that is potentially harmful to health. It may contain incorrect information, have information presented with bias (e.g. a commercial site selling 'cures'), or openly promote poor health choices (e.g. anorexia, suicide). Note the URL. What are the main messages being communicated? How were they communicated? What words, images, colours, and sound were used—and what do those choices communicate? Is the site presented as being more credible than it really is? Does it contain references for scientific information given? Does it contain advertising? What other sites does it link to? Is it clear who wrote it and how you can contact them? How might it harm health?

4 Link to the examples of the Australian social marketing campaign websites listed below. Watch their television advertisements. For each advertisement, answer the following questions: Who do you think the target group is? What is the key message? Note the way the advertisement has been constructed. What do you think the initial research revealed about the target group?

Further reading

Cancer Council Western Australia (2008). *The progress of tobacco control in Western Australia: Achievements, challenges and hopes for the future*. Perth: Cancer Council Western Australia. <www.cancerwa.asn.au/resources/2010-07-07-Tobacco-Control-Monograph.pdf>.

Donovan, R., & Henley, N. (2010). *Principles and practice of social marketing: An international perspective*, 2nd edn. Melbourne: IP Communications.

Howard, C.M., & Mathews, W.K. (2006). *On deadline: Managing media relations*, 4th edn. Long Grove, IL: Waveland Press.

National Cancer Institute (2002). *Making health communication programs work*. Bethesda, MD: National Institutes of Health, US Department of Health and Human Services. <www.cancer.gov/pinkbook>.

O'Shaughnessy, M., & Stadler, J.M. (2008). *Media and society*, 4th edn. Melbourne: Oxford University Press.

Stafford, J., Mitchell, H., Stoneham, M., & Daube, M. (2009). *Advocacy in action: A toolkit for public health professionals*, 2nd edn. Perth: Public Health Advocacy Institute of Western Australia. <www.phaiwa.org.au/index.php/component/attachments/download/35>.

Websites

<www.comminit.com>

The Communication Initiative Network connects people from all over the world so they can share their work in media communication to promote health, peace, and social development.

<www.cdc.gov/healthcommunication>

The Centers for Disease Control and Prevention's 'gateway' to many health communication and social marketing resources.

Center for Communication Programs, Johns Hopkins Bloomberg School of Public Health promotes international public health through partnering organisations to assist them in health communication. This website links to many resources such as downloadable publications/reports and examples of health communication materials.

<www.populationmedia.org>

The Population Media Center works to improve global health through the use of entertainment-education strategies. This website shares their current projects and links to many resources.

<www.communicationforsocialchange.org>

The Communication for Social Change Consortium is a non-profit organisation working globally to help people living in poor communities to communicate in such a way as to influence the change they need in their societies and in their lives.

<www.drinkingnightmare.gov.au>

<www.alcoholthinkagain.com.au>

<www.rta.nsw.gov.au/roadsafety/speedandspeedcameras/campaigns>

<www.ors.wa.gov.au/Campaigns/Pages/campaign.aspx>

<www.drugs.health.gov.au>

<www.quitnow.info.au>

<www.safesexnoregrets.com.au>

<www.findthirtyeveryday.com.au>

<www.drawthelinewa.com.au>

<www.actbelongcommit.org.au>

Interesting examples of Australian social marketing interventions and their media materials.

<http://social-marketing.org>

<www.hc-sc.gc.ca/ahc-asc/activit/marketsoc/index-eng.php>

Useful social marketing sites in the US and Canada.

<www.phaiwa.org.au>

The Public Health Advocacy Institute of WA.

17 | Health and social justice

Ann Taket

TOPICS COVERED

This chapter covers the following topics:
- the relationship between social justice, human rights, and health equity
- the role of human rights in the social and cultural determinants of health
- how progress towards meeting obligations to respect, protect, and fulfil rights relates to progress towards achieving the social and cultural determinants of health and progress towards health equity
- how human rights-based argumentation can provide a strong grounding for public health and health promotion advocacy
- how health and social policy can be scrutinised for its human rights implications

KEY TERMS

Cultural relativism
Equity
Health equity
Human rights

Inequity
Justice
Right
Social justice

Introduction

> Public health should be a way of doing justice, a way of asserting the value and priority of all human life...public health is ultimately and essentially an ethical enterprise committed to the notion that all persons are entitled to protection against the hazards of this world and to the minimisation of death and disability in society. (Beauchamp 1976, p. 13)

The Ottawa Charter (WHO 1986) lists **social justice** and **equity** as among the prerequisites for health, along with peace, shelter, education, food, income, a stable eco-system, and sustainable resources. As Muntaner and colleagues (2009) demonstrate, the report of the Commission on Social Determinants of Health (WHO CSDH 2008) foregrounds social justice and broad political and economic determinants in the world's health agenda. As Venkatapuram and colleagues (2010) discuss, the work of the Commission involved direct engagement with human rights experts and discussion of the close links between **human rights** and the social determinants of health; what remains contested is the extent to which the Commission's final report granted a sufficiently central role to human rights (see e.g. Hunt 2009).

Thus, the achievement of social justice has been closely connected to progress on human rights and the achievement of health equity. Australia, along with most member countries of the UN, has ratified the Universal Declaration on Human Rights and the range of other covenants and conventions covering human rights, thereby acquiring obligations to respect, protect, and fulfil human rights. This chapter examines the role of human rights in the social and cultural determinants of health. Using a series of case studies including Indigenous health and HIV/AIDS, this chapter explores the relationships between health and human rights and introduces readers to a wide range of resources relevant for their application in policy and practice.

Justice, in the sense defined in the Australian Concise Oxford Dictionary, and social justice as defined above, are most closely associated with the theory of justice expounded by liberal philosopher John Rawls (1971), and is consonant with Amartya Sen's important recent contribution on the idea of justice (Sen 2009). Sen's work is particularly valuable for its focus on the question of comparative judgments (comparing social arrangements to identify which is more or less just), rather than focusing on the question of the nature of just institutions and the behavioural norms implicated in these, as Rawls did. Sen's work is also fascinating in exploring a much wider ranges of sources, both Western and non-Western, in support of his argument.

The examination of the nexus between human rights, social justice, and **health equity** (the definition given is paraphrased from that in Braveman and Gruskin 2003, p. 254) provides public health professionals with an exciting opportunity to enter a new and rapidly growing field. Case Study 17.1 introduces this notion by considering the origins of the human rights approach to health. Proponents of human rights approaches to health argue that they are of vital importance in achieving improved health and reducing health inequities. Arguments based on a discourse of rights can provide a strong justification for public health action to tackle health **inequities**, and thus human rights provide a strong foundation for public health advocacy.

Social justice
The improvement of a situation of disadvantage by the redistribution of goods and resources.

Equity Fairness; the application of the principles of justice to correct or supplement rules of law.

Human rights Rights held to be justifiably belonging to any person.

Right A thing one may legally or morally claim.

Justice Fairness.

Health equity
A situation in which groups with different levels of underlying social advantage or disadvantage (wealth, power, or prestige) do not experience health inequalities associated solely with social positioning.

Inequity Inequality resulting from unfairness or bias.

Case Study 17.1   HIV/AIDS: Origins of the human rights approach to health

Jonathon Mann, Director of the Global Program on AIDS at WHO, led WHO work on HIV/AIDS, and is one of the originators of work on human rights approaches to health. The work has its origins in

- abuses of human rights suffered by those living with HIV/AIDS (see also Case Study 17.3)
- evidence that discrimination was resulting in low uptake of HIV/AIDS prevention and care programs.

Mann and Tarantola (1998, p. 5) identify four phases in the history of the response to HIV/AIDS, presenting HIV/AIDS as a

- danger to alert people about
- problem of individual behaviour
- societally contextualised behavioural issue
- human-rights-linked challenge.

The transition from third to fourth phase emerged from the recognition of the important roles of social marginalisation, stigmatisation, and discrimination in vulnerability to HIV/AIDS, and the recognition that a form of analysis focused on the societal basis of vulnerability was required—the focus on social determinants of health within human rights provided a useful framework, vocabulary, and guidance.

See also the case studies on stigma and discrimination in Chapter 15.

The chapter now begins by describing human rights and selected global human rights instruments, discussing common features of human rights, and criteria for assessing when they can justifiably be limited. It moves on to look at the relationships between human rights and the social determinants of health. The responsibilities of governments in respect of human rights are briefly described and tools for public health advocacy and action—human rights approaches to seeking social justice and health equity—are discussed. The chapter concludes with a brief reflection on the value of human rights approaches to health. Limitations of space imposed by a single chapter mean

Stop and Think

- What do you think are our human rights? Jot down your ideas.
- Watch this short video on human rights <www.humanrights.com/what-are-human-rights/brief-history/cyrus-cylinder.html>.
- Reflect on the difference between your answers, what the people interviewed at the start of the video said, and the answers given later in the video.

that the treatment of health equity, social justice, and human rights issues is necessarily brief; they are dealt with at greater length and depth in Taket (2012).

What are our human rights?

Before looking at the contemporary human rights system, it is important to acknowledge the lengthy history of human struggles that have resulted in the creation of this system; for those interested in further coverage of this history see Ishay (2008) and Moyn (2010). Our contemporary system came into being after the Second World War, with the creation of the United Nations, which has the promotion of human rights as a principal purpose according to its charter (United Nations 1945). The UN charter established general obligations that apply to all its member countries, including respect for human rights and dignity.

Three years later, the Universal Declaration of Human Rights (UDHR) was adopted (United Nations 1948). Since then, more than 20 multilateral human rights treaties have been adopted, creating legally binding obligations on the countries that have ratified them. Particularly important treaties are the two covenants: on Civil and Political Rights (ICCPR) and on Economic, Social and Cultural Rights (ICESCR); both were adopted by the UN General Assembly on 16 December 1966. The ICCPR and ICESCR, plus the Universal Declaration of Human Rights and the UN Charter, are often referred to as the 'International Bill of Human Rights'.

The UDHR contains 30 Articles; the box below gives a brief summary of their content. An important feature is the overarching principle of non-discrimination; Article 7 is explicit: 'All are equal before the law and are entitled without any discrimination to equal protection of the law.' Other articles prohibit slavery, torture, and arbitrary detention and protect freedom of expression, assembly, and religion, right to own property, and the right to work and receive an education. Of particular relevance to public health considerations is Article 25, which states, in part: 'Everyone has the right to a standard of living adequate for the health and well-being of himself and his family, including food, clothing, housing and medical care and necessary social services'.

The two covenants aim to make more explicit the content of the UDHR, and set out detail of the reporting and monitoring systems. ICCPR rights include equality, liberty, and security of person, and freedom of movement, religion, expression, and association. ICESCR focuses on well-being, including the right to work, the right to receive fair wages, the right to make a decent living, the right to work under safe and healthy conditions, the right to be free from hunger, the right to education, and the right of everyone to the enjoyment of the highest attainable standard of physical and mental health.

The creation of two covenants, with much overlap (and even more interrelationship) but distinct focuses, deserves some comment. Part of the reason for the division flows from the history of the cold war, but there is also the distinct form and nature of these two sets of rights (Gruskin et al. 2005). Civil and political rights can be seen as 'negative' rights or freedoms, generally requiring states *not* to interfere in the affairs of their citizens (e.g. privacy, freedom of expression, thought, and religion, freedom of movement and assembly, and freedom from torture, arbitrary arrest, and discrimination); these rights are sometimes referred to as 'first generation' rights. In contrast, economic, social, and cultural rights can be considered 'positive' rights, requiring states actively to implement measures to secure these rights (e.g. right to a clean environment, and rights to education, health, welfare assistance, and the right to substantive equality); these are the 'second generation' rights.

Summary content of the articles of the Universal Declaration of Human Rights

1. We are all free and equal
2. Do not discriminate
3. Right to life
4. No slavery
5. No torture
6. You have rights no matter where you go
7. We are all equal before the law
8. Your human rights are protected by law
9. No unfair detainment
10. Right to trial
11. We are always innocent until proven guilty
12. Right to privacy
13. Freedom of movement
14. Right to seek a safe place to live
15. Right to nationality
16. Marriage and family
17. Right to your own things
18. Freedom of thought
19. Freedom of expression
20. Right to public assembly
21. Right to democracy
22. Social security
23. Worker's rights
24. Right to play
25. Food and shelter for all
26. Right to education
27. Copyright
28. A fair and free world
29. Responsibility
30. No one can take away your human rights

Source: Derived from summary given in 'United for Human Rights' video on *The Story of Human Rights*, obtainable at <www.humanrights.com/#/home>

Case Study 17.2   How well is Australia doing in relation to its indigenous population?

We consider this by contrasting conclusions from the earliest and latest set of concluding observations on the Treaty data base (as at January 2011) in relation to Australia from two different monitoring committees.

1993 Concluding Observations of the Committee on Economic, Social and Cultural Rights on Australia E/C. 12/1993/9

Under section D listing the committee's principal subjects of concern, the committee identified

- problems with poor access to education and consequently employment (paragraph 8)
- problem of illiteracy (paragraph 8)
- problems with the lack of sufficient opportunities for involvement in creating awareness of cultural heritage (paragraph 11).

2010 Concluding Observations of the Committee on the Elimination of Racial Discrimination on Australia CERD/C/AUS/CO/15–17

While noting Australia's acknowledgment that Aboriginal and Torres Straits Islanders occupy a special place in its society as the first peoples of Australia and welcoming the establishment of the National Congress of Australia's First Peoples, the Committee

- expressed concern that the National Congress is only an advisory body representing member organisations and individuals and may not be fully representative of Australia's First Peoples
- regretted limited progress towards constitutional acknowledgment of Australia's Indigenous peoples, and slow implementation of the principle of Indigenous people's exercising meaningful control over their affairs
- recommended that the negotiation of a treaty agreement be considered (paragraph 15).

The Committee also expressed concern about the Northern Territory Emergency Response and its discriminatory impact on affected communities, including restrictions on Indigenous rights to land, property, social security, adequate standards of living, cultural development, work, and remedies (paragraph 16).

Source: Extracted from the reports on the Treaty Body Database on the website of the Office of the High Commissioner for Human Rights <www2.ohchr.org>

Each convention or covenant has a date of adoption, when the convention/covenant was opened for signature and ratification, and a later date when it came into force following ratification by a certain number of states. Declarations are not legally binding but carry moral weight by virtue of their adoption by the international community. As well as the UN system, there are also regional human rights treaties, and there may also be national or federal legislation, but there is no space to consider these in any detail here.

Key features of human rights

Human rights are founded on respect for the dignity and worth of each person. They are universal; they apply equally and without discrimination to *all* people. They are also inalienable; no one can have their human rights taken away. Rights can, however, be limited in specific situations (e.g. the right to liberty can be restricted when a person is found guilty of a crime by a court of law); this is considered further in the next section. Perhaps the most important feature of human rights is the notion of universality: that human rights are rights belonging to *all* human beings and are fundamental to every type of society. Each person has the same basic human rights, regardless of gender, age, culture, ethnicity, or religion.

Individual human rights do not exist in isolation from each other; they are indivisible, interrelated, and interdependent. Thus, it is not enough to respect some human rights and not others; violation of one right will often affect respect for several other rights. This does not, however, mean that all rights reinforce one another positively. Rights can affect each other adversely. For example, the right to freedom of expression may interfere with the right to privacy, or with the right to freedom from discrimination. In situations of resource scarcity many rights, such as healthy environment, education, healthcare, and social security may be in competition with each other.

Two different types of rights are distinguished, absolute and relative. Absolute rights are those where restrictions may not be placed on them; even if argued as necessary for some public good, these include the rights to be free from torture, slavery, or servitude; to a fair trial; to freedom of thought. The right to life is not absolute; what is forbidden is arbitrary deprivation of life. Note also that the right to freedom of thought/opinion and the right to hold any opinion does not include unlimited right to free expression of opinion; this is qualified by certain restrictions relating to the protection of the rights of others or in certain specific circumstances. This illustrates the complex interdependence that exists between the achievement of rights of different groups within the same community, and some of the articles in the conventions/covenants provide guidance on when rights can justifiably be restricted. This is discussed in the next subsection.

It is often argued that rights are culturally independent, though not all agree. Cultural relativists argue that the concept of universality is culturally constructed, and that human rights represent the particular belief systems of some cultures and societies rather than those of all cultures and societies. From this viewpoint, some consider the UN human rights as a Western construct of limited application to non-Western nations (see e.g. Kausikan 1996). Space precludes a detailed treatment here, especially as the debate is extremely wide-ranging, but see, for example, Nagengast's careful discussion (1997) of debates on women, minorities, and indigenous peoples; Durrant (2008) who focuses on the issue of physical punishment of children in relation to culture and the rights of children; and finally Bickenbach (2009) who examines the Convention on the Rights of Persons with Disabilities in relation to therapeutic strategies of respecting cultural differences. For an invigorating and critical examination of **cultural relativism** in general see Tilley (2000).

Cultural relativism
The theory or view that morality is relative to culture or that right and wrong vary with cultural norms.

When can rights be restricted or limited?

The interdependence of rights has been noted earlier. Here we look at 'valid' or justifiable limitations on human rights. The UDHR and the two covenants both discuss the issue, setting out the circumstances in which limitation of rights can be justified. They do this in two different ways, first in general articles, and then specifically in relation to particular rights. The form of the limitation varies; of particular interest are limitation on public health grounds, applying to rights such as freedom of movement and association, freedom of expression, and freedom to manifest one's religion or beliefs.

ICCPR Article 4 provides a very important exclusion of any rights limitation that involves discrimination on specific grounds. The corresponding article in the ICESCR is perhaps less precise (and thus less useful) in its formulation. Recognising the difficulty of the judgments that need to be exercised in deciding whether a specific limitation of rights is justified or not, work was carried out to formulate a series of principles to assist such decisions. This resulted in the Siracusa principles which provide criteria for rights limitation to be regarded as legitimate. In the case of restriction on the grounds of protection of public health, Gostin (quoted in Coker 2001) has formulated some specific criteria. Within public health, infectious diseases present one example where restrictions of human rights may need to be considered. Case Study 17.3 considers the issue of restricting the activities of persons who are HIV-positive.

The Siracusa principles

When a government limits the exercise or enjoyment of a right, this action must be taken as a last resort and will only be considered legitimate if the following criteria are met:

- The restriction is provided for and carried out in accordance with the law;
- The restriction is in the interest of a legitimate objective of general interest;
- The restriction is strictly necessary in a democratic society to achieve this objective;
- There are no less intrusive and restrictive means available to reach the same goal; and
- The restriction is not imposed arbitrarily, i.e. in an unreasonable or otherwise discriminatory manner.

Source: ECOSOC (Economic and Social Council) UN Document E/CN.4/1985/4, Annex, UN, Geneva, 1985

Restriction on the grounds of protection of public health

Gostin (quoted in Coker 2001) suggests the following specific criteria:

- Risk posed should be demonstrable and significant;
- Proposed interventions should be demonstrably effective;
- Approach should be cost-effective;
- Sanctions should be least restrictive necessary;
- Policy should be fair and non-discriminatory.

Case Study 17.3   Restricting activities of persons who are HIV-positive

The HIV/AIDS pandemic has provided many instances of restriction of the right to freedom and right to movement (as indeed have SARS and swine flu). As an example, the website 'About AIDS', which provides a wealth of information about living with HIV/AIDS, maintains a regularly updated list of the requirements for HIV testing prior to entry for different countries: <http://aids.about.com/od/legalissues/a/travelindex.htm>. A number of these report refusals of entry to HIV-positive people. The question then becomes which of these can be justified on public health grounds.

For example, Cuba as a country has come in for considerable international criticism over its response to HIV/AIDS for its practice, in the early stages of the pandemic, of quarantining the HIV-positive. Criticism persists to the present day, for example, according to the About AIDS website cited above, the update of 11 August 2010 states: 'Foreign students, foreign workers and long-term foreign residents are screened for HIV; people found to be HIV-positive are reportedly repatriated'. Anderson (2009) presents a very careful rights-based analysis of Cuba's approach to HIV/AIDS, concluding that while Cuba's quarantine period was unnecessarily prolonged in the 1980s, this policy did *not* display discrimination in only targeting particular groups. He concludes that selective criticism of the Cuban program has painted an inaccurate picture overall.

In applying the public health version of the Siracusa criteria, Gostin and Lazzarini (1997, p. 66) argue:

> Significant risk must be determined on a case by case basis through fact specific individual inquiries. Blanket rules or generalizations about a class of persons with HIV infection do not suffice. The risk must be 'significant', not merely speculative or remote. For example, theoretically, a person could transmit HIV by biting, spitting, or splattering blood, but the actual risk is extremely low (approaching zero). Likewise, an HIV-positive health professional who does not perform deeply invasive procedures is highly unlikely to transmit HIV to a patient. Present knowledge does not support screening or excluding that person from the healthcare profession because, lacking a real and substantial possibility of HIV transmission, such policies do not meet the significant risk test.

More recently, Bisaillon (2010) analyses the human rights consequences of the mandatory HIV screening policy for newcomers to Canada, finding a number of problems including unclear objectives and goals for the program, and instances of stigmatisation and discrimination within its operation. She identifies recommendations to address these.

The 'right to health'

One particularly important right for public health practitioners is the 'right to health'. This is directly stated in the preamble to the WHO constitution, article 25 of the UDHR mentions health, and Article 12 of the ICESCR makes it explicit (see the box below). This explicit recognition of the highest attainable standard of health as a 'human right', as opposed to a good or commodity with a charitable construct, provides a very powerful basis for public health advocacy. It is important to note that the Covenant mentions explicitly both mental health and physical health. Other international human rights instruments also address the right to health, both generally and in relation to specific groups.

In discussing the implications of the right to health, Mary Robinson, previous UN High Commissioner for Human Rights, expresses some very important key features:

> The right to health does not mean the right to be healthy, nor does it mean that poor governments must put in place expensive health services for which they have no resources. But it does require governments and public authorities to put in place policies and action plans which will lead to available and accessible healthcare for all in the shortest possible time. To ensure that this happens is the challenge facing both the human rights community and public health professionals. (WHO 2002, p. 9)

To help move towards the right to health, the committee responsible for the ICESCR formulated General Comment 14, and the UN Office of the High Commissioner for Human Rights and WHO

The right to health, statement in ICESCR

1. The States Parties to the present Covenant recognise the right of everyone to the enjoyment of the highest attainable standard of physical and mental health.
1. The steps to be taken by the States Parties to the present Covenant to achieve the full realisation of this right shall include those necessary for:
   a. the provision for the reduction of the stillbirth rate and of infant mortality and for the healthy development of the child
   b. the improvement of all aspects of environmental and industrial hygiene
   c. the prevention, treatment and control of epidemic, endemic, occupational and other diseases
   d. the creation of conditions which would assure to all, medical service and medical attention in the event of sickness.

Source: Article 12, ICESCR

Stop and Think

- What do you think the implications of the right to health are: for governments? for public health practitioners? Jot down your answers.
- Watch the short video where three public health students learn about the right to health: <www.who.int/hhr/activities/videos/en/index.html>.
- Revisit the answers you gave above. Did the video cause you to supplement the answers?

have produced a fact sheet on the right to health (OHCHR/WHO 2008). One of the key normative points about the right to health is that it extends to the underlying determinants of health (General Comment 14, paragraphs 4, 10, 11). Also important is the participation of the population in all health-related decision-making at community, national, and international levels (General Comment 14, paragraphs 11, 17, 34, 54).

Human rights and the social and cultural determinants of health

> There is a powerful synergy between health and rights. By design, neglect or ignorance, health policies and programs can promote and protect or conversely restrict and violate human rights. Similarly, the promotion, protection, restriction or violation of human rights can have direct impacts on health.
> (Brundtland 2005, p. 61)

Here, Gro Harlem Brundtland, the Director-General of WHO at the time, refers to the understanding that the major determinants of better health lie outside the health system, and include the fulfilment of an array of rights that are relevant to, but not intrinsically connected to, the right to health.

Ann Taket

As we will see, in examining the links between human rights and the social and cultural determinants of health, fulfilling human rights is a *necessary prerequisite* for the health of individuals and populations.

See also Chapters 1, 11, 12 & 14 for the social and cultural determinants of health.

Health policies, programs, and practices, in and of themselves, can promote and protect *or* restrict and violate human rights, by design, neglect, or ignorance. Three rather different routes of influence can be distinguished:

1 Human rights violations can directly affect health, for example, harmful traditional practices, torture, slavery, violence against women and children.
2 Vulnerability to ill health can be reduced through the promotion of human rights, for example, the right to health, to education, to food and nutrition, and to freedom from discrimination.
3 Promotion or violation of human rights can occur through health development, for example, promotion through right to participation, freedom from discrimination, right to information, and right to privacy.

Thus, promotion, protection, and restriction or violations of human rights all have direct and indirect impacts on health and well-being; these can also be proximal or distal. Since the 1980s, the HIV/AIDS pandemic and reproductive and sexual health concerns have been instrumental in clarifying the relationships between health and human rights (Gruskin et al. 2007).

Table 17.1 takes this further by showing the major direct links between the social and cultural determinants of health and the rights set out in the UDHR and the major conventions and covenants. Given that both the set of human rights and the social and cultural determinants of health are indivisible and interrelated, it should come as no surprise that there are very few simple one-to-one correspondences set out in the table, and the reader should be warned that the listing is by no means exhaustive.

Table 17.1   Linking human rights and the social and cultural determinants of health

Social and cultural determinants of health	References in UDHR and key conventions
Income and poverty Living conditions, including food, water, sanitation Housing	UDHR, Article 25 (1) Everyone has the right to a standard of living adequate for the health and well-being of himself and of his family, including food, clothing, housing and medical care and necessary social services, and the right to security in the event of unemployment, sickness, disability, widowhood, old age or other lack of livelihood in circumstances beyond his control. (2) Motherhood and childhood are entitled to special care and assistance. All children, whether born in or out of wedlock, shall enjoy the same social protection.
Employment and occupation	UDHR, Article 23 (1) Everyone has the right to work, to free choice of employment, to just and favourable conditions of work and to protection against unemployment. (2) Everyone, without any discrimination, has the right to equal pay for equal work.

(continues)

Social and cultural determinants of health	References in UDHR and key conventions
	(3) Everyone who works has the right to just and favourable remuneration ensuring for himself and his family an existence worthy of human dignity, and supplemented, if necessary, by other means of social protection. (4) Everyone has the right to form and to join trade unions for the protection of his interests. UDHR, Article 24. Everyone has the right to rest and leisure, including reasonable limitation of working hours and periodic holidays with pay.
Education	UDHR, Article 26 (1) Everyone has the right to education. Education shall be free, at least in the elementary and fundamental stages. Elementary education shall be compulsory. Technical and professional education shall be made generally available and higher education shall be equally accessible to all on the basis of merit. (2) Education shall be directed to the full development of the human personality and to the strengthening of respect for human rights and fundamental freedoms. It shall promote understanding, tolerance and friendship among all nations, racial or religious groups, and shall further the activities of the United Nations for the maintenance of peace. (3) Parents have a prior right to choose the kind of education that shall be given to their children. See also ICESCR, Article 13
Transport	None explicitly
Culture and ethnicity Gender and age	UDHR, Article 1 All human beings are born free and equal in dignity and rights. They are endowed with reason and conscience and should act towards one another in a spirit of brotherhood. UDHR, Article 2 Everyone is entitled to all the rights and freedoms set forth in this Declaration, without distinction of any kind, such as race, colour, sex, language, religion, political or other opinion, national or social origin, property, birth or other status. Furthermore, no distinction shall be made on the basis of the political, jurisdictional or international status of the country or territory to which a person belongs, whether it be independent, trust, non-self-governing or under any other limitation of sovereignty. ICCPR, Article 18 (1) Everyone shall have the right to freedom of thought, conscience and religion. This right shall include freedom to have or to adopt a religion or belief of his choice, and freedom, either individually or in community with others and in public or private, to manifest his religion or belief in worship, observance, practice and teaching.

(continues)

Ann Taket

Table 17.1   Linking human rights and the social and cultural determinants of health (*continued*)

Social and cultural determinants of health	References in UDHR and key conventions
	(2) No one shall be subject to coercion which would impair his freedom to have or to adopt a religion or belief of his choice. (3) Freedom to manifest one's religion or beliefs may be subject only to such limitations as are prescribed by law and are necessary to protect public safety, order, health, or morals or the fundamental rights and freedoms of others. (4) The States Parties to the present Covenant undertake to have respect for the liberty of parents and, when applicable, legal guardians to ensure the religious and moral education of their children in conformity with their own convictions.
	ICCPR, Article 26
	All persons are equal before the law and are entitled without any discrimination to the equal protection of the law. In this respect, the law shall prohibit any discrimination and guarantee to all persons equal and effective protection against discrimination on any ground such as race, colour, sex, language, religion, political or other opinion, national or social origin, property, birth or other status. See also Conventions on: Elimination of Racial Discrimination; Elimination of All Forms of Discrimination against Women; Rights of the Child; Rights of Migrant Workers and their Families; Rights of Persons with Disabilities; Protection of All Persons from Enforced Disappearances.
Population-based services and facilities	ICESCR, Article 12

	(1) The States Parties to the present Covenant recognize the right of everyone to the enjoyment of the highest attainable standard of physical and mental health.
	(2) The steps to be taken by the States Parties to the present Covenant to achieve the full realization of this right shall include those necessary for:
	   (a) The provision for the reduction of the stillbirth-rate and of infant mortality and for the healthy development of the child;
	   (b) The improvement of all aspects of environmental and industrial hygiene;
	   (c) The prevention, treatment and control of epidemic, endemic, occupational and other diseases;
	   (d) The creation of conditions which would assure to all medical service and medical attention in the event of sickness.

Social cohesion and social support	UDHR, Article 22
	Everyone, as a member of society, has the right to social security and is entitled to realization, through national effort and international co-operation and in accordance with the organization and resources of each State, of the economic, social and cultural rights indispensable for his dignity and the free development of his personality.

(continues)

Social and cultural determinants of health	References in UDHR and key conventions
	UDHR, Article 29 (1) Everyone has duties to the community in which alone the free and full development of his personality is possible. (2) In the exercise of his rights and freedoms, everyone shall be subject only to such limitations as are determined by law solely for the purpose of securing due recognition and respect for the rights and freedoms of others and of meeting the just requirements of morality, public order and the general welfare in a democratic society. (3) These rights and freedoms may in no case be exercised contrary to the purposes and principles of the United Nations.

To respect, protect, and fulfil...the responsibilities of governments in respect of human rights

Once an instrument is adopted by the General Assembly of the UN or other relevant committee/grouping, it is then opened for signature; countries sign the treaty to indicate their willingness to proceed through the necessary steps to be bound by the treaty. Ratification or accession are the terms used when a country indicates its agreement to be bound by a treaty. If one were cynical, one might suspect that this allows some countries to maintain a façade of compliance by remaining as signatories for a long period or even indefinitely. For example, the ICESCR has been signed but not ratified (as at 21 January 2011) by Belize, Comoros, Cuba, Sao Tome and Principe, South Africa, and the USA. The comment made by Cuba in relation to its signature offers us a specific explanation in referring to the difficulties of making progress while the subject of an economic blockade.

Corresponding to the nine core human rights treaties, there are nine bodies/committees that monitor countries' performance. Secretariat support is provided by the Human Rights Treaties

Mythbuster

As of 14 January 2011, there were 19 human rights covenants, conventions, and optional protocols open for ratification, and 195 member states of the UN.

- The Convention on the Rights of the Child has the greatest number of ratifications and has been ratified by 193 out 195 member states. Which of the following do you think are the two that have NOT ratified it: China, Iran, Somalia, USA?
- Only one member state has ratified all 19 instruments. Is this Australia, Ecuador, the Holy See, or Russia?
- Out of Malaysia, Mexico, Mongolia, and Mynamar, which do you think has ratified the *smallest* number of instruments, and which has ratified the *largest* number of instruments?

You can check your answers at <www2.ohchr.org/english/bodies/treaty/index.htm>, and under Status of Ratifications on the right-hand side of the website, click on 'Click to see the Chart disclosing the status of ratifications of human rights treaties (Excel)'.

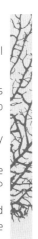

Branch of Office of the High Commissioner for Human Rights (OHCHR) in Geneva. Full details can be found on the OHCHR website, <www2.ohchr.org/english>. Each country is required to submit an initial report on the extent of its compliance with the treaty in question *at the time of the country becoming a party to the treaty*. Subsequently, further reports are submitted at four- or five-yearly intervals. Committees also conduct hearings with government representatives to examine progress. NGOs can submit 'Alternative' Reports to the relevant committees; these may be used during the hearings. The Universal Periodic Review is an additional process which involves a review of the human rights record of each UN member state once every four years.

As well as being responsible for monitoring country progress, some of the committees may receive complaints (usually called 'communications') that human rights violations have occurred. Communications may be from states, but this is rare (Gruskin & Tarantola 2005), or from individuals. Five of the human rights treaty bodies may, under particular circumstances, consider individual complaints from individuals (details can be found on the OHCHR website <www.ohchr.org>). The Convention on Migrant Workers also contains provision for allowing individual communications to be considered by its committee; these provisions will become operative when ten countries have made the necessary declaration under Article 77. A committee's opinions or 'views' relating to individual complaints are not binding in any legal sense. However, as Case Study 17.4 demonstrates, changes in laws or policies may result.

The work of special rapporteurs provides another means of supporting accountability and action. Mandates for special rapporteurs are based on topic and/or situation; they can make country and other visits, send communications to states with regard to alleged human rights violations, and submit annual reports on the activities carried out under the mandate to the Commission and the General Assembly. The first special rapporteur on the right to health was appointed in 2002, with a broad-ranging mandate (see <www2.ohchr.org/english/issues/health/right>).

Case Study 17.4   The UN system helps effect positive change: An example from Australia

1991—Toonen lodges a complaint alleging that the Tasmanian criminal laws on homosexuality violated his rights as a homosexual man.

1994—the Human Rights Committee (monitoring committee for the ICCPR) issued an adverse opinion, holding that the provisions of the Tasmanian legislation violated the articles of the ICCPR in three respects:

*   no distinction is made between sexual activity in public and in private, thus bringing private activity into the public domain;
*   individuals are distinguished in the exercise of their right to privacy on the basis of sexual activity, sexual orientation and sexual identity, i.e. there is discrimination;
*   homosexual activity between consenting homosexual women in private is not outlawed and only some forms of consenting heterosexual activity between adult men and women in private are outlawed.

Reported in United Nations Human Rights Committee Views on Communication, No 488/1992, adopted 31 March 1994.

Australia summarised its response to this in its third report to the Human Rights Committee (CCPR/C/AUS/98/3, pages 4–5, paras 12–14):

Communication 488/1992 N. Toonen v. Australia...

14. In response to the Committee's views, the Federal Attorney-General held discussions with the Tasmanian Premier and Attorney-General. The Tasmanian Government's position was that no action would be taken in response to the Committee's findings. Accordingly, the Federal Government introduced legislation to provide protection for all Australians from arbitrary interferences with sexual privacy. The legislation, entitled the Human Rights (Sexual Conduct) Act, came into force on 19 December 1994. For further details on the Act, the Committee is referred to the commentary on article 17 below.

This laid the basis for a further challenge to the Tasmanian Criminal code, this time in the Australian High Court. Eventually, in 1998 the Tasmanian Anti Discrimination Act passed into law, hailed by Croome (quoted in Bernardi 2001) as 'one of the best pieces of anti-discrimination legislation in the country'.

A full discussion of the case can be found in: Editors (1994) and Bernardi (2001)

Stop and Think

- Do you think there are any countries in which human rights are completely respected?
- Do you think there are any countries in which human rights are completely protected?
- Do you think there are any countries in which human rights are completely promoted?
- Which country do you think displays very good achievements in terms of respecting, protecting, and promoting human rights (write down your answer, you will need it for tutorial exercise 2).

Tools for public health advocacy and action—human rights approaches to seeking social justice and health equity

The previous section has examined the way governments are held to account for their progress towards human rights through the UN system. This section now looks at how public health advocacy and action can support social justice, health equity, and the right to health at the more local level, considering first the use of law at regional or national level, second the use of advocacy, and third the use of human rights analysis to support policy or program planning.

Figure 17.1 Multiple paths for human rights-based accountability and action

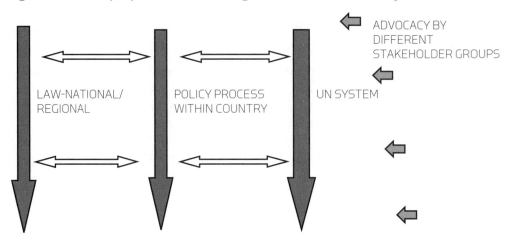

Figure 17.1 depicts the different paths for seeking accountability and action, through the UN systems discussed in the previous section, through regional or national legislative routes, and through the policy process. In each of these different paths, advocacy by relevant stakeholders may be highly significant in affecting the outcome; see Case Study 17.5.

At regional level, the European Court of Human Rights provides a good illustration of possibilities; detailed coverage can be found in Goldhaber (2007). The European Convention on Human Rights (ECHR) was signed in 1950 and entered into force in 1953. The Court, set up in 1959, covers 47 Council of Europe member countries that have ratified the Convention. Individuals or states can apply alleging violation of ECHR, and the judgments are binding on countries concerned. The examples given in the country fact sheets published online (<www.echr.coe.int> and then select reports and then country fact sheets) illustrate the potential in terms of supporting access to healthcare for groups like prisoners, as well as in action against pollution.

Case Study 17.5   Indigenous health: NGO advocacy

NGOs not only use the right to submit communications to the UN about a country's performance, they can also use the very same documents for advocacy within the country. In February 2007, the National Aboriginal Community Controlled Health Organisations made a submission to the Australian Attorney-General's Department's call for comments on the common core documents, incorporating the fifth report under the ICCPR and the fourth report under the ICESCR. A modified extract was also published in the *Medical Journal of Australia* by Couzos and Thiele (2007), focusing on the ICESCR and the right to health and arguing that Australia is not meeting its obligations. The following evidence was cited in support of their argument:

- poor access to primary healthcare for Aboriginal peoples
- Aboriginal and Torres Strait Islander peoples' share of the universal health coverage expenditure is less per person than for other Australians
- failure to monitor mainstream provision to Aboriginal peoples.

Case Study 17.6   Use of national litigation to support the right to health: The case of India

Article 21 of the Indian Constitution guarantees an individual's right to life and is enforceable in court. Although the article does not contain any explicit reference to a right to health, in 1981 the Indian Supreme Court signalled its intention to make the right to health enforceable by inference from the right to life. A sequence of cases (22 separate cases over the period 1980–2002 are described in Singh et al. 2007) has resulted in courts directing provision of particular services to disadvantaged groups in the population and to health-promoting changes in workplaces and working conditions, including:

- installation of safety measures in state-run pencil factories
- improvements in working conditions in state- and private-run asbestos industry
- provision of health services to convicted criminals
- provision of emergency medical care to all free of charge.

Source: Summarised from material in Singh et al. 2007

At the national level, possibilities depend on the position of human rights within the country concerned. In some countries, the right to health or similar rights have been established in national constitutions; others have utilised non-binding policies instead, limiting recourse to courts. As examples of what can be achieved, Singh and colleagues (2007) highlight the health reforms that have been achieved in Argentina, Ecuador, South Africa, and India, the last of which is described in Case Study 17.6. Hogerzeil and colleagues (2006) examined completed court cases in low- and middle-income countries where individuals or groups had sought access to essential medicines, with reference to the right to health. The review identified successful cases in ten countries, eight countries in Central and Latin America, plus India and South Africa. Their interpretation of their findings is that litigation can help ensure governments fulfil their human rights obligations in this respect, but they suggest that the courts should be used as a last resort and that it is better to ensure that human rights considerations are planned into policy and programs.

Human rights analysis: Assessing policies and programs for their human rights implications

The past 30 years have seen the development of a wealth of different approaches and tools for the task of ensuring that health policies and programs respect, protect, and promote human rights. In a recent review Worm (2010) examines no fewer than 17 different approaches. The box below summarises a seven-stage approach that is the earliest specific human rights assessment tool to appear in the health literature. Originating in some of the early work on human rights and HIV/AIDS (Gostin et al. 1994), the tool has been applied to analyse a wide range of policies and programs across the globe. Ford and associates (2010) present an analysis of when to start antiretroviral therapy in resource-limited settings. In relation to specific policies or programs, Taket (2012) contains a number of examples of analysis: at national level the MindMatters program implemented in secondary schools in Australia to promote mental health and well-being in students, and a peer education-based HIV/AIDS prevention program for adolescents in South Africa (the GOLD program); and at regional level the midday meal scheme implemented in the Indian state of Madhya Pradesh, and the Styrian Tobacco Prevention Strategy in Austria.

In terms of program planning, Case Study 17.7 looks at the example of Care International and the evaluation they carried out into the use of their rights-based approach. Jonsson (2003)

A seven-stage approach to human rights analysis

1. What is the specific intended purpose of the policy or program?
2. What are the ways in which and the extent to which the policy or program may impact positively and negatively on health?
3. Using the relevant international human rights documents, what and whose rights are affected positively and negatively by the policy or the program?
4. Does the policy or program necessitate the restriction of human rights?
5. If so, have the criteria/preconditions to restrict rights been met?
6. Are the health and other relevant structures and services capable of effectively implementing the policy or program?
7. What system of monitoring, evaluation, accountability, and redress exist to ensure that the policy or program is progressing towards the intended effect and that adverse effects can be acted upon?

Source: Gostin et al. 1994; Gruskin & Tarantola 2005

Case Study 17.7 CARE International, a human rights-based organisation

CARE International is one of the world's largest independent relief and development organisations, working in more than 70 countries and benefiting over 45 million poor and marginalised people. It is a practical, hands-on organisation with programs around the world dealing with a wide range of issues that keep people trapped in poverty—HIV/AIDS, discrimination, a lack of clean water, lack of employment, lack of housing, i.e. tackling the social determinants of health and working towards social justice. As they put it in their organisational mission: 'We seek a world of hope, tolerance and social justice, where poverty has been overcome and people live in dignity and security.' While CARE is a large international organisation, with more than 12,000 employees worldwide, they have a strong local presence. More than 90% of the staff are citizens of the countries where programs are run. CARE has no political or religious affiliation.

In 2003, they moved to adopt an explicit human rights-based approach in their work, comprising six program principles. They carried out a self-evaluation of the application of this approach in practice, examining 16 projects from Bangladesh, Bolivia, Burundi, Cambodia, Guatemala, Honduras, India, Peru, Rwanda, Sierra Leone, Somalia, and Thailand. For each project they measured achievements against each of the six principles and local outcomes.

Not all the projects were equally successful, but analysis of their different experiences offered some useful findings:

- Obtaining the support of key stakeholders was not always possible at the outset, and required persistence, advocacy, transparency, and negotiation. Any effort to raise awareness of rights and responsibilities relating to the problems facing marginalised groups *must* include rights holders and duty bearers, both of whom are equally capable of transformation.
- A rights-based approach needs variety and flexibility in the use of participatory methods for analysing needs, diagnosing problems, generating and appraising options, and decision-making.
- Need for systematic examination of inequities. This extends to disaggregating within marginalised or excluded groups by gender and other relevant categories. This type of investigation is fundamental and relies for its validity on the participation of marginalised groups.
- Use of human rights language and legislation. The examples spanned a spectrum of rights: from moral rights (to be heard), and economic, social, and cultural rights (to live in dignity and well-being), to legal rights (individual human rights or rights as a citizen). Not all projects perceived the need to invoke human rights legislation or frameworks. Explicit use was made by programs that incorporated human rights into community education, or that were aimed specifically at achieving the legal rights of citizens. In other examples, rights language was minimised in favour of tapping into the values, beliefs, and principles of the culture to achieve more equitable treatment of excluded groups.

The evaluation found promising signs of change: duty bearers who responded to pressures or demands of marginalised groups; a greater ability in CARE to broach and discuss issues of inequity with clients and partners; whole communities that have taken control over decision-making processes; and myriad instances of marginalised groups who are no longer voiceless or faceless. Questions about longer-term sustainability were raised.

Source: Summarised from CARE International UK's website <www.careinternational.org.uk> and Picard 2005.

describes the United Nations Children's Fund (UNICEF)'s rights-based approach to development programming, and Chopra and Ford (2005) consider a human rights approach to health promotion, drawing on the UNICEF approach. Most recently, the United Nations Population Fund (UNFPA) and Harvard School of Public Health have jointly authored a guide to a human rights-based approach to programming (UNFPA 2010).

The importance of human rights for public health practice: Rhetoric or reality?

Overall, human rights may benefit work in the area of public health by providing....

A tool to enhance health outcomes through using a human rights approach to designing, implementing and evaluating health policies and programmes;

Ann Taket

An 'empowering' strategy for health which includes vulnerable and marginalized groups engaged as meaningful and active participants;

A useful framework, vocabulary and form of guidance to identify, analyse and respond to underlying determinants of health;

A powerful authoritative basis for advocacy and cooperation with governments, international organizations, international financial institutions, and in building of partnerships with relevant actors in civil society. (WHO 2002b, p. 18)

WHO thus argues that human rights approaches provide a lever for seeking actions that protect and promote public health and provide important tools for tackling health inequity. But is this merely rhetoric? Many examples of successful use of rights-based approaches can be found, and the chapter has introduced some of these. There are many areas that the chapter has not touched on where such approaches have been successfully applied, and where the work that is being carried out illustrates untapped potential for the future. In this closing section, there is space to mention only a few.

Internationally, there has been a lot of successful work supporting the availability of essential medicines at low or no cost, for example, Brazil's work in championing improved access to antiretrovirals (Galvao 2005; Nunn et al. 2009). Reproductive health is another area where much has been achieved; Cabal and colleagues (2003) examine the work of the Center for Reproductive Rights, in Latin America, which, through legal advocacy, brought cases before the Inter-American Commission on Human Rights and the UN Human Rights Committee, as well as in courts of various countries. Taken together, the cases they discuss illustrate how international human rights litigation can help raise awareness of reproductive rights at national and international levels; they have also led to important change in legal and policy practice. Cook and colleagues (2003) provide a wealth of case studies in reproductive and sexual health at the individual care level.

Jacobson and Banerjee (2005) consider how tobacco control strategies can use human rights framing in voluntary non-smoking strategies to their advantage, and Fox (2005) examines how public health needs to frame its efforts to counter the tobacco industry's use of 'rights argumentation' to position itself as the protector of individual rights. In the field of harm reduction, Fry and colleagues (2005) and Keane (2003) both offer distinctive critiques of the role of human rights approaches in harm reduction. In relation to specific population groups, Morgan and David (2002) discuss the usefulness of human rights principles for ageing advocacy and public education efforts. Finally, Case Study 17.8 considers domestic violence, an example of an underrecognised major public health problem, which it is useful to view using a human rights framework.

After reading this chapter it should be clear that nothing represents a magic bullet to ensure social justice and the removal of health inequity under all circumstances, but there are many different examples of where rights-based approaches have been useful and also others where success has been more qualified. As the work of CARE International explicitly demonstrated, there may well be situations where it is not considered appropriate to use the language of rights. The question of using human rights approaches in addressing the social determinants of health has received much recent attention in the wake of the CSDH's final report. In a single issue of the journal *Health and Human Rights*, Venkatapuram and colleagues (2010) and Rasanathan and colleagues (2010) provide thoughtful discussions of some of the challenges and opportunities in taking this work further in the future. In remains to be seen exactly how far the potential provided by rights-based approaches can assist public health practitioners in working for health and social justice.

Case Study 17.8   Domestic violence, a major public health and human rights issue

Abuse against women by intimate partners is a major public health problem, globally (Garcia-Moreno et al. 2005), nationally (NCRVWC 2009), and in Victoria (Office of Women's Policy 2009). It occurs in all countries irrespective of culture, socio-economic status, or religion, and occurs in all types of relationships, both same-sex and heterosexual (Krug et al. 2002). The context and severity of violence by men against women makes domestic violence against women a much larger problem in public health terms (WHO 1997b; Krug et al. 2002).

Intimate partner abuse is the major cause of death, disability, and illness among women aged between 15 and 44 years in Victoria (VicHealth 2004; Vos et al. 2006). Intimate partner abuse has severe short- and long-term health consequences, both physical and mental, for the partner experiencing abuse and for any children in the family (Itzin et al. 2010). The problem has major societal costs in both social and economic terms; the annual cost of domestic violence in Australia was estimated at $8.1 billion for the year 2002–03 (Access Economics 2004).

A frequent characteristic of domestic violence is that the perpetrator often blames his abuse on the woman and her behaviour, and uses the abuse to assert control over the woman and her life. The woman experiencing abuse is often made to feel inadequate, a failure, and that she deserves the abuse. Sometimes her movements are curtailed and she is kept a virtual prisoner in the house. These characteristics have led to domestic violence being viewed legally as a human rights issue (Chapman 1990), and to cases being brought under the UN and regional systems for the protection of human rights. One of the earliest was in 1998, when a petition was presented to the Inter American Commission on Human Rights (IACHR) bringing the case of a Brazilian woman who had suffered years of abuse from her husband. Despite numerous reports to various authorities within the country, no action was taken. The Commission held the Brazilian Government responsible for violation of the woman's rights, and made a number of specific recommendations (a full report of the case can be found at <www.cidh.oas.org/annualrep/2000eng/ChapterIII/Merits/Brazil12.051.htm>). The IACHR, in its latest annual report for 2010, finds that the state of Brazil has implemented only some of the recommendations made (IACHR 2011, pp. 95–6), and urges the government to continue implementing public policies so as to prevent, punish, and eradicate violence against women; the IACHR will continue to monitor implementation of the recommendations into the future.

For a further example of the value of a human rights framework in domestic violence, this time in addressing a different range of social and cultural factors that come into play in the case of refugee women in Australia who experience domestic violence, see the paper by Rees (2004).

Summary

Human rights approaches are of great potential importance in providing grounding for public health policy and practice that seeks social justice in the health arena. There are considerable overlaps between the social determinants of health and human rights, and consequently inextricable links between the achievement of social justice, health equity, and human rights. An understanding of the UN human rights system, the various human rights instruments, and the monitoring and reporting system is thus of great relevance to public health professionals. There are a number of different routes by which governments can be held accountable for their achievements or lack of them, and action to address social injustice and health inequities supported through the UN system, through national/ regional legislation, and through the policy and programming process. Advocacy by concerned actors such as NGOs can play an important role in each of these three routes.

Tutorial exercises

1   As well as international human rights instruments, regions, countries, states, and territories also have produced a variety of other human rights instruments. One such is the Victorian Charter of Rights and Responsibilities, which became law in the State of Victoria in 2006. Read and compare the Universal Declaration of Human Rights and the Victorian Charter of Rights and Responsibilities (see Websites for sources for each).

   »   Which is more comprehensive?
   »   What are the differences between them in their coverage of the social and cultural determinants of health?
   »   Which gives the strongest foundation for advocacy to ensure health equity?

2   Earlier you were encouraged to stop and think about what country or countries had the best performance in terms of protecting, promoting, and fulfilling human rights. Pick one of these countries. At the website of the Office of the High Commissioner for Human Rights <www2. ohchr.org/english> scroll down until you find the selection box for 'human rights by country', use the drop-down menu to select your country and then click GO. In the centre of the screen you'll find links to the most recent reports on the country. Check them and see if your original assessment was accurate; update it where necessary.

Further reading

Bankston, C.L. III. (2010). Social justice: Cultural origins of a theory and a perspective. *Independent Review*, 15(2), 165–78.

Braveman, P. (2010). Social conditions, health equity, and human rights. *Health and Human Rights*, 12(2), 31–48.

Chapman, A.R. (2010). The social determinants of health, health equity, and human rights. *Health and Human Rights*, 12(2), 17–30.

Gruskin. S., Mills, E.J., & Tarantola, D. (2007). History, principles and practice of health and human rights. *The Lancet* 370, 449–55.

O'Flaherty, M., & Ulrich, G. (2010). The professionalization of human rights field work. *Journal of Human Rights Practice*, 2(1), 1–27.

OHCHR/WHO Office of the United Nations High Commissioner for Human Rights and World Health Organization (2008). The Right to Health, Fact Sheet No. 31. <www.who.int/hhr/ activities/factsheets/en/index.html>.

Rasanathan, K., Norenhag, J., & Valentine, N. (2010). Realizing human rights-based approaches for action on the social determinants of health. *Health and Human Rights*, 12(2), 49–59.

Sen, A. (2009). *The idea of justice*. London: Penguin.

Taket, A. (2012). *Health equity, social justice and human rights*. London: Routledge.

Venkatapuram, S., Bell, R., & Marmot, M. (2010). The right to sutures: Social epidemiology, human rights, and social justice. *Health and Human Rights*, 12(2), 3–16.

World Health Organization (2002). *25 questions and answers on health and human rights*. Geneva: WHO. <www.who.int/hhr/activities/publications/en>.

Websites

<www.un.org/en/documents/udhr>

<www.un.org/cyberschoolbus/humanrights/resources/plain.asp>

This website provides a source for the Universal Declaration of Human Rights. The UDHR is available in English and other languages. For a plain language version see the website given above.

<www.who.int/hhr/readings/regional/en/index.html>

This website gives an up-to-date list of regional instruments relevant to health and human rights.

<www.escr-net.org>

International Network for Economic, Social and Cultural Rights: Runs a general listserv and a variety of discussion groups, including Discussion Group on the Human Right to Health.

<www.phmovement.org/en/campaigns/145/page>

People's health movement campaign on right to health.

<www.phmovement.org/en/campaigns/33/page>

People's health movement campaign on women's access to health.

<www.glballawyersandphysicians.org>

Global Lawyers and Physicians–Working Together for Human Rights. Global Lawyers and Physicians is a not-for-profit non-government organisation that focuses on health and human rights issues. Their website contains much in the way of publications, etc., and a health and human rights database, with a vast set of links.

<www.equalopportunitycommission.vic.gov.au/pdf/The%20Charter%20of%20Human%20Rights%20and%20Responsibilities%20-%20Protection%20of%20freedoms%20and%20rights%20for%20everyone%20in%20Victoria.pdf>

This website provides a source for the Victorian Charter of Human Rights and Responsibilities. Notice what a long complicated web address is required to access it. You might wish to consider why you think this might be. The Charter became law in Victoria in 2006; the corresponding legislation is at: <www.austlii.edu.au/au/legis/vic/consol_act/cohrara2006433>

18 | The economics of health and disease

Rob Carter

TOPICS COVERED

This chapter covers the following topics:

- why economics is relevant to the field of public health
- the role and content of economic analysis—key tasks of 'description', 'explanation', 'prediction', and 'evaluation'
- the important distinction between 'positive economics' and 'normative economics'
- markets, 'economic rationalism', and reasons justifying government intervention
- what role 'efficiency' should play in healthcare
- 'best practice' from an economic perspective
- the socio-economic determinants of health
- links between economics and other disciplines

KEY TERMS

Burden of disease study
Cost of illness study
DALY
Demand
Decision rule
Direct cost
Efficiency
Economic rationalism
Government failure
Indirect cost
Intangible cost

ICER
Market failure
Merit goods
Normative economics
Opportunity cost
Population Attributable Risk
Positive economics
Relative risk
Spillover effects
Supply-induced demand

Introduction

This chapter explains why the discipline of health economics is relevant to the field of public health. The starting point is to appreciate that all societies are organised around markets where decisions are made about what is produced, how it is produced, and who gets access to the goods and services produced. While markets will vary from country to country in their complexity and characteristics, they will all address these three questions. Sometimes governments choose to intervene in the free operation of markets either because markets are not working properly (**market failure**) or for reasons of social justice (they believe access should be on the basis of *need* rather than *ability to pay*). When governments choose to intervene in markets (through regulations, taxes, subsidies, or directing the provision of services), economics also has a role to play in guarding against **government failure** (McPake & Normand 2008).

The relevance of economic thinking to public health rests on two important notions, those of *scarcity* and the consequent need to make choices. The reality of the need to make choices, sometimes difficult choices, leads to the relevance of **efficiency** as an objective to guide choice. Efficiency is essentially about the relationship between costs and benefits. In considering the concept of efficiency, three terms are important—allocative efficiency, technical efficiency and distributive equity.

Allocative efficiency focuses on value for money or what products/services should be produced. It involves best allocation of resources in the health system such that the allocated inputs yield the best or most valued possible outcomes. An allocatively efficient health system produces an optimal mix of health interventions. *Technical efficiency* focuses on how goods or services are produced. It refers to that production function where output is achieved at minimum resource cost, or when no further output can be achieved with available inputs. *Distributive equity* focuses on whether the distribution of a chosen outcome (e.g. health status, income) or service (healthcare, education, employment) is considered 'fair' or just. In the context of markets, it involves the question of whether it is acceptable for access to services to be based on *demand* (ability and willingness to pay) as opposed to *need* (as defined by a third-party expert, such as a clinician).

It is essential to note that efficiency is not only about costs, but also about how we define benefits and the underlying principle of **opportunity cost**. The concept of opportunity cost focuses on what benefits we receive from what we chose to do, compared to what benefits we could have got had we done something different. To put it another way, what do Australians want from their healthcare system? How do we juggle competing objectives such as maximising the health status of the population, achieving equity of access and health outcomes, achieving an affordable system, and gaining acceptability from all the various stakeholders? These challenges and trade-offs are central to the study of health economics (Wonderling et al. 2005).

In addressing these challenges, economists carry out four separate but interrelated tasks: *description, prediction, evaluation, and explanation* (Moodie & Carter 2010, p. 167). Unfortunately, researchers and policymakers often confuse which task is appropriate to answer which research or policy question. Related confusions are seeing the aims of efficiency and affordability as the same thing, thinking that value

Market failure The situation where free markets do not achieve *allocative efficiency* and/or *technical efficiency*. Common sources of market failure include spillover effects; insufficient information to allow consumers to make good choices; supply-induced demand; and merit goods. Health economists see the health sector as having many of these characteristics.

Government failure The adverse consequences of ineffective or inefficient government intervention in markets through activities such as taxes/subsidies, regulation of market entry, direct provision of services, etc.

Efficiency Maximising the benefits (whatever we define them to be) from the resources available. It involves minimising the *opportunity cost* involved with resource allocation decisions.

Opportunity cost The benefit or value of the best alternative use of a resource that is forgone as a result of its current use. Minimising opportunity cost is the key rationale underlying an economic approach to decision-making.

Positive economics
Economic theory and methods that focus on a description of current practice and the characteristics or functioning of markets and the general economy.

Normative economics
Economic theory and methods that evaluate policies and ideas for change (what ought to be done).

judgments can somehow be excluded by the sophistication of the technical analysis, and not distinguishing between the tasks of *prioritising problems* and *prioritising solutions* (Moodie & Carter 2010). Central to understanding economics is the important distinction between **positive economics** and **normative economics** and its significance for policy prescriptions about what constitutes value (in notions of value for money) and the rationale for government intervention in our markets (McPake & Normand 2008, p. 3).

In this chapter, these various terms will be defined, the issues involved will be clarified, and case studies will be provided to illustrate key concepts. The material presented is intended to give readers an introduction to health economics as a way of thinking and as a way of contributing to decision-making and policy formulation. It provides the economic perspective on how 'best practice' can be determined and funding priorities set. It is intended to give readers the building blocks for understanding why and when you need to consult health economists—or indeed why you may even want to become one.

Why health economics is relevant to public health

> I think a lot of the suspicion about health economics, and about health economists, is the belief that our view of people is simply that they are (potentially) productive resources, that their value stems solely from that attribute, and therefore that the most cost-effective way of caring for the elderly (or the mentally or physically handicapped) is to kill them off as quickly and cheaply as possible. If that were in fact our position, we should undoubtedly deserve any hostility that came our way, but fortunately it isn't. (Williams 1987, p. 1)

Why should economists work in the field of public health? What wisdom could they bring to bear on public health issues that could make a difference to the prevention of illness and/or to promoting good health in the community? To assess the credentials of health economics to make a useful contribution, one must first appreciate what economics is about and the roles it performs. The fundamental problem addressed by economists is the allocation of available resources between competing **demands** in a way that maximises community welfare. While this is obviously an important mission, it is not enough in itself to clarify the potential contribution of economics.

Demand The quantity of a service or product sold in the marketplace at a specified price. *Demand* is distinguished from *wants* in economics by consumers' preparedness to actually purchase the good or service—that is, demonstrating their willingness to pay.

The relevance of economic thinking rests on the existence of two other important things: resource scarcity and the consequent need for choice (McPake & Normand 2008). If our resources were unlimited, then economics would be irrelevant—you would only need those disciplines that answered whether healthcare services were effective (e.g. epidemiology, medicine) and acceptable (e.g. behavioural science, ethics, political science). Unfortunately, resources are limited, particularly in relation to the almost unlimited range of *wants*, *demands*, and *needs* that we have. Individuals, institutions, and governments must therefore make choices about how to use their available resources and which wants to satisfy. The reality of scarcity is familiar to all those who work in public health or healthcare today: there are simply not enough resources (staff, equipment, facilities, and so on) to do all the very useful and important things that could be done. Resource scarcity leads to the relevance of *efficiency* as an objective to guide choice.

Simply put, efficiency means maximising the benefits obtained from the resources available. It involves a consideration of how we define benefit and the underlying principle of *opportunity cost* (Wonderling et al. 2005). The opportunity cost of using resources in one way is the benefit we forgo in its best alternative use. Investment in care for children, for example, may involve forgoing care for the elderly; investment in care for cancer patients may involve forgoing care for heart disease patients; or investment in immunisation may involve forgoing cancer screening programs. To make these choices we need to define what we mean by benefit: is it just about maximising health gain or do we care about who receives that health gain? Is it more important to help children than elderly people; should those with severe illness be helped before those with mild problems; should special needs groups (e.g. low-income; rural/remote; Indigenous Australians) receive special consideration? Put another way, what do we as a community want from our healthcare system and how much are we prepared to pay for it? What share of national income should go to the health sector, versus education, defence, transport, the arts, sport, and so on?

Stop and Think

» In your own life, have you been conscious of what economists call the principle of opportunity cost—that in choosing to buy that car to get to university you could not afford the overseas trip with your mates to Bali; that in choosing to go out on the town you compromised the savings plan; or in going to the beach on Sunday you lost the study time you needed to finish the essay?

» Can you see how minimising the opportunity cost of your choices might be useful, might lead to better decision-making? In 'economics-speak', this would be called 'maximising your welfare' or satisfaction.

Mythbuster

Consider why health economists may find the following statements really annoying:

I worry about the application of economics to public health—it is just about cost-cutting!

Economists are no different to accountants—they just focus on money, finances, and issues of affordability.

Economics is immoral—it pays no regard to the importance of human life!

For economists, such views ignore the fundamental point that economics is about maximising benefits with the resources available—the key issue is how we define benefit. Far from being immoral, ethicists are on side with health economists that we need clarity about what we want from our healthcare system. In health economics, the measurement of costs is just a means to an end—it enables us to work out how much benefit we can achieve from our different choices. It is for this reason that some economists have argued that 'cost-benefit analysis' should really be renamed 'benefit-benefit forgone analysis'!

Rob Carter

In addressing these challenges, economists carry out the four tasks noted above: *description*, *prediction*, *evaluation*, and *explanation* (Moodie & Carter 2010, p. 167). Before turning to these tasks, however, it is important to make one more preliminary comment about the discipline of economics: it concerns the important distinction between *positive economics* and *normative economics*.

'Positive economics' and 'normative economics'

Economics as a discipline distinguishes between *positive economics* and *normative economics*, with the former covering 'what is' and the latter 'what ought to be' (McPake & Normand 2008, p. 3). Positive economics is meant to be as value-free as possible and is dominated by the task of description. There are unavoidable value judgments that data is worth collecting and that particular definitions are appropriate; but beyond this, positive economics strives to be as value-free as possible. Examples of *positive economics* include our statistics on Gross Domestic Product (GDP); unemployment and workforce participation rates; average weekly earnings; health expenditure; health status; infant mortality rates; hospital occupancy rates; smoking prevalence; and the incidence of cancer.

Normative economics, on the other hand, is quite consciously based on value judgments of what 'better' means—of why things should be changed. We should do A rather than B because A is 'more effective', or 'more cost-effective', or 'more just', or 'more affordable', or 'more feasible', and so on. The failure of policymakers (and some economists) to make their value judgments transparent can lead to confusion on whether recommendations for policy change are based on economic theory or political ideology (Rice 2003). This is illustrated in Case Study 18.1 about Professor Milton Friedman, a well-known Nobel Prize–winning economist. As the case study illustrates, the reliance on the free market by economic rationalists embodies the value judgment that it is acceptable for access to healthcare to be determined by the consumer's ability and willingness to pay. Alternative notions of social justice embody the judgment that access to health services should be based on need and give rise to government involvement through public health insurance. Some goods (e.g. health and education) are considered so important (i.e. **merit goods**) that they are made available on terms more generous than in the marketplace, often as a fundamental part of citizenship. Case Study 18.2 is about why governments get involved in healthcare markets, drawing on arguments presented in the health economics literature (Rice 2002; Olsen 2009; Folland et al. 2010; Phelps 2010).

Merit goods Goods or services where the state has an interest in its citizens consuming the good or service. The benefit to the state of a healthy educated population may be such as to override the principle of 'consumer sovereignty' (consumers knowing what's best for them).

Case Study 18.1   Ideology versus economic theory

Consider the use of the word 'efficiency' in the following statement by Milton Friedman. He was attacking the US Government's Medicare program (for the elderly) and Medicaid program (for the poor and disabled) in a presidential campaign.

> The *inefficiency*, high cost and inequitable character of our medical system can be fundamentally remedied in only one way: by moving in the other direction, towards re-privatising medical care....The [proposed] reform has two major steps: (1) End

both Medicare and Medicaid and replace them with a requirement that every US family unit have a major medical insurance policy with a high deductible, say $20,000 a year or 30% of the unit's income during the prior two years, whichever is lower; and (2) end the tax exemption of employer provided medical care...Each individual or family would, of course, be free to buy supplementary insurance, if it so desired. (*Wall Street Journal*, 12 November 1991, p. A21)

The hidden value system is that market-based healthcare systems are inherently superior (i.e. more efficient) to government-based healthcare systems, with all that that implies in terms of access to care on a needs basis as opposed to an ability-to-pay basis. Note that the poorer or sicker members of US society would almost surely have to pay the full deductible before insurance sets in (a high percentage of their income), while richer or healthier members would be unlikely to reach the deductible (a smaller percentage of their income).

Stop and Think

» Think about the ideologies that characterise our own political system in Australia. For example, the Liberal Party focus on 'personal responsibility' and free markets ('libertarianism') and the Labor Party focus on 'equality of opportunity' and government involvement ('egalitarianism').

» Consider how economics often gets caught up in the rhetoric of politics and whether you or your parents could disentangle them. A basic understanding of the strengths and limitations of economics might help.

Case Study 18.2 Government involvement in health

Over the last 20–30 years there has been a surge of interest in reforming the organisation and delivery of healthcare systems around the world by replacing government regulation and provision with a greater reliance on market forces. This led several health economists, particularly Thomas Rice (2002), to review the traditional market model, its underlying assumptions, and its applicability to health. Rice argues that several of the key assumptions behind efficient markets simply do not hold in health because of the reliance of patients on clinicians (**supply-induced demand**) and the existence of **spillover effects** (such as herd immunity through immunisation), together with various limitations on the supply side. The net effect is that demand and supply are not independently determined and that consumers are not always the best judge of their own welfare in relation to consumption of health goods and services.

Rice argues that the free market cannot be relied upon to allocate health resources efficiently and that there is an *efficiency rationale* for governments to

Supply-induced demand The situation where supply and demand are not independently determined (a requirement for competition). Usually occurs where consumers lack sufficient knowledge to know what services they require and are therefore dependent on the provider to guide their choices.

Spillover effects The situation where either costs or outcomes are not captured by the price of a good or service. Spillover effects may be either positive (e.g. herd immunity from immunisation) or negative (e.g. pollution).

intervene in the funding and provision of healthcare. Rice challenges in particular the implicit assumption behind the resurgence of interest in market competition: that 'economic theory' demonstrates that competition in healthcare will automatically lead to superior social outcomes (i.e. improvements in community welfare). Note that Rice is not saying there is no role for competition in healthcare, just that there is also an important place for government. Many, but not all, health economists support Rice's views (see also Jacobs 1997; Feldstein 2005; Morris et al. 2007; Olsen 2009; Folland et al. 2010; Phelps 2010).

It is also important to recognise that while 'market failure' may provide an efficiency rationale for government intervention in the health sector, it is by and large not the main reason why governments become involved (Olsen 2009). Rather than pursuing efficiency, most governments intervene for reasons associated with equity and social justice. Market-based systems ration access to healthcare on the basis of people's ability to pay and/or acquire health insurance. Most countries choose not to rely on this system as the primary approach to *merit goods* such as health and education. Thus, in all developed countries a form of public healthcare insurance is made available, and in most countries there is also government intervention, albeit to different extents, to regulate the production and distribution of healthcare. Having intervened initially for reasons of equity and social justice, most governments would then seek to avoid and/or minimise the possibility of *government failure* (e.g. government regulation creating distortions in the market—such as a shortage of registered GPs).

Burden of disease study (BoD) A type of descriptive analysis that summarises the health impact of a chosen disease or risk factor. The health impact of disease can be reported in many ways: incidence, prevalence, premature deaths; or mortality and morbidity impacts combined.

Cost of illness study (COI) A type of descriptive analysis that summarises the cost impact of a chosen disease or risk factor. Most COI studies include all 'direct' and 'indirect' costs. Some may also put a dollar cost on pain and suffering ('intangibles').

Description in health economics

It was mentioned above that health economists carry out four separate but interrelated tasks (*description, prediction, evaluation,* and *explanation*). With *description* the task is to measure and report on current activities, resources, attributes, behaviours, system effects, and so on. This can range from broad socio-economic data (such as income, employment, education, social support, and housing) to descriptions of the financing and organisation of the health sector (Duckett 2000; Palmer & Short 2000), to disease and injury impacts, or to healthcare expenditure patterns. The Australian Bureau of Statistics and the Australian Institute of Health and Welfare are major providers in Australia of this type of information. Other useful sources include the Commonwealth and state/territory health departments, the Health Insurance Commission, and various research institutions. Some relevant websites that will give you a sense of the wide range of information available are listed below.

The task of description naturally involves a heavy emphasis on empirical studies and associated data collections. Health economists often work hand in hand with other disciplines when undertaking the descriptive analysis—such as epidemiologists for disease patterns, demographers for population trends, clinicians for treatment pathways, behaviourial scientists for survey data, biostatisticians for data analysis, and accountants for cost records. Three types of descriptive data are particularly popular in public health: **burden of disease studies (BoD), cost of illness studies (COI),** and socio-economic studies. Table 18.1 and Figure 18.1 provide examples

Table 18.1   Leading causes of burden by sex, Australia 2003

Rank	Males	DALYs	% of total	Females	DALYs	% of total
1	Ischaemic heart disease	151,107	11.0	Anxiety & depression	126,455	10.0
2	Type 2 diabetes	76,886	5.6	Ischaemic heart disease	112,385	8.9
3	Anxiety & depression	65,323	4.8	Stroke	65,166	5.2
4	Lung cancer	55,028	4.0	Dementia	60,734	4.8
5	Stroke	53,296	3.9	Breast cancer	60,517	4.8
6	Chronic obstructive pulmonary disease	49,201	3.6	Type 2 diabetes	55,737	4.4
7	Adult-onset hearing loss	42,653	3.1	Chronic obstructive pulmonary disease	37,548	3.0
8	Suicide	38,717	2.8	Lung cancer	33,876	2.7
9	Prostate cancer	36,547	2.7	Asthma	33,827	2.7
10	Colorectal cancer	34,643	2.5	Colorectal cancer	28,961	2.3

Source: Vos 2010, p. 2

Figure 18.1   Disease burden attributable to 14 risk factors by sex, Australia 2003

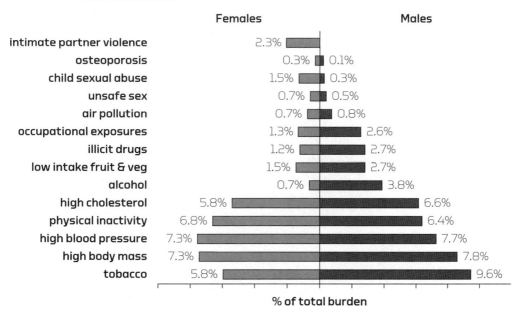

Source: Vos 2010, p. 2

Rob Carter

DALY Stands for *Disabilty Adjusted Life Year*. The DALY is a summary measure of illness that combines: years of life lost due to illness (YLL) against a specified life expectancy; and years of life lived with disability (YLD).

Decision rule An agreed guideline where analysts specify in advance what result is correct or acceptable. It is used to answer what 'value for money' means. In Australia, a common rule of thumb is to specify '$50,000 per QALY/DALY prevented' as the benchmark for what constitutes a cost-effective use of healthcare resources.

Direct cost In health economics, those resources whose consumption is wholly attributable to the provision and use of the health service in question. Direct cost is usually measured in terms of expenditure categories such as salary and wages, capital, consumables, repairs and maintenance, and overheads.

Indirect cost In health economics, focuses on productivity impacts in the general economy, due to existing morbidity/mortality patterns, as well as the introduction of health services. If the introduction of a national screening program, for example, involved attendance during work hours, this would have a negative productivity impact in the short term but a positive impact in the longer term due to the reduction in disease incidence and/or severity.

of BoD data being used to describe leading causes of premature death and disability using the **DALY** measure.

It is important to note that such descriptive studies in health are generally focusing on the nature and size of the problem, rather than on solutions. While descriptive studies can certainly feed into analyses that evaluate solutions, they should not be confused as being the same thing. This takes us back to the distinction between normative and positive economics. Health economists are critical when the rationale for resource allocation is the 'size of the problem' (description) rather than the cost-effectiveness of solutions to address the problem (evaluation). Economists use the value judgment of improved efficiency (implemented through **decision rules** associated with economic evaluation) to justify their recommendations (Drummond et al. 2007). One of the important skills for students to develop is to be able to tease out and assess the appropriateness of the different rationales on which decisions are based. Such rationales can vary from simple historical precedent ('always done it this way'); to feasibility (cheapest or easiest to do); to effectiveness (works best); to equity (fair go for all); or to cost-effectiveness posed by economists ('best buys' approach).

Case Study 18.3 illustrates typical COI and BoD data developed in the context of obesity prevention—now one of our major public health concerns. From a research perspective, it is important to note that description usually involves the construction of particular concepts (such as what 'being overweight or obese' means or how is 'cost' defined), and that this process of construction may involve particular assumptions and definitions that need to be recognised. In our obesity case study, for example, certain diseases were not included because the evidence of causality was not strong enough (e.g. respiratory disease, anxiety and depression, gout, and cancer of the uterus). Further, in establishing the cost of a particular disease or illness, assumptions are required concerning the elements that represent a 'cost'. All COI studies will estimate the **direct cost** of disease management and care, while some will also try to estimate the **indirect costs** of lost production in the broader

Stop and Think

- Is the rationale that we have a 'significant problem' (described either in terms of health burden, cost of care, or public opinion) enough to justify government funding?
- Many economists argue that the focus for funding should be on effective and cost-effective solutions and not the size of the problem. Do you agree?
- Should we take both aspects into account—look for cost-effective solutions to the large problems first?

economy, or even try to impute a cost to pain and suffering (**intangibles**). In Case Study 18.3, only the direct costs of healthcare were included.

Limitations of COI studies

Existing expenditure on a disease, no matter how large, is not sufficient in itself to justify further expenditure (i.e. description is not evaluation, but may be input into evaluation). It is not so much the size of the disease burden per se that should guide resource allocation, but rather the efficiency of specific interventions designed to reduce the disease burden (Mathers, Penm et al. 1998; Mathers, Stevenson et al. 1998).

Case Study 18.3   Is obesity an important public health problem: What is its health and cost impact?

COI and BoD studies are often used to flag the importance of a particular risk factor or disease. Studies that look at risk factors try to estimate the share of our national health burden and national healthcare expenditure that is caused by the chosen risk factor. Key steps include: 1) identifying those diseases that are causally related to the risk factor; 2) estimating the total health burden and total healthcare expenditure of these diseases; and 3) attributing a share of these costs and health impacts to the risk factor (using concepts of **relative risk** and **population attributable fractions** from the discipline of epidemiology). Set out below are a series of tables that illustrate these steps taken from a study of obesity (Carter & Moodie 2005, pp. 178–81).

The first table (Table 18.2) reports the results from steps 1 and 2: estimating the total health burden and cost impact of relevant diseases. Note that the health burden is reported in terms of both mortality (deaths) and a combined mortality/morbidity measure (DALYs). DALYs capture premature death (as they are estimated against a nominated life expectancy) and its implications for quality of life.

The next two tables (Table 18.3 and Table 18.4) report the third step: What part of these health and cost impacts can be attributed to people being overweight or obese? If we add the deaths for women and men from overweight/obesity together, we see that there are a substantial number of premature deaths (6000 per year) that are preventable. As a percentage of our total health burden (DALYs), this is approximately 5% for both men and women. This DALY percentage may look a little small, but in public health terms, changes of this magnitude are very significant. Readers will note that this preventable health burden also has significant cost implications for the health sector—over $1.6 billion per year. This raises the key policy issue—what can we do about preventing obesity?

Intangible costs The pain and suffering imposed by disease and/or its treatment, which are typically very difficult to quantify in dollar terms. Some COI studies include them and some forms of economic evaluation (e.g. cost-benefit analysis) also measure health outcomes in dollar terms.

Relative risk A measure used to predict the likelihood of disease in exposed individuals relative to those who are unexposed.

Population attributable risk (PAR) A measure that captures the excess rate of disease in the total study population of exposed and unexposed individuals that is attributable to the exposure. The PAR is important in public health as it is used to measure the benefits of risk factor reduction.

Rob Carter

Table 18.2   Total health burden and total recurrent direct healthcare expenditure for adults in selected diseases causally related to overweight/obesity (Steps 1 and 2)

Diseases	Deaths Men	Deaths Women	DALYs 1 Men	DALYs 1 Women	Healthcare AUD$M Men	Expenditure 2 AUD$M Women
Diabetes	1,616	1,479	35,792	31,694	262.76	296.92
Gallbladder disease	116	120	1,357	1,882	39.35	39.35
CHD < age 65	4,508	1,541	76,971	29,587	841.09	504.89
CHD > age 65	12,755	13,877	103,659	101,113	–	–
Stroke (ischaemic)	5,216	7,623	64,330	72,248	423.93	524.91
Hypertension	618	1,025	4,999	8,042	503.84	746.73
H'cholesterolaemia	0	0	n/a	n/a	125.51	174.42
Breast cancer (women 50–69)	–	1,184	–	23,677	–	56.73
Bowel cancer	2,674	2,299	35,511	31,440	93.76	93.76
Kidney cancer	510	510	6,475	4,937	18.42	12.28
Endometrial cancer	–	325	–	6,045	–	12.79
Osteoarthritis	25	71	22,610	33,695	352.15	586.91
Back problems	5	5	4,390	3,501	384.20	447.11
Totals	**28,043**	**30,059**	**356,094**	**347,861**	**$3,045.00**	**$3,496.80**

Notes: 1. The DALYs are for Australia in the year 1996 and may therefore underestimate the number of DALYs in the reference year of this study (2000). 2. The estimates of healthcare expenditure for each disease are based on the AIHW Disease Costs and Impacts database (DCIS) and associated publications (Mathers Penm et al. 1998).

Table 18.3   The health burden attributable to overweight and obesity (Step 3)

Diseases	Deaths Due to Overweight		DALYs Due to Overweight		Deaths Due to Obesity		DALYs Due to Obesity	
	Men	Women	Men	Women	Men	Women	Men	Women
Diabetes	450	288	9,975	6,167	478	479	10,590	10,273
Gallbladder disease	23	16	264	247	21	26	262	403
CHD < age 65	652	166	11,130	3,189	598	276	10,202	5,296
CHD > age 65	0	0	0	0	469	717	3,814	5,226
Stroke (ischaemic)	123	223	1,517	2,118	145	318	1,792	3,018
Hypertension	100	110	809	867	127	233	1,025	1,829
H'cholesterolaemia	0	0	n/a	n/a	0	0	n/a	n/a
Breast cancer (women 50-69)	-	0	-	0	-	73	-	1,466
Bowel cancer	236	131	3,128	1,791	190	184	2,520	2,522
Kidney cancer	0	0	0	0	0	50	0	485
Endometrial cancer	-	0	-	0	-	46	-	849
Osteoarthritis	4	7	3,270	3,221	5	17	4,770	7,879
Back problems	0	0	404	103	0	0	383	181
TOTAL	1,588	941	30,490	17,703	2,035	2,420	35,358	39,427
% of total deaths/ DALYs in men or women	2.33%	1.56%	2.29%	1.50%	2.98%	4.00%	2.66%	3.34%

Table 18.4   Healthcare expenditure attributable to overweight/obesity (Step 3)

Diseases	Expenditure Due to Overweight AUD$M (2000)		Expenditure Due to Obesity AUD$M (2000)		Total Obesity and Expenditure Overweight	
	Men	**Women**	**Men**	**Women**	**Men**	**Women**
Diabetes	73.23	57.78	77.74	96.24	150.97	154.02
Gallbladder disease	7.66	5.16	7.58	8.43	15.24	13.59
CHD < age 65	121.63	54.42	111.48	90.37	233.11	144.78
CHD > age 65						
Stroke (ischaemic)	10.004	15.39	11.81	21.93	21.80	37.32
Hypertension	81.58	80.48	103.28	169.79	184.86	250.28
H'cholesterolaemia	10.04	5.11	3.95	3.72	13.99	8.83
Breast cancer (women 50–69)	–	0	–	3.51	–	3.51
Bowel cancer	8.26	5.34	6.65	7.52	14.91	12.86
Kidney cancer	–	0	–	1.21	–	1.21
Endometrial cancer	–	0	–	1.80	–	1.80
Osteoarthritis	50.92	56.11	74.30	137.24	125.22	193.35
Back problems	35.38	13.11	33.49	23.11	68.87	36.21
TOTAL	**398.69**	**292.89**	**430.29**	**564.87**	**828.98**	**857.76**
% total recurrent health expenditure	**0.77%**	**0.56%**	**0.83%**	**1.08%**	**1.59%**	**1.65%**

Care should be taken in interpreting direct costs associated with disease treatment as an estimate of financial savings that would result from prevention of disease. Conversion of such potential cost savings into actual savings involves a number of practical issues (such as workforce restructuring, professional interests, management policies, and public reaction) as well as theoretical issues (such as the mix between 'fixed' and 'variable' costs and 'lumpiness' in the expansion/contraction of capital equipment and assets) (Mathers, Penm et al. 1998).

Underlying COI studies are several conceptual and methodological issues that affect the estimates produced. The choice of study perspective, for example, has an important impact on inclusion/exclusion criteria for cost categories. Similarly, it is important to appreciate whether a prevalence-based or incidence-based approach to costing is being employed. Data sources are also important, particularly whether a top-down approach (using broad aggregate data sets that are attributed to individual diseases) or a bottom-up approach (with specified care pathways based on patient level data) is being used (Mathers, Penm et al. 1998).

Prediction in health economics

With *prediction* the task is to estimate future trends in risk factors, health status, and resource use. As the research question moves from describing the status quo (i.e. what happens now) to predicting future trends, it becomes increasingly important for assumptions to be clearly specified. The task of prediction focuses attention on the quality of the evidence base for estimating what will happen in the future, as well as the associated question of the need for *uncertainty analysis* to support the estimates. Policymakers usually want know two key things: 1) what is the estimate, for example, is it a good or bad number? and 2) can they believe it?

Case Study 18.4 includes important predictions that have been completed on expected disease and expenditure trends for Australia between 2003 and 2033. The projection model used here combines demographic factors of population ageing and population growth, together with non-demographic factors of changes in disease rates, volume of services per treated case, treatment proportions (the proportion of cases that receive treatment), and excess price inflation (i.e. the difference between inflation in the health sector and inflation in the general economy). This type of projection work is worth doing, not so much for the final numbers it produces, but because it analyses what drives

Case Study 18.4   Is our healthcare system sustainable?

In Australia, recent projections by the Australian Institute of Health and Welfare (AIHW 2008a) have total health and residential aged care expenditure growing by 189% over the 2003–33 period; increasing from $85 billion to $246 billion (an increase of $161 billion). This growth would increase health expenditure as a proportion of GDP from 9.3% to 12.4%. These estimates, while challenging in their own right, are lower than earlier estimates from the federal Treasury (Treasury 2007). The projected increase of $161 billion (Table 18.5) in health expenditure is driven by an increase in the 'volume of services per case' ($81.3 billion), largely because of introduction of new technologies and changes in treatment practices, and this is expected to continue; an ageing population ($37.8 billion) and population growth ($34.4 billion) (Figure 18.2).

Table 18.5 and Figure 18.2 illustrate health expenditure projections.

Figure 18.2   Breakdown by cost driver of projected change in total health and residential aged care expenditure, 2012-13 to 2032-33

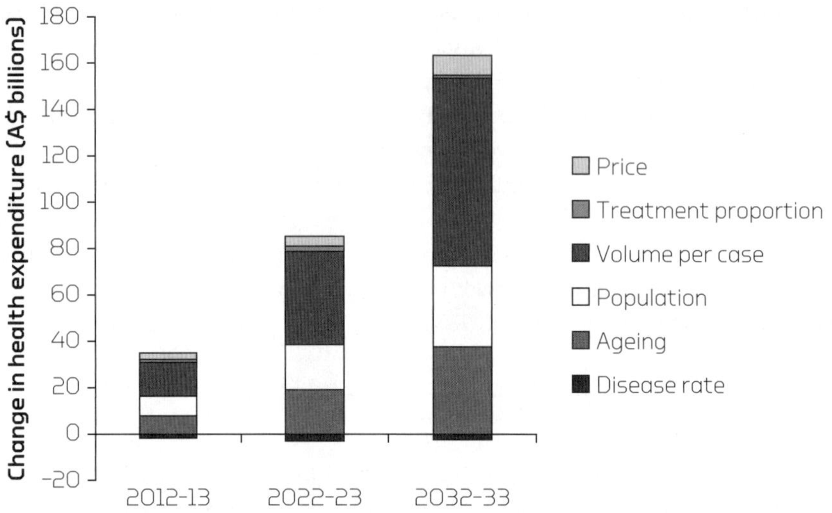

Source: AIHW 2008a, pp. 11-14

Table 18.5   Projected total health expenditure (2002-03 dollars) by cause, Australia, 2002-03 to 2032-33

	Expenditure by Year ($billion)		Change 2003-2033
Cause	2002-03	2032-33	Per cent
Cardiovascular	9.3	22.6	143%
Respiratory	7.2	22.0	206%
Injuries	6.7	14.4	115%
Dental	5.9	14.9	153%
Mental	5.2	12.1	133%
Digestive	4.9	16.5	237%
Neurological	4.7	21.5	357%
Musculoskeletal	4.4	14.2	223%
Genitourinary	3.7	10.9	195%
Cancer	3.5	10.1	189%
Diabetes	1.6	8.6	438%
Other[b]	28	78.3	180%
Total health expenditure	**85.1**	**246.1**	**189%**

Source: AIHW 2008a, pp. 11-14

growth in healthcare expenditure; and because the models developed can be used to ask 'what if' questions to test the impact of different policies and changes in the socio-economic environment.

These projections, however, and the underlying demographic, burden of disease, and treatment practice assumptions all reflect a 'business as usual' scenario. There is a growing appreciation among governments and their advisers that informed purchasing is central to efforts to harness this expenditure growth and to use available budgets more efficiently. In short, governments desperately need reliable information on the costs and health outcomes of current practice and of options for change that will enable them to direct available resources towards *best-practice* cost-effective services. This brings us to the evaluation task.

Stop and Think

Projections are usually centred on a careful analysis of past trends in disease rates and associated healthcare expenditure.

» Can you think of reasons why the simple extrapolation of past trends might be problematic the further out you go into the future?

Evaluation in health economics

While the tasks of *description* and *prediction* can be challenging and have their contentious aspects, it is the third task of *evaluation*—with its central role of assessing value—that is the most debated and often the most misunderstood contribution of economics. Evaluation in economics has distinctive characteristics that separate it from evaluation as practised by other disciplines (Fox-Rushby & Cairns 2005; Drummond 2007). Evaluation in economics involves both a comparison of alternatives (one of which is usually current practice and the other an option for change), and importantly, has regard to both their costs and benefits. The key task of economic evaluation is to address the question: What difference will the proposed intervention or option for change make compared to what's happening now? Evaluation often involves both *description* (e.g. clearly describing current practice, the current health burden, the elements of the new intervention, and its efficacy credentials) and *prediction* (e.g. estimating the cost, cost offsets, and health impacts through time, often until death of the patient cohort); but importantly, it also involves a value judgment (implied or hopefully explicit) about the 'appropriate' use of healthcare resources.

In economics, the issue of appropriateness is guided by *decision rules* on the relationship between *incremental benefit* achieved (i.e. benefit from intervention versus benefit from current practice) and *incremental cost* (i.e. cost of intervention versus cost of current practice). This is called an 'incremental cost-effectiveness ratio' or **ICER**. Different types of economic evaluation are distinguished by how they measure benefits. In cost–benefit analysis (CBA) outcomes are measured in dollar terms; in cost-utility analysis (CUA) outcomes are measured as quality-adjusted life years (QALYs/DALYs); while in cost-effectiveness analysis (CEA) outcomes are measured in physical units that have clinical significance (such as 'cancer detected' or 'pain-free day'). Quality of life measures are often preferred as the measure of outcome

ICER 'Incremental Cost-effectiveness Ratio'. The results of economic evaluations in the health sector are generally expressed as a ratio that summarises the additional cost of the intervention compared to current practice (incremental cost), over the additional health gain compared to current practice (incremental benefit).

in economic evaluation because they combine both mortality and morbidity effects and allow comparsion between very different interventions (e.g. an intervention to achieve pain relief from severe arthritis versus an anti-smoking campaign to prevent premature death). The way economic evaluations are used to guide policy is to specify a decision threshold that represents value for money. In Australia, any intervention that costs less than $50,000 per QALY is considered good value for money (Vos et al. 2010).

The task of economic evaluation is thus intimately linked to the contribution of health economics to health service planning and priority-setting. It is this third plank of economics that moves the contribution from a problem-focused activity to a solutions-based activity. Irrespective of their views about the merits of COI/BoD in policy development, all economists would agree that economic evaluation has the potential to make important contributions to policy. The most important example of this from a public health perspective is the recent ACE-Prevention study, described in Case Study 18.5.

Case Study 18.5   The ACE-Prevention study

ACE-Prevention (Vos et al. 2010) was a five-year NHMRC-funded study that evaluated 123 preventive interventions and 27 treatment interventions for the general population. The models were also adapted to estimate the cost-effectiveness of 21 interventions for the Indigenous population. ACE-Prevention was a significant achievement, more than doubling the published economic appraisal research on health promotion/illness prevention in Australia. While not purporting to be exhaustive, ACE-Prevention provides an extensive and balanced coverage of the available evidence base for priority-setting in the prevention of non-communicable disease in Australia. Such information enables governments to:

- direct available resources towards best-practice cost-effective services;
- modify inefficient services to improve their cost-effectiveness;
- discontinue inefficient services that cannot be made more cost-effective or be justified on other compelling grounds;
- target services to those in need, as opposed to people with low-risk profiles who are unlikely to benefit in a cost-effective manner.

The main messages from ACE-Prevention are:

- Many interventions for prevention have very strong cost-effectiveness credentials (43 that are either dominant or cost less than $10,000 per DALY prevented). Such interventions should only be ignored if decision makers have very serious reservations about the evidence base or are facing insurmountable problems in relation to stakeholder acceptability or feasibility of implementation.
- Another group of preventive interventions (31) are good value for money compared to the decision threshold of less than $50,000 per DALY prevented.
- There are also interventions for prevention that have poor cost-effectiveness credentials (38); have an insufficient evidence base (4); are associated with more harm than benefit ('dominated': 2); or are dominated by more cost-effective alternatives (2). It is vital to recognise that prevention is not always value for money and is not always 'better than the cure'.

- A large impact on population health (i.e. >100,000 DALYs prevented per intervention) can be achieved by a limited number of cost-effective interventions: taxation of tobacco, alcohol, and unhealthy foods; regulating the salt content of processed food; improving the efficiency of blood pressure and cholesterol-lowering drugs; gastric banding for severe obesity; and an intensive SunSmart campaign.
- There are more cost-effective interventions with a moderate impact on population health (between 10,000 and 100,000 DALYs prevented per intervention). The main missed opportunities at the national level among these are screening programs for pre-diabetes, chronic kidney disease, and low bone mineral density in elderly women. Smoking cessation aids, pedometers, and mass media for physical activity are other approaches with moderate impact on population health.
- Of the cost-effective interventions with a smaller population health impact (<10,000 DALYs per intervention), the growing list of potential preventive measures for mental disorders deserves special mention.

Stop and Think

Sometimes public health advocates are very wary of economic evaluation and see it as a natural enemy of public health. They are worried that it is somehow synonymous with **economic rationalism**, which advocates a minimalist government role in healthcare.

Economists on the other hand see it as unethical not to evaluate public health proposals to ensure that they are effective and cost-effective—particularly those programs that offer public health services (screening, immunisation, behaviour change) to the general public who have not sought out such help.

» Do you understand where public health advocates are coming from (i.e. wanting to see services they believe in get implemented) and do you also see that economists have a valid case? How would you arbitrate a divergence of views like this if you were the decision-maker?

Economic rationalism
A term used to describe those economists who advocate a predominant role for markets and a minimal role for government. Economic rationalists advocate minimal government interference in the free operation of markets and stress the potential for government failure.

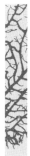

Mythbuster

Over the years, as advocates for public health have struggled to gain funding to implement their programs, a rationale has evolved that 'prevention is always better than cure!'

Do you support this rather ideological view, or can you see that perhaps this is not always so? Do you agree with those who argue that if you offer services to people not seeking them (which often differentiates prevention from care), there is an even greater ethical imperative to ensure that such services are efficacious and do no harm?

From an economic perspective the recent ACE-Prevention study has clearly shown that not all prevention is value for money and that while there is a strong case for more funding for public health, we need to spend our public health budgets wisely.

Rob Carter

Explanation in health economics

The fourth task in health economics focuses on establishing causality. While economists have their own techniques for analysing causation (e.g. econometrics), they also work with statisticians and epidemiologists in establishing correlation and causation.

As covered in other chapters of this textbook, a person's health and well-being has many facets that result from a complex interplay between societal, environmental, socio-economic, biological, and lifestyle factors, nearly all of which can be modified to some extent by healthcare and other interventions. Measuring and and monitoring determinants (the description task) helps to explain trends in health (the prediction task). This information can then be used to help us understand why some groups have poorer health than others. An important issue in public health is the impact of socio-economic factors such as income, employment, education, social support, and housing. These factors help to explain many of the health inequalities in Australia today. In general, relatively disadvantaged members of the community live shorter lives and have higher rates of illness, disability, and death than those relatively advantaged. This pattern occurs consistently within countries across the world, despite vast differences between them in their overall wealth (AIHW 2006b). A study of people living in areas of relatively low socio-economic status in Australia, for example, reported that they experienced a 32% greater burden of disease than people living in high socio-economic areas (Begg et al. 2007).

See also Chapter 19 on the healthcare system as a structural determinant of health.

See Chapter 1 on socio-economic status.

The box below illustrates socio-economic characteristics that have been shown to be determinants of health; that is, they play some causal role in health status. The most recent Australian data is presented based on AIHW reports. The clear importance of socio-economic status has important implications for health policy and the nature and design of healthcare services. This in turn should be reflected in the economic evaluation of new interventions. While conceptually different, there are thus natural synergies and interconnections between the tasks of description, prediction, evaluation, and explanation.

Socio-economic status as a determinant of health

Much of Australia's burden of disease can be attributed to lifestyle factors such as smoking, physical inactivity, and being overweight or obese (Begg et al. 2007). Results from the 2007–08 National Health Survey (2008) indicate that these factors are generally more common as socio-economic status declines. In particular, the prevalence of smoking in the lower SES group was over twice that of the highest group. These SES patterns were also evident among Indigenous Australians. Figure 18.3 and Table 18.6, produced by the AIHW (2010a), illustrate these associations.

Studies of death rates in Australia reveal substantial socio-economic inequality (Draper et al. 2004). The Draper study found a life expectancy gap between the highest and lowest SES groups of four years for males and two years for females. Studies considering death from specific health conditions confirmed similar socio-economic gradients for cardiovascular disease (AIHW 2006b), diabetes (AIHW 2008a), and injuries among young Australians (AIHW 2008c).

Figure 18.3   Premature deaths at ages 15-64 years, by sex and socio-economic status, 2002-06

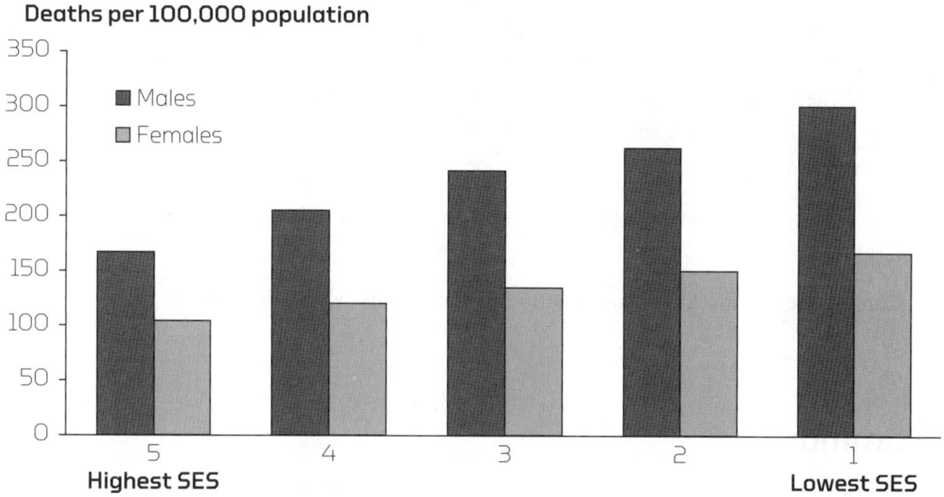

SES Socio-economic status.

Source: AIHW 2010a, pp. 254-5

Table 18.6   Prevalence of selected health measures by socio-economic status, 2007-08 (%)

Characteristics	Highest SES:5	4	3	2	Lowest SES:1
Health risk factors					
Daily smoking	11.1	15.1	18.8	21.1	28.6
Sedentary exercise level	24.9	31.0	38.1	38.8	45.4
Risky or high-risk alcohol consumption	12.7	12.6	13.3	13.6	10.1
Overweight or obese	37.9	41.2	42.7	42.2	42.5
Health condition					
Depression	3.5	3.3	3.5	4.0	4.4
Diabetes (Type 2)	2.9	3.7	4.1	4.3	6.2
Chronic respiratory disease	2.2	2.7	2.8	3.1	3.3
Cardiovascular disease	17.3	17.1	21.0	22.2	23.8
Severe/profound disability	2.9	4.1	4.6	5.3	6.1

1. Data are based on persons aged 15 years and over, except smoking and alcohol consumption (18 years and over).
2. Data are age-standardised to the 2001 Australian population.

Source: AIHW 2010a, pp. 254-5

Rob Carter

Stop and Think

» The role and significance of education and income on health are now well recognised. Can you see how these factors might interact—how education will impact on employment opportunities and knowledge of the healthcare system; how low income will impact on education opportunities, housing, and lifestyle; how lifestyle associated with poor income and education may compromise good health?

» Can you see why disadvantaged people tend to come from disadvantaged families?

» Can you see why low SES is more common among people with a disability?

Summary

The relevance of economic thinking to public health rests on the existence of resource scarcity and the consequent need to make choices. These factors lead to the relevance of efficiency as a policy objective. Efficiency is essentially about the relationship between resource use and the benefits flowing from their application. The examination of resource use is simply a means to an end: to maximise benefits from our choices. A key issue that arises is how we define benefit—what do we want from our healthcare system? The fundamental concept of opportunity cost focuses on what benefits we receive from what we chose to do, compared with what benefits we sacrifice from forgone alternatives.

In applying the key principle of minimising opportunity cost, economists carry out four separate but related tasks: description, prediction, evaluation, and explanation. While conceptually different, there are natural synergies and connections between these tasks. While descriptive studies can certainly feed into analyses that evaluate solutions, they should not be confused as being the same thing. Health economists are critical when the rationale for resource allocation is the 'size of the problem' (description) rather than the cost-effectiveness of solutions to address the problem (evaluation). Economists use the value judgment of improved efficiency (implemented through decision rules associated with economic evaluation) to justify their recommendations.

One of the important skills for students to develop is to be able to tease out and assess the appropriateness of the different rationales on which decisions are based. Such rationales can vary from simple historical precedent (i.e. 'always done it this way'), to feasibility (cheapest or easiest to do), to effectiveness (works best), to equity (fair go for all), or to the cost-effectiveness posed by economists ('best buys' approach).

Tutorial exercises

As a group discuss and try to answer the following questions without referring back to the text (at least in your first go at it):

1   Why does health economics matter to public health?

2   Why is it important to distinguish between methods that help you prioritise problems and those that help you prioritise solutions?

3 What rationales do you and your classmates believe to be the most important in guiding resource allocation in public health?

Further reading

Drummond. M.F., Sculpher, M.J., Torrance, G.W., O'Brien, B.J., & Stoddart, G.L. (2007). *Methods for the economic evaluation of healthcare programmes*, 3rd edn. Oxford: Oxford University Press.

Duckett, S.J. (2000). *The Australian healthcare system*. Melbourne: Oxford University Press.

Feldstein, P.J. (2005). *Healthcare economics*, 6th edn. New York: Delmar Cengage Learning.

Folland, S., Goodman A.C., & Stano, M. (2010). *The economics of health and healthcare*, 6th edn. New Jersey: Prentice Hall.

Fox-Rushby, J., & Cairns, J. (2005). *Economic evaluation*. New York: Open University Press.

Jacobs, P. (1997). *The economics of health and medical care*, 4th edn. Frederick, MD: Aspen Publications.

Kernick, D. (2002). *Getting health economics into practice*. Oxford: Radcliffe Medical Press.

McPake, B., & Normand C. (2008). *Health economics: An international perspective*, 2nd edn. London: Routledge.

Mooney, G., & Scotton R. (1999). *Economics and Australian health policy*. Sydney: Allen & Unwin.

Morris, S., Devlin, N., & Parkin, D. (2007). *Economic analysis in healthcare*. West Sussex: John Wiley & Sons.

Olsen, J.A. (2009). *Principles in health economics and policy*. New York: Oxford University Press.

Palmer, G.R., & Short S.D. (2000). *Healthcare & public policy*, 3rd edn. Melbourne: Macmillan Publishers.

Phelps, C.E. (2010). *Health economics*, 4th edn. New York: Addison Wesley.

Wonderling, D., Gruen, R., & Black, B. (2005). *Introduction to health economics*. New York: Open University Press.

Websites

<www.deakin.edu.au/strategic-research/population-health/deakin-health-economics/index.ph>

Deakin Health Economics (DHE) was established in late 2006 and forms part of a Strategic Research Centre in Population Health at Deakin University. The expertise and standing of the research team is affirmed by an impressive track record in both competitive grants (national and international), commissioned research and publications. With a staff of 16 health economists, including nine senior researchers, DHE is a strong centre of excellence in applied economic appraisal. The site describes the research program and links to publications, and provides staff to contact for further information.

<www.buseco.monash.edu.au/centres/ch>

The Centre for Health Economics (CHE), Faculty of Business and Economics, Monash University, has been at the forefront of health economics teaching and research in Australia for more than 13 years. Its more than 600 publications represent a significant part of the country's total health economics output. The overriding goal of the Centre is to undertake and promote high-quality health economics research and teaching activities, with both a national and international focus.

<www.chere.usyd.edu.au>

The Centre for Health Economics Research and Evaluation (CHERE) is a Key University Research Centre of the University of Technology, Sydney. CHERE is a joint initiative of the Faculties of Business and Nursing, Midwifery and Health at the University of Technology, Sydney, in collaboration with Sydney South West Area Health Service. It was established as a UTS Centre in February 2002. CHERE's aim is to contribute to the development and application of health economics and health services research through research, teaching and policy support. CHERE is recognised nationally and internationally as a centre of excellence in health economics and health services research.

<www.york.ac.uk/inst/ch>

The UK Centre for Health Economics (CHE-UK) is a specialist health economics research unit within the University of York. CHE was established in 1983 and has continually expanded since its inception. Providing research of worldwide repute, its principal areas of activity include economic evaluation of health technologies, outcome measurement, primary care, and resource allocation.

<http://cebm.jr2.ox.ac.uk>

The Centre for Evidence-Based Medicine (CEBM) has been established in Oxford as the first of several centres around the UK whose broad aim is to promote evidence-based healthcare and provide support and resources to anyone who wants to make use of them. Their prospectus outlines the specific aims of the Centre and the goals they have identified, as well as the means they propose to use in achieving those goals.

<www.york.ac.uk/inst/crd/welcome.htm>

The Centre for Reviews and Dissemination (CRD) was established in January 1994 to provide the UK National Health Service (NHS) with important information on the effectiveness of treatments and the delivery and organisation of healthcare. The CRD, by offering rigorous and systematic reviews on selected topics, a database of good-quality reviews, a dissemination service, and an information service, helps to promote research-based practice in the NHS. CRD collaborates with a number of health research and information organisations across the world and is a UK member of the International Network of Agencies for Health Technology Assessment (INAHTA). CRD produces a database of HTA projects and publications.

<http://http1.brunel.ac.uk:8080/departments/herg/home.html>

The Health Economics Research Group (HERG) at Brunel University, UK, aims to undertake high-quality, policy-relevant research and to contribute to the development of evaluation methodologies. The current research program has a unifying focus on economic evaluation of health technologies.

<www.aihw.gov.au>

The Australian Institute of Health and Welfare is Australia's national agency for health and welfare statistics and information. It publishes many reports and discussion papers, drawing on a wide range of data collections–its two flagship publications, 'Australia's Welfare' and 'Australia's Health', are published bi-annually. These publications provide a comprehensive review of health statistics in Australia. Many of these publications are available on the website.

<www.health.gov.au>

The Australian Department of Health and Ageing (DHA) website provides information on Commonwealth Government policies and programs as well as links to related national and international health sites. Many publications, including annual reports and budget papers, are available on the website free of charge. In addition, there is a service that provides links to the most requested information for student assignments.

<www.dhs.vic.gov.au>

Like the Australian Department of Health and Ageing, the Victorian Department of Human Services (DHS) also has a very useful publications area which is often worth a look. Other state departments of health would also have useful publications available on their websites.

<www.abs.gov.au>

The Australian Bureau of Statistics (ABS) website provides access to a range of health and non-health statistics, publications, and papers. For example, Australia's current key economic and social indicators, including the Consumer Price Index and Average Weekly Earnings, are widely used in economic analysis. Another service is AusStats, a web-based service providing the full standard ABS product range (both free and charged material).

<www.hic.gov.au>

The Health Insurance Commission (HIC) is Australia's primary health information management and payment agency. This site contains information about HIC, including its Charter of Care, information on HIC's global services, recent media releases, and recruitment information. In addition, pharmaceutical expenditure data and other health-related statistics are available on the website.

Rob Carter

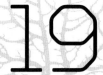

19

The social determinants and the healthcare system

Yvonne Parry and Eileen Willis

TOPICS COVERED

This chapter covers the following topics:
• the healthcare system as a structural determinant of health
• models of healthcare and the social determinants of health
• access to healthcare as an intermediary determinant of health
• the Australian healthcare system and the social determinants of health
• policy initiatives for promoting the social determinants of health

KEY TERMS

Bulk billing
Health access
Intermediary determinants
of health
Interest groups
Market-based model
Public policy

Quintile
Role substitution
Separation rates
Structural determinants of
health
Welfare state

Introduction

Many of the chapters in this book have stressed that social factors, rather than biological or genetic ones, determine people's health. In this chapter, one specific social factor is examined and analysed for how it impacts on the health of individuals and population groups. This socio-political factor is the type of healthcare system available to a nation's citizens. In previous chapters, the authors have identified a range of social, cultural (including media), environmental, economic, and discriminatory practices that impact on the health of individuals and populations, including the way people may be stigmatised and suffer discrimination. In this chapter, the focus is on how the provision of health services and access to these services can be seen as a social determinant of health. The chapter will argue that access to consistent, timely, and appropriate health services is necessary to maintain and promote effective health outcomes for individuals and populations, especially disadvantaged groups.

In order to demonstrate how a nation's healthcare system can be understood as a social determinant of health, the chapter will draw on the World Health Organization's CSDH framework (2007), particularly the work of Solar and Irwin (2007). The first section of the chapter will summarise the CSDH argument that the healthcare system is a structural determinant of health and access to health services is an intermediary determinant of health. Second, it will describe the Australian healthcare system, specifically Medicare. It will then identify those features of the Australian healthcare system that are positive social determinants of health, and those features that contribute to and maintain inequalities in health. In the final section, examples of public policy that might contribute to good health outcomes and overcome some of the structural and intermediary determinants of health are provided.

The social determinants of health

The Commission on Social Determinants of Health (WHO 2007) has divided the social determinants of health into two broad categories: the structurally determined or 'upstream' factors, and the intermediary or 'downstream' factors. The **structural determinants of health** refer to those factors that impact on people's socio-economic position. These include such factors as an individual's income, occupation, and education. Other factors include welfare and taxation policies, or policies that allow equal opportunity for all groups regardless of gender, race, disability, or class. These social factors impact on life chances, which in turn impact on the health status of individuals. The evidence is that an individual's socio-economic position, in interaction with the overall socio-political climate of a country, determines health outcomes such as life expectancy (mortality) or rates of illness (morbidity) (Wilkinson & Pickett 2009). Individuals cannot control the socio-political context of a country, although groups such as political parties or **interest groups** or social movements might be able to bring about policy changes to improve health status.

The **intermediary determinants of health** are shaped by the structural determinants. They can best be understood as the way the structural determinants

See Chapter 11 on the social determinants of health.

Structural determinants of health Those aspects of a society that influence an individual's health. These include the provision and availability of welfare services such as free healthcare, redistributive taxation practices, and policies to ensure that groups are not discriminated against.

See also Chapters 1 & 11 for a broad coverage of the social determinants of health.

Interest groups Groups of citizens that organise to influence government or public policy.

Intermediary determinants of health Those factors such as social position, access to healthcare, type of housing, or psychosocial risks in the environment or workplace that impact on health status.

impact on individuals and the way they react to these determinants. They include factors such as access to healthcare, transport, adequate and safe housing, and safe working conditions (Solar & Irwin 2007). For example, populations in outer, lower socio-economic suburbs of large cities may not have access to the same efficient transport as people in inner suburbs. These people may react to this by not seeking specialist healthcare when it is needed. The intermediary determinants create a causal chain of influence over a person's life span and include factors such as their material circumstances, social position, environmental risks, and housing stress (Solar & Irwin 2007). For example, many social democratic countries have **public policies** around employment that protect workers who are made redundant from sinking into poverty by providing unemployment benefits to tide the worker over until they get a new job. Such welfare polices are part of the structural determinant of health and a key component of the **welfare state**. At the intermediary level, occupational health and safety policies ensure that individuals do not get injured on the job and are able to work in healthy environments. However, the intermediary determinant requires the individual worker to engage in a two-way process of adhering to work safety policies through appropriate workplace behaviour. Because the intermediary determinants of health include individual behaviours they also provide the means of direct delivery of interventions. In the above example, this might include health promotion campaigns directed at safety at work. Figure 19.1 illustrates the two social determinants.

Public policy
Policies brought in by governments to administer education, healthcare, water, sanitation, etc.

Welfare state Provision by government of social services such as education, healthcare, old-age pensions. Usually free and funded through taxation.

Figure 19.1   The structural and intermediary social determinants of health

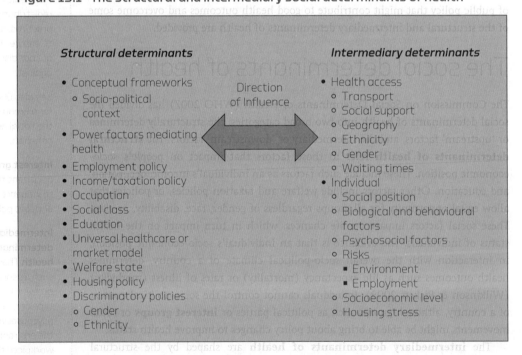

Source: Parry 2009

Stop and Think

Wilkinson and Pickett (2009) in their book *The Spirit Level* provide an evidence-based comparison of the richest 23 countries globally (with populations of over 3 million). They establish that it is more than income, both individually and nationally, that determines the health and social well-being of a population.

Health and social problems are linked to the size of the inequality within a nation, or the gap between rich and poor. Those countries that have smaller gaps between the haves and the have nots and provide support for their people, are more equal, and have fewer health and social problems overall. Conversely, those countries with large gaps have many more social and health problems to tackle. For example, the USA, one of the world's richest nations, has poorer outcomes across a range of health and social issues than many less wealthy countries.

The ability of a country to provide health and social services to its populace in an equitable manner also has a profound influence on population outcomes and the problems faced by the society as a whole. This is captured by the quote below:

> First, the differences between more and less equal societies are large—problems are anything from three to ten times as common in the more unequal societies. Second, these differences are not differences between high- and low-risk groups within populations which might apply only to a small proportion of the population, or just to the poor. Rather, they are differences between the prevalence of different problems which apply to the whole population. (Wilkinson & Pickett 2009, p. 173)

» How can this be? This seems counter-intuitive as surely those countries with more income and with affluent populations have fewer health problems.

» Do you have a view on why this is so?

The healthcare system as a structural determinant of health

As illustrated in Figure 19.1, the structural determinants of health go beyond income, occupation, and education to include the values and social policies in place in a country. This includes the kind of healthcare system. For example, if the government sees health as a human right, rather than an individual responsibility, it is likely to have some form of universal and free healthcare. If the prevailing value is individual rights, the healthcare system may be a user pays or private one.

The type of healthcare system a country has is a structural determinant of health, but as you can see, so too are our values.

Health policies, including the healthcare system, are maintained because they serve the interests of particular powerful interest groups who have sets of values about what they see as important. Besides the government in power, other powerful interest groups might include employer associations, private health insurers, unions, and health professional associations who all have ideas on how healthcare should be organised. Depending on their power, these groups are able to promote and maintain their interests because of their access to powerful decision-makers in government. These groups prevail upon the government to change or alter health policy in their interest or in the interest of members. This can be either positive or negative for particular populations. For example, a public free healthcare system is positive for low socio-economic groups, but a private user pays system may suit the needs of wealthier population groups who can afford private health insurance.

Types of healthcare systems and impact on access

One way of examining how the healthcare system is a structural determinant of health is to examine how the service is financed and whether this system allows for universal and relatively free coverage for all citizens. According to Docteur and Oxley (2003), there are three basic models of health delivery and financing. These healthcare systems differ in several ways: whether the funding is public or private, whether the care is provided by private practitioners or publicly paid providers, and who accepts responsibility for the provision and management of public or private healthcare.

The first is the *public-integrated model*. In countries that have this model, public hospitals and services are funded by the government as part of the welfare state. This makes it a *welfare-based model*. They do not separate insurance and provision functions. Doctors and other health professionals can be either public employees paid on a salary, or if in private practice contracting their services to the government. There is universal population coverage, regardless of income, and this

Health access The opportunity or right to receive affordable, timely, and appropriate healthcare in a manner that promotes optimum health.

coverage is simple to provide. Thus, **health access** is not dependent on the person's ability to buy health, but on the government's responsibility to provide healthcare as a right for all citizens. Healthcare is paid for through taxation. Those earning more income pay higher taxes and levies towards the healthcare system. Costs and the delivery of the system are directly covered by the government (Docteur & Oxley 2003; Davis et al. 2010). In this system, growth of overall health costs is easier to contain as the government provides both the universal coverage and the provision of services

free from competition. The model is used in Australia (in the public hospital sector), Greece, Ireland, Italy, New Zealand, and Spain. Public hospitals are central to the provision of care in this model (Docteur & Oxley 2003).

The limitations of this model include the lack of incentives to increase productivity or efficiency or to be responsive to patient's needs since the health professionals are waged. There is also a limit on the degree of consumer choice for the provider of services (Docteur & Oxley 2003).

The second approach is the *public-contract service delivery* model. This approach to healthcare funding uses public funds to contract private companies to provide healthcare (Docteur & Oxley 2003). An example of this in Australia is the primary healthcare services provided by general practitioners.

GPs are private providers paid on a fee-for-service basis by the Commonwealth through Medicare (NHHRC 2009a). The public contract model does provide incentives to prevent ill health and can be very responsive to patient needs. For example, in Australia the Commonwealth is able to provide incentives for GPs to become more efficient, increase their productivity, and offer new services. As there is only one funding body, this model is efficient, with low administration costs (Docteur & Oxley 2003). This model is also used in Germany, France, Netherlands, the UK (GP Trusts), and Japan. It requires high levels of government regulation and control to protect public funds and consumer health outcomes (Docteur & Oxley 2003), but despite this has the limitation of not being able to completely control service provider fees. As a consequence, access can be limited by the fact that the patient may have to make a co-payment or pay a gap fee.

The third and final model, the *private insurance model*, is an insurance-based system where delivery relies on the private sector, with the insurance and services delivered by private companies. In some countries, such as Switzerland, it is compulsory to take out private health insurance, while in others it is voluntary, as in the USA (Docteur & Oxley 2003).

There is a high degree of choice in this system and responsiveness to the patient's needs such as very short waiting lists or none. However, there is little or no cost control by government, insurance companies, providers, or individuals. Private insurance companies charge what the market will pay and in some instances limit access to care depending on the type of insurance cover. Affordability for the consumer is an issue with this model. In the 1990s, in an effort to manage increasing costs, the USA introduced managed care plans (Docteur & Oxley 2003). This change allowed insurers to select clients and providers and restrict patient treatments and service access (Docteur & Oxley 2003; Davis et al. 2010). More recent reforms by President Obama have attempted to ensure people are fully insured by private insurers, although how successful this will be is yet to be determined. Where private health insurance is the major form of health cover, unless the government provides some members of the society with healthcare, such as the poor and elderly, large segments of the population may not be covered by any form of health insurance and therefore have limited access to health. Examples of countries using this system include Switzerland (compulsory insurance), USA (voluntary insurance, although health insurance is a standard benefit of employment including in many minimum wages jobs), and Australia, where 50% of Australians have some form of private health insurance (Medicare Australia 2011). Table 19.1 summarises some of the differences in the three models around issues of access such as funding source, the extent of coverage, choice of practitioner, and waiting times.

Table 19.1   Models of healthcare access

Model	Funding Source	Health Access	Cost	Coverage	Choice	Waiting Lists
Public-integrated	General taxation	Universal primary and acute	Relatively free	Universal	No	Yes
Public-contract	General taxation or levy	Universal primary and acute	Relatively free, but may have gap fees	Restricted	Some	Yes

(continues)

Table 19.1   Models of healthcare access (*continued*)

Model	Funding Source	Health Access	Cost	Coverage	Choice	Waiting Lists
Private insurance	Consumer pays	Can be universal where legislated	Based on insurance premium costs and type of cover	Limited	Yes but restricted	No

Source: Adapted from Docteur & Oxley 2003; Davis et al. 2010

Mythbuster

Consider the claim that the USA has the best healthcare system in the world.

» *From the data presented so far why might this be an accurate statement? Why might this be an inaccurate statement?*

Health access as an intermediary determinant of health

Health access is defined as the opportunity or right to receive affordable, consistent, timely, and appropriate healthcare in a manner that promotes optimum health (Mahnken 2001). The particular model of healthcare impacts on access, but there are also intermediary factors such as waiting times for services, the number and amount of co-payments, barriers to particular services such as dental care, geographical isolation, or obstacles linked to gender, ethnicity, or age.

When people do not have access to good healthcare there are a number of negative consequences. These are not just limited to individuals, but include the entire population. They go beyond health to include negative outcomes for an individual's education, employment, and engagement in the social life of a community. For example, limited access to healthcare services is associated with a significant increase in infant mortality and morbidity (Frankenberg 1995; Sandiford et al. 1995; INDEPTH Network 2007), poorer economic outcomes and poverty (Wadsworth & Butterworth 2006; McCally et al. 2008), lower levels of social and community support (Hendryx et al. 2002), and lower education attainment (Solar & Irwin 2007; Doley et al. 2008). Further, limited access to healthcare in childhood is thought to cause disengagement from schooling (Doley et al. 2008), deleterious adult physical and psychological health outcomes (Wadsworth & Butterworth 2006), an increased incidence of poverty (Wadsworth & Butterworth 2006; McCally et al. 2008), and decreased participation in society, including the capacity to produce and consume goods (Hendryx et al. 2002; Shaw et al. 2006; Solar & Irwin 2007).

Limited health access can also lead to further health problems or deterioration in an existing condition (Bartley et al. 2005, 2006). This in turn may impact on a child's education, or an adult's income, or their capacity to care for their children. It may prevent them from returning to work, or increase the number of sick days they take. Accessing healthcare services is presumed to be an individual responsibility and behaviour; this is why the CDSH defines it as an intermediary determinant. However, as the case study below notes, while deciding to go to the doctor is an individual one, the factors that influence this decision may be out of the person's control. The case study illustrates one way in which health access, the cost of paying for medical care, impacts on a family's health.

Stop and Think

Research in Australia of patients admitted to hospital for a pre-existing condition found that 16.6% of the admissions were 'preventable but not prevented' (Hart 2006, p. 85). These patients had illness conditions that could have been prevented had they sought earlier medical care. If these patients had accessed appropriate primary healthcare services in a consistent, timely manner almost a fifth of the admissions would not have been necessary. Accessing healthcare and services in a manner that enables the cycle of illness to be interrupted or prevented is not only cost-effective, it is also less physically and psychologically tiring for those suffering illness episodes (Hart 2006).

Case Study 19.1   Access to healthcare by different social groups in Australia

In research conducted on access to primary care services, Parry (2011) interviewed a number of parents who took their children to the Emergency Department of a large public hospital for illnesses that were not life-threatening, instead of seeking more appropriate care from their local GP. Parry found that cost was a major factor in parents' decisions on seeking care for their children and themselves.

In the quote below, Gail, a single mother of two children, explains why she takes her child to a hospital Emergency Department rather than the more appropriate local GP clinic, and in her own case puts off consulting a medical specialist for several years.

> I just really wish the doctors wouldn't charge that big a gap, because that's the problem I have with the whole thing and that's why I wait years to get anything done. If I had the money I could see a specialist. My GP knows I'm a single parent and have a Healthcare Card and he still charges a gap fee to see the kids if I arrive at the surgery after 4 p.m. Sometimes you can't get an appointment before then, then there's a gap fee...They charge the gap they want, it's not fair.

In this case, the GP charges low-income patients a fee for a medical consultation. The clinic does **bulk-bill** if parents make an appointment before 4 p.m., but as Gail notes this is not always possible, particularly as she works. These high gap charges (intermediary determinant of health) are outside Gail's control. The Medicare model of service provision limits Gail's access to care because costs cannot be controlled by the government. In this case study Gail does not delay accessing healthcare when her children are sick; she either takes them after 4 p.m. to the clinic and has to pay a gap fee, or travels to the

Bulk billing The practice whereby the doctor accepts the Medicare scheduled fee rebate from the Commonwealth Government as the sole payment for a service rather than the additional cost of a gap fee.

> Emergency Department of a public hospital where it is free. However, she does delay accessing healthcare for herself because of the high gap fees for medical specialist care. Delaying care can exacerbate an illness.
>
> Adapted from Parry 2011

The Australian healthcare system

Market-based model A system where access to education, health, and housing must be paid for by the individual, or those who are sick or incapacitated must provide for their own income protection.

As we noted above, healthcare systems around the world can be divided into three broad categories, the first two welfare-based models and the third a **market-based model**. A welfare-based model assumes that health is a basic human right and that all citizens should have equal and timely access to healthcare. As a consequence, governments usually take some responsibility for organising and funding the healthcare system. A market model argues that in a democracy citizens should be able to choose how much and what kind of healthcare they wish to purchase. Under the market model, citizens pay for healthcare; under the welfare model, the government provides and manages the care through a state-run system or the funding of an insurance scheme. Pure market or pure welfare models do not exist. Most countries have a mix of both.

The Australian healthcare system is a mixture of market (private insurance model) and welfare provision (public-integrated and public-contract models). The foundation of the current Australian healthcare system is Medicare. It was established in 1984 by the Hawke Federal Labor Government at a time when up to 35% of Australians had no health cover (Willis 2009a). In recent years, funding has extended to some allied health and nursing services for people with chronic illness (Willis 2009a). The first point to note about Medicare is that it is a compulsory (everyone must be in the scheme), universal (everyone is covered by the scheme regardless of income), health insurance scheme based on the principle of equal access for all Australians. It is funded through taxation and a progressive levy on all taxpayers. This levy is set at 1.5% of each person's income or 2.5% for people on higher incomes who do not have private health insurance. The Medicare levy does not cover the full cost of healthcare, so in reality most Medicare-related health costs are funded through taxation (Leeder 1999; AIHW 2009).

Medicare is divided into two distinct parts: funding for hospitals and funding for primary care and other medical, allied health, and nursing services. Funding for hospitals can be viewed under the public integration model. The Commonwealth funds all public hospitals to around 50% of costs through tied grants to the state and territory governments, who must provide free and timely access to healthcare for all Australians and other eligible persons (Commonwealth of Australia 1993). While not a national health service, this component of Medicare effectively provides free hospital care to all Australians and as a healthcare policy is illustrative of a positive structural determinant of health. For example, if you were involved in a motor vehicle accident, had a heart attack, or a mental health event a state-funded ambulance would convey you free of charge immediately to a public hospital where you would receive free hospital, medical, nursing, and allied healthcare, including free pharmaceuticals during your hospital stay. Follow-up care in rehabilitation or part of the hospital's outpatient clinics would also be free, although you might have to pay a small charge for ongoing pharmaceuticals and wait several weeks or months for an outpatient appointment.

Similarly, if you required elective surgery such as a hip replacement this could be provided in a public hospital free of charge.

The second part of Medicare, also funded by the Commonwealth, provides funding for the patient to cover primary care from a medical practitioner, and some allied health and nursing services. This aspect of Medicare conforms to the public contract model. When the Hawke Labor Government introduced Medicare in 1984 they hoped funding for these medical services would be free through bulk billing. The Commonwealth sets the scheduled fee for all medical services and pays the doctors 85% of this fee. If the doctor bulk-bills the patient is not charged the gap fee, so the service is effectively free, but the doctor only receives 85% of the estimated cost of the service. If the doctor charges the scheduled fee the patient pays the additional 15%. This is called a gap payment. In its original design Medicare provided relatively free access to primary medical care with a low gap fee. Underlying both features of Medicare is an acknowledgment that health and access to affordable care is a basic human right that should be managed and provided by government and paid for through taxation or some form of universal insurance. These aspects of Medicare make it a positive structural determinant of health and in theory should ensure health access.

The limits of access to hospital care

The original 1984 Medicare agreements between the state and territory governments and the Commonwealth noted that hospital care must be timely. Timely care is defined as care that is offered within a clinically appropriate period. For example, as noted above, if you had a heart attack you would receive immediate care. But since not all medical conditions need to be treated straight away, some patients are assigned to elective surgery or outpatient waiting lists. While waiting lists must be made public, and the patient must not wait beyond what is considered safe, this is an area where health access becomes problematic. There are three problems associated with timely access to hospital care that illustrate the complexity of access to healthcare as a social determinant of health even in systems that take as a premise that health is a human right. The first problem is the increase in the population requiring care either as an emergency admission or for elective surgery. The increased pressure on public hospitals is partly explained as a result of population growth, the increase in the percentage of people living into their seventies and beyond requiring care for chronic conditions, the increase in education which leads people to demand quality healthcare, the drop in the number of people with private health insurance, and the high cost of medical care. As a result, elective surgery in public hospitals may not always be as timely as needed for the patient's comfort or convenience. This can impact on people's general well-being, but also on their capacity to earn their living and function in everyday life. The high demand for healthcare services may lead governments with publicly funded hospital systems to use a quota system to restrict the number of procedures as a cost containment strategy, since price is not a deterrent to patients (Hurst & Siciliani 2003). While there is logic to this strategy, it assumes that considerable numbers of patients demand, and their doctors perform, unnecessary surgery.

A second factor is geography. Not all Australians have equal access to public hospitals providing emergency or elective care. Examples include those living in rural and remote areas, particularly Indigenous Australians, and even those living in outer suburbs. Travelling to the city for hospital care brings with it added expenses, although the Patient Admission Transport Scheme, a welfare scheme that reimburses patients from rural and remote areas for their travel and accommodation costs while in a city hospital, provides some additional financial assistance. A major problem for these populations is that it is difficult to entice health professionals to work in isolated communities, or the population may be so low that it is not economically efficient for governments to provide the service. The model of healthcare is a factor here in influencing governments to provide the service.

A third factor relates to socio-economic status, including cultural and ethnic disparities in health access. Over 26% of those admitted to a public hospital for elective surgery come from the *Most Disadvantaged* quintile, while only 13% come from the *Most Advantaged quintile* (AIHW 2010d, p. 131). However, the disadvantage does not stop here. People in higher income brackets have higher rates of elective surgery. Sixty-nine per 1000 persons accessed elective surgery from the

Quintile A quintile represents 20% (a fifth) of the population. The lowest quintile is the poorest group; the highest group is the wealthiest.

highest **quintile**, while only 38 per 1000 did in the lowest quintile (AIHW 2009, p. xv). This points to an underlying problem with the mixed nature of the Australian healthcare system. Those with private health insurance are able to seek timely and usually quick elective surgery or medical care in a private hospital with the doctor of their choice. Waiting lists are not as long in private hospital. People without private health insurance must wait until their name comes to the top of a public hospital waiting list. The problem is that in many cases emergency admissions take precedence over elective surgery, the lists of people needing surgery are long, and the number of procedures a hospital may perform in any one year may be capped.

Being poor, and therefore likely to be sicker, is not the only difficulty for low socio-economic populations. Their access to healthcare is also stratified. For example, data from the Australian Institute of Health (AIHW 2010d, p. 131) shows that the median waiting time for patients on public hospital waiting lists was 34 days. However, those in the second lowest quintile (or *Second Most Disadvantaged*) waited 37 days, while those in the highest quintile (*Most Advantaged*) only waited 24 days (AIHW 2010d, p. 261).

Figure 19.2   Separations per 1000 population for public and private elective surgery, by remoteness of area of usual residence

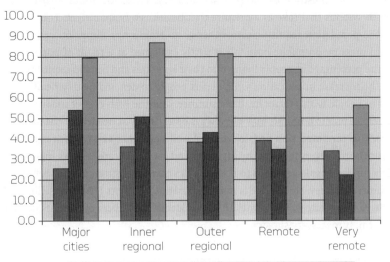

Source: AIHW 2010d

The impact of disadvantage can be examined through **separation rates** for elective surgery, this time looking at the issue of remoteness. Data from the 2008–09 report on Australian hospital statistics 2008–09 (AIHW 2010d) illustrates the impact of remoteness on access to elective surgery for people in the cities, outer suburbs, rural, and remote regions (Figure 19.2).

Separation rates The percentage of people who leave hospital before midnight on any one day either discharged, transferred to another facility, or who die.

Stop and Think

We know that geography makes a difference to rates of illness. People in rural areas in Australia have higher rates of illness, yet the graph above indicates that they are disadvantaged in access to elective surgery. This is partly because they do not have access to private hospitals as there are few in regional, rural, or remote areas.

» If you were Minister for Health how might you go about remedying this disadvantage?

Presumably, access to timely acute care should simply be a matter of increasing resources to the public system. However, how funds are allocated is a political issue that reflects the values of a society and the power of particular interest groups. For example, in order to encourage people to take out private health insurance, the Howard Federal Coalition Government introduced a 30% rebate for individuals and families with private health insurance. This policy decision diverted resources from the public health system to providing financial incentive to wealthier people. It increased the percentage of people with private health insurance, which in turn increased profits for private insurers, private hospitals, and doctors in private practice (Laris et al. 2008), but of course it may

Figure 19.3   Percentage of persons with private health insurance by quintile for Adelaide, South Australia

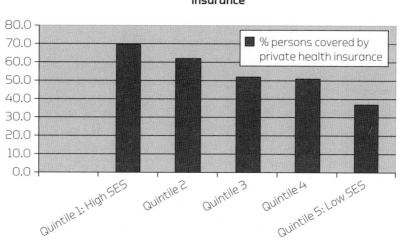

Source: PHIDU 2010

also have increased timely access to care for this population. Data on private health insurance shows that those in the *Most Disadvantaged* quintile have lower rates of private health insurance. Figure 19.3 provides the figures for Adelaide in South Australia by quintile. Readers can readily see that people in the *Most Disadvantaged* quintile have lower rates of health insurance. This means that elective, surgical, acute short-term health access is funded in the private sector, in favour of chronic, emergency, and costly health services provided in the public sector (Laris et al. 2008), given that 75% of the doctor's fee is covered through Medicare. Attempts by the Federal Labor Government to reduce this rebate have been politically difficult, indicating the power of interest groups to maintain health policy that supports the rich over the poor.

The limits of access to primary care

Just as access to hospitals can be problematic, so too is access to primary medical care. Costs, distance, and the problem of supply are major barriers to accessing primary care such as GP services. When Medicare was first introduced it was hoped that the majority of doctors would bulk-bill. However, as the story of Gail (Case Study 19.1) notes, doctors are free to charge any fee they like and many charge above the scheduled fee, leaving patients with an additional gap fee. To assist low-income individuals and families to manage the costs of primary care various Commonwealth governments have introduced safety nets to assist individuals and families manage the rising cost of co-payments. The first is the Family Safety Net. In 2010 the gap fee was $388.80 for an individual or family, after which point Medicare reimburses the individual or family the full scheduled fee. However, since many doctors charge above the schedule fee (Willis 2009b) the patient may still have a high gap fee to pay. To counter this a second safety gap, called the Extended Medicare Safety Net, was introduced by the Howard Government (1996–2007) to cover this gap. In early 2010, the safety net was $562.90 for disadvantaged individuals and families and $1126 for other families and individuals. Thus, disadvantaged families on low incomes or Commonwealth Benefits need to spend $562.90 in Extended gap fees before the rebate is provided. This rebate then provides for 80% of out-of-pocket expenses (Medicare Australia 2011).

The issue of fees for primary medical care is further complicated by the corporatisation of medicine (White 2001). Many small GP clinics have amalgamated to form large multi-purpose clinics either controlled by the doctors themselves or multinational firms. These clinics provide access to care without an appointment, so attract patients who cannot access a family doctor. However, access to the same doctor is not guaranteed. While the positive side of this development means patients can access the diagnostic tests they may need on-site, and get immediate medical care, the profit motive for owners has led to increased charges and a lack of continuity of care. For example, some large multi-purpose medical clinics that previously bulk-billed patients now require a co-payment or charge a significantly high gap fee that may mean that people on low incomes may put off seeking medical care that could prevent further illness (Vaughan & Harvy 2009). The issue of continuity of care goes to the heart of primary medical care. Wong and Regan (2009, p. 6) conducted research into client's experiences of access including the quality and consistency of healthcare they received. Patients in their research identified three types of continuity:

> i) relational—the ongoing therapeutic relationship between a consumer and
> provider; ii) informational—the use of information on past events and personal

characteristics to make care appropriate; and iii) management—a consistent and coherent approach to the management of a health condition. Participants believed that the inability to maintain a continuous relationship with a provider contributed to challenges in maintaining people's health.

Their data provides the basis for improvements to be incorporated into any future policy and health provision changes, and increasing compliance with treatment.

Distance, supply, and access

In addition to costs, distance and the shortages of GPs and medical specialists in rural and outer suburbs in Australia creates access problems. The problem manifests in two ways. First, there are fewer health professionals per population working in rural and remote regions, and second, the structure of the primary care component of Medicare (public contract model) means that health services in rural and remote regions are anti-competitive. For example, in rural and remote areas the number of GPs per population is considerably less than the higher-income densely populated urban areas of the capital cities. The low populations in rural areas create regional monopolies as the rural GPs are self-employed practitioners with no or restricted competition. This gives these medical practitioners the significant advantage of charging gap fees strengthened by medical shortages, professional dominance, and limited alternatives for services (Kenny 2004). The result is significant disparity in health access between rural and urban populations (Kenny 2004).

This inequity in access also extends to some urban populations. For example, many outer suburban areas have limited health access. This limits after-hours access and places a strain on other services (PHCIS 2006). Areas of socio-economic disadvantage also have higher numbers of patients per GP. Table 19.2 gives examples for five suburbs or towns in South Australia. Since Salisbury has a fertility rate of 2–3 children per women, while the Adelaide metropolitan area average is 1.61 (PHCIS 2006), there is a higher percentage of families with children in these areas with limited or no access to GPs. This table also shows that people living in Burnside have greater access to GP services than those living in outer suburbs or in rural and remote areas. The likely outcome for people in the Flinders Ranges or Salisbury is that they will have to wait for an appointment, whereas people in Burnside may be able to get a same-day appointment.

Table 19.2   Ratio of GP to population; selected SLA, South Australia

Statistical Local Area	1 Gp Per Head of Population	Designation
Burnside	659	Urban–inner
Playford	2,883	Urban–outer
Salisbury	2,883	Urban–outer
Mallala	4,172	Rural
Flinders Ranges	6,340	Remote
SA Average	**1,126**	

Source: Adapted from PHIDU 2006

Cost, access, distance, undersupply, and long waits for an appointment can deter people from accessing primary care, or they may seek inappropriate care such as attending a public hospital emergency department. For example, in 2009–10, 44% of presentations to public hospital emergency departments were for what is referred to as GP-type presentations. These are for illnesses that could be dealt with more effectively by the patient's family doctor. For large public hospitals this rate rose to 51% of all presentations (AIHW 2010d, p. 13). What this data indicates is that between 40% and 50% of people who present at a public hospital emergency department for primary care should really have seen their local GP. While it is not clear exactly why these people do not seek primary care from their GP, the research does show that low socio-economic groups the world over cannot afford appropriate primary medical care or do not have access to it. From this, we can assume that the key to health access is cost; this might be the cost to the consumer or the impact on profits made by the provider (Bell et al. 2007; Kelaher et al. 2008).

Health access reform

Most Western countries have attempted to deal with the problems of health access over the last 20 years through a series of reforms. In the early 1990s, these reforms focused on increasing productivity and efficiency of existing services by setting targets that attempted to ensure better access. Examples included providing hospitals with incentive funding if patients on elective surgery waiting lists did not have long waits. In Australia, public hospitals have to publish waiting times so that the public can see how efficient they are (Willis 2009b). More recent reforms to increase patient access have included increasing the number of health professionals educated and trained, and extending the skills and practice of health professionals other than doctors through a process of **role substitution**. Nurse practitioners are one example of this. Nurse practitioners can prescribe a limited number of drugs and order diagnostic tests. Another strategy has been to design new models of care. Case Study 19.2 provides information on GP Plus and Super Clinics—two policy initiatives aimed at reducing costs and ensuring speedy access to care.

Role substitution The process whereby one profession takes up the role and skills of another.

This discussion on health access has assumed that all sick people need is access to a GP and a hospital. This is not always the case. Comprehensive healthcare also means access to pharmaceuticals, dental care, and ongoing services for those with a mental illness or a chronic condition and for the elderly. Where these services are not provided in a free and timely manner, because they are outside the remit of the welfare state, some populations will have reduced life chances. Of course even where there is excellent health access, if populations do not have access to employment, education, or housing their health status will deteriorate.

Case Study 19.2   GP Plus and GP Super Clinics: Policy futures

In an attempt to improve access to health in areas where there is high need and limited services, the South Australian Government has introduced GP Plus Centres in low socio-economic suburbs and the Commonwealth will fund a number of GP Super Clinics around the country. These clinics were developed in conjunction with service providers to improve access and decrease the inappropriate use of services such as emergency departments for primary healthcare conditions. These services are located in areas of high need and low GP coverage.

The GP Plus clinics provide allied health and community support services such as parenting and counselling sessions. They may also provide access to speech pathologists, community paediatricians, mental health services providers, and kindy gym classes. The clinics are also able to provide after-hours access to GP services provided there is no alternative GP practice in that area. Where after-hours GPs are provided by the GP Plus Clinic all patients are bulk-billed if they have a Medicare card ensuring free access.

In addition, the GP Plus Centre also provides x-ray, blood screening, and other pathology services in order to decrease the need for patients to access acute care services for diagnostic purposes. However, GP after-hours services are not provided if the community has alternative access to a GP. For example, one GP Plus Centre in Adelaide is co-located with a daytime and after-hours private GP service. As a consequence, no GP services are provided by the GP Plus Centre until the private service closes each day at 5.30 p.m. The GP private service only bulk-bills healthcare card holders. Other patients need to pay an upfront gap fee of between $30 and $60 before seeing a GP. This has the potential to limit access and divert patients to emergency departments where the services are free.

Stop and Think

The establishment of GP Plus and GP Super Clinics is an attempt by state and Commonwealth governments to increase patient access to free primary care. However, the way in which Medicare is organised means that the profits of doctors must be safeguarded. Aspects of the Australian Constitution do not allow governments to insist that doctors become salaried employees.

» If you were Minister of Health, how might you go about remedying this disadvantage?

Summary

The social determinants of health are divided into the structural and intermediary. Health access is an intermediary determinant of health. An examination of health access as a social determinant of health requires understanding what kind of healthcare a particular country has in place. Most countries in the developed world have one of three types of healthcare systems. The first is the public-integrated model, which is usually funded by government. The second is the public-contract service delivery model, which uses public funds to contract private companies to provide healthcare. Both models have the capacity to provide universal and relatively free access to healthcare. The third model is the private fee-for-service approach. This model limits health access to those who can afford the care. The type of healthcare system a nation has is influenced by the values of that society, the kind of government, and its social policies. Health access as a social determinant is also underpinned by an understanding of health as a social right, rather than health as an individual responsibility.

In order to examine the health access of a particular system it is necessary to investigate the policies governing the provision of healthcare. In Australia, for example, Medicare both facilitates and limits access to healthcare. Access to GPs is based on the public-contract service delivery model whereby GPs are paid to deliver the service as private providers. As a consequence, they may not offer after-hours services or services to people in remote or rural areas. An example of recent policy initiatives to overcome this is the establishment of Medicare Locals across Australia. These will have a brief to ensure there are after-hours services in their region.

Tutorial exercises

1   Go to <www.equalitytrust.org.uk/why>.

Read the front page. Watch the video report. On the right-hand corner at the bottom is a PowerPoint show. Watch this. Select a social determinant of health and see the results. The places will be either countries, or states in the USA. Bring some observations that you make to the class for discussion.

2   Go to the interactive features/graph on the website below. The biennial report compares healthcare system performance over several OECD countries. Review the results with the class.

3   Read the report *Mirror, Mirror on the Wall: How the Performance of the U.S. Health System Compares Internationally*, <www.commonwealthfund.org/Content/Publications/Fund-Reports/2010/Jun/Mirror-Mirror-Update.aspx?page=all>.

This website provides a set of interactive graphs that discuss patient satisfaction, health system performance, and quality and safety issues in health systems. The US health system as a private insurance system is the most responsive to patient needs. So, why does it score so poorly on patient satisfaction, etc.? Discuss.

4   Identify those aspects of the social determinants of health that are part of the healthcare system. Identify those factors that are not part of the healthcare system. Discuss what can be done by health professionals to address the social determinants of health. What limitations do health professionals face?

5   What are the strengths and weaknesses of the Australian health system in terms of its approach to the social determinants of health?

Further reading

Davis, K., Schoen, C., & Stemikis, K. (2010). *Mirror, mirror on the wall: How the performance of the U.S. health system compares internationally.* The Commonwealth Fund. Report No 1400. <www.commonwealthfund.org/Content/Publications/Fund-Reports/2010/Jun/Mirror-Mirror-Update.aspx?page=all>.

Docteur, E., & Oxley, H. (2003). *Health-care systems: Lessons from the reform experience. OECD Health Working Paper 9.* Paris: OECD.

Hart, J.T. (2006). *The political economy of healthcare: A clinical perspective.* Bristol, UK: Policy Press.

Hendryx, M., Ahern, A., Lovrich, N., & McCurdy, A. (2002). Access to healthcare and community social capital. *Health Services Research*, 37(1), 85–101.

Marmot, M., & Wilkinson, R.G. (eds) (2006). *Social determinants of health*, 2nd edn. Oxford: Oxford University Press.

Websites

<www.phcris.org.au>

This website is the home of the Primary Healthcare Research and Information Centre. You can use it to keep up to date with policy reforms in general practice in Australia.

<www.publichealth.gov.au>

This web page is the home of the Public Health Information Development Unit. You can use it to access data on socio-economic status and health in Australia.

<www.who.int/social_determinants/thecommission/finalreport/en/index.html>

This is the home page for the WHO Commission on Social Determinants of Health.

Yvonne Parry and Eileen Willis

Glossary

Active ageing
Optimising health, participation, and security to enhance quality of life.

Adaptation
Taking action to minimise the current and expected impacts of climate change.

Anthropogenic change
Caused by human activity.

Baby boomers
Those born during the post-Second World War baby boom. They are usually defined as those born between 1946 and 1964.

Behavioural factors
Risk factors such as diet, exercise, smoking, and alcohol consumption and their effects on the incidence of chronic illness.

Best practice
Theoretically based activities and/or practices that have a rigorous and systematic evidence base to support their recognition as effective and appropriate means for delivering programs or services.

Biological basis
The genetic basis of chronic illness, and also refers to the effects of ageing.

Biological determinants
The inner physiological aspect of health and disease. Genes play a crucial role in underlying biological differences between individuals.

Biomedical model of ageing
Emphasises the role of age-related biological changes and chronic illness (morbidity) on the ageing process.

Biomedical model of health
Suggests that illness results from a malfunction of the body (i.e. germs or disease) and that each disease affects the body in a predictable way.

Built environment
All the buildings, structures, infrastructure, etc. created by human beings in an effort to improve their living environment.

Bulk billing
The practice whereby the doctor accepts the Medicare scheduled fee rebate from the Commonwealth Government as the sole payment for a service rather than the additional cost of a gap fee.

Burden of disease study (BoD)
A type of descriptive analysis that summarises the health impact of a chosen disease or risk factor. The health impact of disease can be reported in many ways: incidence, prevalence, premature deaths; or mortality and morbidity impacts combined.

Chromosomes
Threadlike structures of DNA (deoxyribonucleic acid) within cells that carry genetic information in the form of genes.

Chronic disease
A disease that cannot be transmitted from person to person, is usually long lasting and may not be amenable to cure. Many chronic diseases are associated with certain lifestyles or behaviours.

Climate
The average weather, encompassing natural variability and extremes.

Climate change
A variation in climate that is attributable to either natural environmental changes or stemming from human action (anthropogenic change).

Climate change literacy
General knowledge or awareness of the concepts, cause, and effects of climate change.

Cohort
A group who share the same experiences, in the same time, in the same sequence.

Collaboration
A process involving different parties who are committed to working interdependently to achieve a common goal or address a common issue.

Communicable disease
The transmission of an infectious agent from one person to another.

Communicable disease, contagious disease
Alternative terms for *infectious disease*.

Cost of illness study (COI)
A type of descriptive analysis that summarises the cost impact of a chosen disease or risk factor. Most COI studies include all 'direct' and 'indirect' costs. Some may also put a dollar cost on pain and suffering ('intangibles').

Cultural competency
The ability to work effectively with people from different cultural and language backgrounds.

Cultural relativism
The theory or view that morality is relative to culture or that right and wrong vary with cultural norms.

Culture
A system of shared ideas, attitudes, and practices that defines the social system of its members.

DALY
Stands for *Disabilty Adjusted Life Year*. The DALY is a summary measure of illness that combines: years of life lost due to illness (YLL) against a specified life expectancy; and years of life lived with disability (YLD).

Decision rule
An agreed guideline where analysts specify in advance what result is correct or acceptable. It is used to answer what 'value for money' means. In Australia, a common rule of thumb is to specify

'$50,000 per QALY/DALY prevented' as the benchmark for what constitutes a cost-effective use of healthcare resources.

Defences against infection—adaptive (also known as specific) defences
Antibodies and cells that act against unique antigens, that is, against the identifiers of specific pathogens or parasites, ultimately enabling their destruction and removal. Adaptive defences are acquired in response to exposure to these unique antigens, but depend on our inherited capacity to respond to them.

Defences against infection—innate (also known as non-specific) defences
Structures and functions that are present from birth, and that act immediately to prevent any foreign material either from entering the body or from establishing an infectious disease should one have already gained entry.

Demand
The quantity of a service or product sold in the marketplace at a specified price. *Demand* is distinguished from *wants* in economics by consumers' preparedness to actually purchase the good or service—that is, demonstrating their willingness to pay. In so doing, consumers are said to reveal what value they place on different products or services by how they use their available income.

Determinants of health
A range of individual, social, economic, environmental, and cultural conditions that have the potential to contribute to or detract from the health of individuals, communities, or whole populations.

Deviance
Behaviour that transgresses social expectations and is likely to attract sanctions from other members of the society.

Difference
Used when an individual possesses characteristics that are dissimilar to or behave differently from the majority of people within a society.

Direct cost
Cost in health economics refers to the resources consumed during the provision of healthcare. Direct cost refers to those resources whose consumption is wholly attributable to the provision and use of the health service in question. Direct cost is usually measured in terms of expenditure categories such as salary and wages, capital, consumables, repairs and maintenance, and overheads.

Discrimination
The idea that someone is of less value and should be excluded from social networks and the benefits of society.

Disease
A condition adversely affecting health that has measurable (clinical) symptoms.

Disease genetics
The search for gene mutations thought to cause ill health conditions.

Economic rationalism
A term used to describe those economists who advocate a predominant role for markets and a minimal role for government (i.e. government to have only key functions such as defence, law, and

safety). Economic rationalists advocate minimal government interference in the free operation of markets and stress the potential for government failure.

Efficiency
Maximising the benefits (whatever we define them to be) from the resources available. It involves minimising the *opportunity cost* involved with resource allocation decisions.

Emergency management
A systematic approach based on science and undertaken by experts. It focuses on planning, organising, directing, and controlling emergency situations and it is collaborative and intersectoral in implementation.

Emerging disease
A disease that has not previously been observed in human populations.

Endemic
Always present in a particular environment; often used to refer to a disease or the organism that causes a disease.

Entertainment-education
A mass media 'vehicle' which is designed to entertain a wide general audience while changing societal attitudes and norms. It models and normalises behaviour change that promotes health and social development.

Environmental determinants
Effects of factors in both the physical and social environment. These include air quality related to pollution, chemicals, water quality, and outcomes of climate change and global warming.

Environmental health
The assessment, correction, control, and prevention of those aspects of human health, including quality of life, that are determined by physical, chemical, biological, and psychosocial factors in the environment.

Epidemic
A higher than usual number of cases of a disease or condition in a particular geographic area; there are no requirements for number of cases.

Epidemiology
The study of the distribution and determinants of disease.

Equity
In healthcare can be defined as the absence of systematic disparities in health (or in the major social determinants of health) between social groups who have different levels of underlying social advantage/disadvantage.

Ethnicity
Refers to a shared cultural background which is a characteristic of a group within a society.

Evidence-based
Using good-quality information to develop a policy, position, strategy, or action.

Food security
Having access to sufficient food that is nutritionally and culturally appropriate.

Functional health
Is seen as well-being, not merely as the avoidance of disease and disability.

Gender
Socially and culturally constructed categories reflecting what it means to be 'masculine' and 'feminine' and associated expectations of roles and behaviours of men and women.

Gene mutations
Thought to cause particular ill health conditions.

Gene therapy
The insertion of DNA into cells to correct genetic defects. This involves supplementing or replacing a gene where its abnormality or absence leads to a disease.

Genes
Basic units in the body's cells which contain the genetic material that codes for heredity as well as health, growth, and development.

Genetic condition
A condition or disorder caused by a genetic mutation that affects how body systems develop or function.

Genetic determinism
The belief that a person's health and behaviour are predetermined by their genetic makeup.

Genetic discrimination
The unfair treatment of an asymptomatic person on the basis of their genetic characteristics or makeup.

Genetic mutation
A permanent change in a gene that prevents the cell from accurately reading the genetic code. Genetic mutations can occur naturally or they can result from exposure to chemical or physical agents; they can also sometimes be inherited.

Genetic reductionism
Attempts to understand and present complex sets of relationships/precursors to disease by genetic explanations only. By focusing on these, important social and related factors which can contribute to illness are ignored.

Genetic risk
The probability that a trait, condition, or disorder will occur or recur in an individual or family more frequently than it occurs by chance.

Geneticisation
Explanations of social, cultural, or health phenomena with reference to genetic frameworks.

Genome
All the genetic material in the cells of a living organism.

Genotype
A person's genetic constitution.

Global warming
The rise in global temperature observed during the 20th century and projected to continue into the future.

Government failure
The adverse consequences of ineffective or inefficient government intervention in markets through activities such as taxes/subsidies, regulation of market entry, direct provision of services, etc.

Greenhouse gas
A gas that contributes to trapping heat in the atmosphere, warming the earth. These gases are both naturally occurring and released into the atmosphere by humans.

Health
There is no definite meaning of health. Its meaning can be different depending on individuals, social groups, and cultures and can differ at different times. In general, it means not just the absence of illness or disease but a total sense of well-being.

Health access
The opportunity or right to receive affordable, timely, and appropriate healthcare in a manner that promotes optimum health.

Health equity
A situation in which groups with different levels of underlying social advantage or disadvantage (wealth, power, or prestige) do not experience health inequalities associated solely with social positioning.

Health literacy
The individual's ability to successfully seek out, identify, interpret, and act on health information so as to protect and improve their health.

Health promotion
A discipline that takes a holistic approach to positively maintaining and improving the health and well-being of individuals, communities, and whole populations.

Health sociology
A discipline that recognises that health and illness are influenced by a range of social determinants and focuses on the social patterns of health and illness.

Healthy ageing
The process of achieving optimal health and well-being through active adaptation to ageing processes.

HIV/AIDS
Human Immunodeficiency Virus (HIV) and Acquired Immunodeficiency Syndrome (AIDS) emerged as a major public health issue in 1981 in North America. It has now affected gay men, injecting drug users, women, and newborn babies in many parts of the world. It is a highly stigmatised illness because it is seen to be associated with individuals who engage in deviant sexual behaviour or anti-social behaviour of other kinds.

Human agency
Our ability to negotiate the social structures and a way to account for individual differences in the life course.

Human Genome Project
An international research project begun in 1990 and completed in 2003 which aimed to map all chromosomes and sequence all genes in the human being.

Human rights
Rights held to be justifiably belonging to any person.

ICER
Stands for 'incremental cost-effectiveness ratio'. The results of economic evaluations in the health sector are generally expressed as a ratio that summarises the additional cost of the intervention compared to current practice (incremental cost), over the additional health gain compared to current practice (incremental benefit). The resulting ratio is then compared with a decision rule to decide whether the option for change is value for money.

Ideology
A collection of beliefs or ideas particular to a group or discipline.

Illness
A condition adversely affecting health as perceived by the individual in question.

Illness behaviour
The socially acceptable way to act when sick.

Immunisation
The acquisition of adaptive immunity to an infectious disease, including both humoral and cellular immunity. Humoral immunity (antibodies in plasma and other body fluids) can be active or passive. Immunisation can be naturally acquired following exposure to a pathogen, or artificially acquired as a result of vaccination.

Incidence
The occurrence of new cases of a disease or condition in a particular population during a period of interest.

Indirect cost
In health economics, this term refers to productivity impacts in the general economy (paid and/or unpaid), due to existing morbidity/mortality patterns, as well as the introduction of health services. If the introduction of a national screening program, for example, involved attendance during work hours, this would have a negative productivity impact in the short term. If the screening program prevented disease, however, this would have an important positive productivity impact in the longer term.

Individual ageing
The biological, psychological, and social changes in an individual over time.

Inequity
Inequality resulting from unfairness or bias.

Infection
The presence of pathogens or parasites on or in body tissues and/or fluids with the result that they cause disease.

Infectious disease
A disease that can be transmitted from person to person, either directly through the spread of a disease-causing agent or indirectly such as by a vector.

Intangible costs
The pain and suffering imposed by disease and/or its treatment, which are typically very difficult to quantify in dollar terms. Some COI studies include them and some forms of economic evaluation (e.g. cost–benefit analysis) also measure health outcomes in dollar terms.

Interest groups
Groups of citizens that organise to influence government or public policy.

Intermediary determinants of health
Those factors such as social position, access to healthcare, type of housing, or psychosocial risks in the environment or workplace that impact on health status.

Justice
Fairness.

Labelling theory
The process of labelling a person with stigma, which through the process of social interaction will eventually lead the person to change their self-perception and lose social opportunity.

Life and historical times
A way of accounting for cohort effects and how they affect the individual now and in the future.

Life course perspective
The cumulative effects of events from earlier life on later life.

Life expectancy
The average life span at birth for a given society.

Life event
Abrupt and sudden change in life resulting in significant change in trajectory and stress.

Linked lives
The interdependence we have with others in our social networks and relationships and how these affect our life course.

Living environment
The surroundings in which we live, work, and participate; everything that is external to the human body that incorporates social, cultural, and political processes, built and natural elements, and the interaction of these as one ecosystem.

Local government
Australia has three tiers of government, with local government being the closest to the people, providing local public services such as rubbish collection and immunisation, and facilities such as parks and community buildings within a particular area.

Longevity
The length of one's life, often used to describe the state of someone who has lived beyond their natural life expectancy.

Market-based model
A system where access to education, health, and housing must be paid for by the individual, or those who are sick or incapacitated must provide for their own income protection.

Market failure
The situation where free markets do not achieve *allocative efficiency* and/or *technical efficiency*. Common sources of market failure include spillover effects; insufficient information to allow consumers to make good choices; supply-induced demand; and merit goods. Health economists see the health sector as having many of these characteristics.

Marketing
The strategies used by commercial or non-profit enterprises—including the use of persuasive communications such as advertising—that aim to change attitudes so that the consumer feels positive towards, and decides to buy or use, the advertised product or service.

Mass media
The means by which messages are communicated throughout a society, transmitting the same message to large numbers of people over a large geographical area at the same time, e.g. television, cinema, radio, the internet, newspapers, and magazines.

Media advocacy
Aims to stimulate public support—and obtain the attention and sympathy of policymakers and legislators—to gain changes in law and policy which impact on public health.

Merit goods
A term used to define goods or services where the state has an interest in its citizens consuming the good or service. In the case of merit goods, such as healthcare and education, the benefit to the state of a healthy educated population may be such as to override the principle of 'consumer sovereignty' (consumers knowing what's best for them).

Mitigation
Taking action to reduce greenhouse gas emissions.

Moral career
A process when a stigmatised individual initially makes sense of their social position within the society and later acquires a set idea of what it would be like to hold a specific characteristic.

Morbidity
Having to do with disease; the morbidity rate is the rate of a particular disease in a given population during a period of interest; the relative incidence of a particular disease.

Mortality
Having to do with death; the mortality rate is the rate of death from a particular cause in a given population during a period of interest.

Multi-factorial disorders
Genetic disorders that are caused by a combination of factors including genetic mutations and environmental factors; examples are familial breast, ovarian, and bowel cancers.

Municipal Health and Well-being Plans
Planning documents designed to ensure that LG strategic planning and decision-making considers impacts on health using the social model of health perspective.

New Urbanism
An urban design movement that is scaled for the pedestrian, yet capable of accommodating public transport and cars; it contains a range of housing and job types, with a high-quality public realm, and is strongly influenced by urban design standards prominent before the rise of the car.

Non-communicable disease
A term applied to a diverse group of diseases. These diseases do not involve infectious agents, so cannot be passed from person to person, but tend to be ongoing and to have persistent symptoms. The term 'chronic disease' is often used interchangeably with non-communicable disease.

Normal flora
The microorganisms that live, without detriment, on or in regions of the body that communicate with the external environment; they help to control populations of potential pathogens; also known as commensal organisms.

Normative economics
Economic theory and methods that evaluate policies and ideas for change (what ought to be done).

Old-old population
Refers to that segment of the population aged 85 years and above.

Older adults
Refers to that segment of the population that is aged 65 years and above.

Opportunity cost
The benefit or value of the best alternative use of a resource that is forgone as a result of its current use. Minimising opportunity cost is the key rationale underlying an economic approach to decision-making.

Outbreak
An unusual cluster of cases of a disease or condition in a particular geographic area; there are no requirements for number of cases.

Parasite
Any single- or multi-cellular organism that obtains nourishment from the host that it lives on or in.

Pathogen
A microorganism that can cause disease.

Phenotype
A person's physical appearance.

Population ageing
The increase in proportion of older people in a population caused by mortality, fertility, and migration.

Population attributable risk (PAR)
A measure that captures the excess rate of disease in the total study population of exposed and unexposed individuals that is attributable to the exposure. The PAR is important in public health as it is used to measure the benefits of risk factor reduction.

Population density
The number of people per square unit of land; often reported as some number of people per square mile or square kilometre.

Population health
An approach to improving the health of populations by introducing interventions that have the potential to affect everyone.

Positive ageing
Refers to numerous concepts such as one's ability to live to an old age with little or no disability prior to death as well as attitudes towards ageing, e.g. having a positive attitude towards older people.

Positive economics
Economic theory and methods that focus on a description of current practice and the characteristics or functioning of markets and the general economy.

Predictive genetic test
A DNA test to establish the statistical probability that a person has inherited an increased risk of developing a multi-factorial condition.

Pre-symptomatic genetic test
A DNA test to establish if a person has or has not inherited a faulty gene associated with developing a single-gene disorder.

Prevalence
The number of all cases of a disease or condition in a particular population during a period of interest.

Primary prevention
Inhibiting the development of disease.

Productive ageing
Refers to an individual's or population's ability to maintain productivity and participate actively in the social and economic advancement of the nation.

Psychosocial factors
Aspects of the living environment that have the potential to affect people's feelings, perceptions, and cognitive state.

Psychosocial models of ageing
Acknowledge the importance of psychological resilience and adaptation, mental health, life satisfaction, and social environments including social support and social networks.

Public health communication
Uses a variety of carefully developed communication strategies to improve or maintain the health of a population.

Public health genomics
An emerging scientific field that aims to understand genetics in the contexts of populations and public health.

Public policy
Policies brought in by governments to administer education, healthcare, water, sanitation, etc.

Quintile
A quintile represents 20% (a fifth) of the population. The lowest quintile is the poorest group; the highest group is the wealthiest.

Rate
A proportion for which a particular time period is specified.

Relative risk
A measure used to predict the likelihood of disease in exposed individuals relative to those who are unexposed.

Right
A thing one may legally or morally claim.

Risk
The probability or likelihood of a particular effect occurring in a particular population during a period of interest.

Role substitution
The process whereby one profession takes up the role and skills of another.

Secondary prevention
Strategies that enable populations to deal with risks and threats.

Semiotics
The study of the meaning of signs and symbols (e.g. images and colours) within a particular culture and how they communicate specific information and influence the interpretation of messages.

Separation rates
The percentage of people who leave hospital before midnight on any one day either discharged, transferred to another facility, or who die.

Single-gene disorders
Genetic disorders caused by the inheritance of a mutation in a single gene; an example is Huntington's disease.

Social capital
The intangible factors that create networks and linkages among groups and individuals; includes things like trust in others, reciprocity, and group membership.

Social class
The position of a person in a system of structured inequality; it is grounded in unequal distribution of income, wealth, status, and power.

Social construction of health
Refers to a range of social forces that combine to create and modify the experience of health, such as social groups, social institutions, and the wider culture.

Social determinants
Socio-economic factors such as income, education, and location that affect the incidence of chronic illness.

Social ecological model
A nested systems model that represents the social, environmental, cultural, behavioural, and economic systems which impact on an individual's health.

Social epidemiology
The systematic and comprehensive study of health, well-being, social conditions or problems, and diseases and their determinants, using epidemiology and social science methods to develop

interventions, programs, policies, and institutions that may reduce the extent, adverse impact, or incidence of a health or social problem and promote health.

Social exclusion
A shorthand label for what can happen when individuals or areas suffer from a combination of linked problems such as unemployment, poor skills, low incomes, poor housing, high crime environments, bad health, and family breakdown.

Social gradient
Life expectancy is shorter and most diseases are more common further down the social ladder in each society.

Social inclusion
Used to describe strategies and policies designed to create a socially inclusive society, and also the experience of belonging to such a society.

Social justice
The improvement of a situation of disadvantage by the redistribution of goods and resources.

Social marketing
The application of commercial marketing communication techniques to the promotion of health and other socially desirable outcomes.

Social model of health
Suggests that health is influenced by a dynamic set of social structures and aims to identify the factors within a society that inhibit the health of individuals.

Social norms
Rules or standards that guide or constrain individuals' actions or behaviour.

Social Skeleton: health, illness and structure agency model
Represents the social structures individuals are part of and demonstrates how social groups, social institutions, and the wider culture influence perceptions of health, illness, and well-being.

Socially inclusive society
One where all people feel valued, their differences are respected, and their basic needs are met, so they can live in dignity.

Socio-economic status
Represents how individuals and groups are 'placed' in a society, and how social and economic factors interact to affect health. These factors include social prestige, education, occupation, material resources, housing, and working conditions.

Sociolinguistics
The study of language in the social/cultural context.

Spillover effects
The situation where either costs or outcomes are not captured by the price of a good or service. Spillover effects may be either positive (e.g. herd immunity from immunisation) or negative (e.g. pollution).

Stereotype
A conventional, formulaic, and oversimplified conception, opinion, or image; one that is regarded as embodying or conforming to a set image or type.

Stigma
An attribute or characteristic that separates people from one another. It is used by individuals to interpret specific attributes of others as 'discreditable or unworthy' and this results in the stigmatised person becoming devalued.

Stigmatisation
The process of stigmatising a person.

Structural determinants of health
Those aspects of a society that influence an individual's health. These include the provision and availability of welfare services such as free healthcare, redistributive taxation practices, and policies to ensure that groups are not discriminated against.

Successful ageing
Ageing is said to be successful when an individual stays free of illness and disability into old age, and is likely to function well physically, mentally, and socially (Rowe & Kahn 1997).

Supply-induced demand
The situation where supply and demand are not independently determined (a requirement for competition). Usually occurs where consumers lack sufficient knowledge to know what services they require and are therefore dependent on the provider to guide their choices.

Timing of lives
An account for the age-graded perspective of social markers, roles, and events.

Town planning
The direction of the development and use of land to serve the economic and social welfare of the community, as well as to protect and enhance the natural environment.

Trajectory
A life course leading to a particular social or health state.

Transition
Moving from one life stage to another, or from one life event to another.

Turning point
A crucial point in time that leads to significant change of direction.

Urbanisation
The increasing concentration of human population, activities, and services in towns and cities.

Vaccination
Administration of substances that will normally induce adaptive immunity in a person, including memory cells.

Vector-borne
A disease spread by an insect (mosquitoes, ticks, lice, etc.) that transmits the disease to humans or other animals.

Vulnerability
Limited access to resources to adapt to changing conditions.

Welfare state
Provision by government of social services such as education, healthcare, old-age pensions. Usually free and funded through taxation.

Well-being
A positive conceptualisation of health: feeling healthy, happy, or doing well in life. It can be completely separated from the objectively measured health or disease status of an individual.

Zoonosis
A disease that originated in an animal species but that has adapted such that it can affect human beings.

References

Abercrombie, N., Hill, S., & Turner, B.S. (1994). *The Penguin dictionary of sociology*. London: Penguin.

Abrahams, J. (2001). Disaster management in Australia: The National Emergency Management System. *Emergency Medicine*, 13, 165–73.

Abrams, H.K. (2001). A short history of occupational health. *Journal of Public Health Policy*, 22(1), 34–80.

ABS (Australian Bureau of Statistics) (2005). *Population projections, Australia, 2004 to 2101*. <www.abs.gov.au/AUSSTATS/abs@.nsf/Lookup/3222.0Main+Features12004%20to%20 2101?OpenDocument>.

ABS (2006). *Health of older people in Australia: A snapshot, 2004-05*. <www.abs.gov.au/ausstats/ abs@.nsf/mf/4833.0.55.001>.

ABS (2008). *Year Book Australia*. <www.abs.gov.au/ausstats/abs@.nsf/0/FF4D0275EFAC806FCA 2573D2001101CE?opendocument>.

ABS (2009a). *Deaths, Australia, 2009*. Cat. No. 3302.0, ABS: Canberra. <www.abs.gov.au>.

ABS (2009b). *Experimental life tables for Aboriginal and Torres Strait Islander Australians 2005-2007*. Cat. No. 3302.0.55.003. Canberra: ABS.

ABS (2010a). *Births, Australia 2009*. Canberra: ABS. <www.abs.gov.au/ausstats/abs@.nsf/ Products/F57D30403E4EBD9BCA2577CF000DEFBD?opendocument>.

ABS (2010b). *Deaths, Australia 2009*. Canberra: ABS. <www.abs.gov.au/ausstats/abs@.nsf/Products/ 70D796FF9A6BF6A2CA2577D600109EE2?opendocument>.

Access Economics (2004). *The cost of domestic violence to the Australian economy: Part 1*. Canberra: Access Economics.

Adams, J., Lui, C-W., & McLaughlin, D. (2009). The use of complementary and alternative medicine in later life. *Reviews in Clinical Gerontology*, 19(4), 227–36.

Adeghate, E., Schattner, P., & Dunn, E. (2006). An update on the epidemiology and etiology of diabetes mellitus. *Annals of the New York Academy of Science*, 1084, 1–29.

Agyeman, J., & Evans, B. (2002). Editorial: Environmental quality and human equality. *Local Environment*, 7(1), 5–6.

AIHW (Australian Institute of Health and Welfare) (2004). *Health inequalities in Australia: Mortality*. Canberra: Queensland University of Technology and AIHW.

AIHW (2005). *Diabetes in culturally and linguistically diverse Australians: Identification of communities at high risk*. Canberra: AIHW.

AIHW (2006a). *Australia's health 2006*. Canberra: AIHW.

AIHW (2006b). *Socioeconomic inequalities in cardiovascular disease in Australia: Current picture and trends since the 1990s*. Bulletin No. PHE 123. Canberra: AIHW.

AIHW (2008a). *Indicators of chronic diseases and their determinants*. Canberra: AIHW. <www.aihw. gov.au/publications/phe/ifcdtd08/ifcdtd08-c01.pdf>.

AIHW (2008b). *Diabetes: Australian facts 2008*. Diabetes Series No. 8, Cat. No. CVD 40. Canberra: AIHW.

AIHW (2008c). *Injury among young Australians*. Bulletin No. 60, Cat. No. 102. Canberra: AIHW.

AIHW (2008d). *Projection of the Australian health care expenditure by disease, 2003 to 2033*. Health and Welfare Expenditure Series No. 36. Canberra: AIHW.

AIHW (2009). *Australian hospital statistics 2007–2008*. Health Service Series No. 33, Cat. No. 71. Canberra: AIHW.

AIHW (2010a). *Australia's health 2010*. Australia's Health series No. 12. Cat No. AUS 122. Canberra: AIHW.

AIHW (2010b). *Chronic diseases*. Canberra: AIHW. <www.aihw.gov.au/cdarf/index.cfm>.

AIHW (2010c). *Prevalence of risk factors for chronic disease*. Canberra: AIHW. <www.aihw.gov.au/cdarf/data_pages/prevalence_risk_factors/index.cfm>.

AIHW (2010d). *Australian hospital statistics 2008–2009*. Health Service Series No. 34, Cat. No. 84. Canberra: AIHW.

AIHW (2011). *Indigenous health*. Canberra: AIHW. <www.aihw.gov.au/indigenous-health>.

AIHW (n.d.). *Indigenous life expectancy*. <www.aihw.gov.au/mortality/life_expectancy/indig.cfm>.

Almeida, O., Norman, P., Hankey, G., Jamrozik, K., & Flicker, L. (2006). Successful mental health ageing: Results from a longitudinal study of older Australian men. *American Journal of Geriatric Psychiatry*, 14, 27–35.

Alper, J.S., Ard, C., Asch A., Beckwith, J., Conrad, P., & Geller, L.N. (eds) (2002). *The double-edged helix: Social implications of genetics in a diverse society*. Baltimore: Johns Hopkins University Press.

ALRC (Australian Law Reform Commission) (2004). *Genes and ingenuity: Gene patenting and human health*. <www.alrc.gov.au/publications/report-99>.

ALRC/AHEC (Australian Law Reform Commission and Australian Health Ethics Committee) (2003). *Essentially yours: The protection of human genetic privacy in Australia*. <www.alrc.gov.au/publications/report-96>.

Alston, M., & Kent, J. (2004). *Social impact of drought. Report to NSW Agriculture*. Centre for Rural Social Research, Charles Sturt University, Wagga Wagga, NSW.

Altman, D. (1994). *Power and community: Organizational and cultural responses to AIDS*. London: Taylor & Francis.

American Diabetes Association (2011). Diabetes A-Z. <www.diabetes.org/diabetes-basics/genetics-of-diabetes.html>.

Ames, M. (2005). *Going postal: Rage, murder, and rebellion from Reagan's workplaces to Clinton's Columbine and more*. Berkeley, CA: Soft Skull Press.

Amos, A., McCarty, D., & Zimmet, P. (2010). The rising global burden of diabetes and its complications: Estimates and projections to the year 2010. *Diabetic Medicine*, 14, S1–S85.

Anderson, M., Elam, G., Gerver, S., Solarin, I., Fenton, K., & Easterbrook, P. (2008). HIV/AIDS-related stigma and discrimination: Accounts of HIV-positive Caribbean people in the United Kingdom. *Social Science and Medicine*, 67(5), 790–8.

Anderson, T. (2009). HIV/AIDS in Cuba: A rights-based analysis. *Health and Human Rights in Practice*, 11(1), 93–0104.

Andreasen, A. (1995). *Marketing social change: Changing behaviour to promote health, social development, and the environment*. San Francisco: Jossey-Bass.

Andrews, A. (2002). *National strategy for an ageing Australia: An older Australia, challenges and opportunities for all*. Canberra: Commonwealth of Australia.

Angus, D. (1998). Recent developments in emergency management. *Australian Journal of Emergency Management*, Autumn, 34–8.

Angus, J., & Reeve, P. (2006). Ageism: A threat to 'aging well' in the 21st century. *Journal of Applied Gerontology*, 25, 137–52.

Annandale, E., & Hunt, K. (eds) (2000). *Gender inequalities and health*. Buckingham, UK: Open University Press.

Anson, D., Smith, G., & Parsons, D. (2006). Gene therapy for cystic fibrosis airway disease: Is clinical success imminent? *Current Gene Therapies*, 6(2), 161–79.

Anspach, R. (1979). From stigma to identity politics: Political activism among the physically disabled and former mental patients. *Social Science and Medicine*, 13, 765–73.

Antonovksy, A. (1996). The salutogenic model as a theory to guide health promotion. *Health Promotion International*, 11(1), 11–18.

Apinundecha, C., Laohasiriwong, W., Cameron, M.P., & Lim, S. (2007). A community participation intervention to reduce HIV/AIDS stigma, Nakhon Ratchasima province, northeast Thailand. *AIDS Care*, 19(9), 1157–65.

Arnold, R.G., Carpenter, D.O., Kirk, D., Koh, D., Armour, M-A., Cebrian, M., et al. (2007). Meeting report: Threats to human health and environmental sustainability in the Pacific Basin. *Environmental Health Perspectives*, 115(12), 1770–5.

Atkinson, A.B., & Leigh, A. (2006). *The distribution of top incomes in Australia*. The Australian National University Centre for Economic Policy Research: *Discussion Paper*. <http://people.anu.edu.au/andrew.leigh/pdf/TopIncomesAustralia.pdf>.

Auffrey, L. (2008). Turning to the environment for answers. *The Canadian Nurse*, 104(2), 3.

Australian Government (2009). *Closing the gap on Indigenous disadvantage*. Canberra: Australian Government.

Australian Government (2010). *Social inclusion*. <www.socialinclusion.gov.au/Pages/default.aspx>.

Australian Government (2011). *Social inclusion pinciples*. Canberra: Australian Government. <www.socialinclusion.gov.au/SIAgenda/Principles/Pages/default.aspx>.

Australian Government Department of Health and Ageing, *Arbovirus and malaria surveillance*. <www.health.gov.au/internet/main/publishing.nsf/content/arbovirus+and+malaria+surveillance-2>.

Australian Government Department of Health and Ageing (2010). *Immunise Australia program*. <www.immunise.health.gov.au>.

Australian Government Department of Health and Ageing and NHMRC (2008). *The Australian immunisation handbook*, 9th edn. <http://immunise.health.gov.au/internet/immunise/publishing.nsf/Content/handbook-home>.

Australian Local Government Association (2006). *Local government and the national emergency management* agenda. <www.alga.asn.au/newsroom/speeches/2006/20060529.php>.

Australian Productivity Commission (2011). *Caring for older Australians*. <www.pc.gov.au/__data/assets/pdf_file/0011/104879/aged-care-draft.pdf>.

Australian Treasury (2010). *The intergenerational report 2010: Australia to 2050: Future challenges*. Canberra: Commonwealth of Australia.

Baer, H., & Singer, M. (2009). *Global warming and the political ecology of health*. Walnut Creek, CA: Left Coast Press.

Balfour, J., & Kaplan, G. (2002). Neighborhood environment and loss of physical function in older adults: Evidence from the Alameda County Study. *American Journal of Epidemiology*, 155(6), 507–15.

Baltes, P., & Baltes, M. (1990). *Successful aging: Perspectives from the behavioral sciences*. Cambridge: Cambridge University Press.

Baltes, P.B., Dittmann-Kohli, F., & Dixon, R.A. (1984). New perspectives on the development of intelligence in adulthood: Toward a dual-process conception and a model of selective optimization with compensation. In P.B. Baltes & O.G.J. Brim (eds), *Life-span development and behaviour*, vol. 6. New York: Academic Press, 33–76.

Bankston, C.L. III. (2010). Social justice: Cultural origins of a theory and a perspective. *Independent Review*, 15(2), 165–78.

Barker, K. (2005). Sex, soap, and social change: The Sabido methodology. In M. Haider (ed.), *Global public health communication: Challenges, perspectives, and strategies*. Subury, MA: Jones & Bartlett Publishers, 113–53.

Barling, J., Dupré, K.E., & Kelloway, E.K. (2009). Predicting workplace violence and aggression. *Annual Review of Psychology*, 60, 671–92.

Barnes, E. (2005). *Diseases and human evolution*. Albuquerque, NM: University of New Mexico Press.

Baron, S., Field, J., & Schuller, T. (2000). *Social capital: Critical perspectives*. Oxford: Oxford University Press.

Barrett, T. (1999). Morbillivirus infections, with special emphasis on morbilliviruses of carnivores. *Veterinary Microbiology*, 69, 3–13.

Bartley, M., & Owen, C. (1996). Relation between socioeconomic status, employment and health during economic change 1973–93. *British Medical Journal*, 313, 445–9.

Bartley, M., Blane, D., & Davey-Smith, G. (2005). The sociology of health inequalities. *Sociology of Health and Illness*, 20(5), 1–8.

Bartley, M., Blane, D., & Montgomery, S. (1997). Socioeconomic determinants of health: Health and the life course: Why safety nets matter. *British Medical Journal*, 314, 1194–5.

Bartley, M., Ferrie, J., & Montgomery, S.M. (2006). Health and labour market disadvantage: Unemployment, non-employment and job insecurity. In M. Marmot & R. Wilkinson (eds), *Social determinants of health*. Oxford: Oxford University Press, 78–96.

Bates, B. (1992). *Bargaining for life: A social history of tuberculosis*. Philadelphia: University of Pennsylvania Press.

Baum, F. (2008). *The new public health*, 3rd edn. Melbourne: Oxford University Press.

Bauman, Z. (1999). *In search of politics*. Stanford: Stanford University Press.

Baydar, N., Brooks-Gunn, J., & Furstenberg, F.F. (1993). Early warning signs of functional literacy: Predictors in childhood and adolescence. *Child Development*, 64(3), 815–29.

Bayer, R. (2008). Stigma and the ethics of public health: Not can we but should we. *Social Science and Medicine*, 67, 463–72.

Bayer, R., & Stuber, J. (2006). Tobacco control, stigma, and public health: Rethinking the relations. *American Journal of Public Health*, 96, 47–50.

Beauchamp, D.E. (1976). Public health as social justice. *Inquiry*, 13(1), 3–14.

Beauchamp, D. (1996). Public health as social justice. In D. Beauchamp & B. Steinbeck (eds), *New ethics for the public's health*. New York: Oxford University Press, 105–14.

Becker, H.S. (1963a). *Perspectives on deviance: The other side*. Toronto: Macmillan.

Becker, H.S. (1963b). *Outsiders: Studies in the sociology of deviance*. New York: Free Press.

Becker, M.H. (1993). A medical sociologist looks at health promotion. *Journal of Health and Social Behavior*, 34, 1–6.

Begg, S., Vos, T., Barker, B., Stevenson, C., Stanley, L., & Lopez, A. (2007). *The burden of disease and injury in Australia 2003*. Cat. No. PHE82. Canberra: AIHW.

Bell, N., Schuurman, N., & Hayes, M.V. (2007). Using GIS-based methods of multicriteria analysis to construct socio-economic deprivation indices. *International Journal of Health Geographics*, 6(17), 20–39.

Bell, S. (2002). Environmental health: Victorian anachronism or dynamic discipline. *Environmental Health*, 2(4), 23–33.

Bellwood, P. (2005). *The first farmers: The origins of agricultural societies*. Oxford: Blackwell.

Bengston, V.L., Gans, D., Putney, N., & Silverstein, M. (eds) (2009). *Handbook of theories of aging*, 2nd edn. New York: Springer.

Ben-Shlomo, Y., & Kuh, D. (2002). A life course approach to chronic disease epidemiology: Conceptual models, empirical challenges, and interdisciplinary perspectives. *International Journal of Epidemiology*, 31, 285–93.

Berenson, A. (ed.) (1990). *Control of communicable diseases of man*. Washington, DC: American Public Health Association.

Berger, J.T. (1998). Culture and ethnicity in clinical care. *Archives of Internal Medicine*, 159(12), 2085–90.

Bernardi, G. (2001). From conflict to convergence: The evolution of Tasmanian Anti-discrimination Law. *Australian Journal of Human Rights*. <www.austlii.edu.au/au/journals/AJHR/2001/6.html>.

Bernhardt, J.M. (2004). Communication is at the core of effective public health. *American Journal of Public Health*, 94(12), 2051–2.

Betancourt, J.R., Green, A.R., Carillo, J.E., & Owusu, A-F. (2003). Defining cultural competence: A practical framework for addressing racial/ethnic disparities in health and health care. *Public Health Reports*, 118, 293–302.

Betancourt, J.R., Green, A.R., Carillo, J.E., & Park, E.R. (2005). Cultural competence and health care disparities: Key perspectives and trends. *Health Affairs*, 24(2), 499–505.

Better Health Channel (2010a). *Chlamydia*. <www.betterhealth.vic.gov.au/bhcv2/bhcarticles.nsf/pages/Chlamydia>.

Better Health Channel (2010b). *Pinworms*. <www.betterhealth.vic.gov.au/bhcv2/bhcpdf.nsf/ByPDF/Worms_pinworms/$File/Worms_pinworms.pdf>.

Better Health Channel (2010c). *Tapeworms and hydatid disease*. <www.betterhealth.vic.gov.au/bhcv2/bhcarticles.nsf/pages/Tapeworms_and_hydatid_disease>.

Bhugra, D., & Jacob, K.S. (1997). Culture bound syndromes. In D. Bhugra & A. Munro (eds), *Troublesome disguises*. Oxford: Blackwell, 296–334.

Bhui, K., & Dinos, S. (2008). Health beliefs and culture: Essential considerations for outcome measurement. *Disease Management and Health Outcomes*, 16(6), 411–19.

Bickenbach, J.E. (2009). Disability, culture and the UN convention. *Disability and Rehabilitation*, 31(14), 1111–24.

Bisaillon, L.M. (2010). Human rights consequences of mandatory HIV screening policy of newcomers to Canada. *Health and Human Rights*, 12(2), 119–34.

Bishop, B. (1999a). *The National Strategy for an Ageing Australia: Healthy aging discussion paper*. Canberra: Commonwealth of Australia.

Bishop, B. (1999b). *The National Strategy for an Ageing Australia: Background paper*. Canberra: Commonwealth of Australia.

Black, D. (1980). *Inequalities in health: The Black report*. Harmondsworth: Penguin.

Black, F.L. (1966). Measles endemicity in insular populations: Critical community size and its evolutionary implications. *Journal of Theoretical Biology*, 11, 207–11.

Black, F.L. (1997). Measles. In A.S. Evans & R.A. Kaslow (eds), *Viral infections of humans: Epidemiology and control*, 4th edn. New York: Plenum, 507–29.

Blake, J., & Davis, K. (1964). Norm, values, and sanctions. In R.E.L. Faris (ed.), *Handbook of modern sociology*. Chicago: Rand McNally, 456–84.

Blane, D. (2006). The life course, social gradient and health. In M. Marmot & R.G. Wilkinson (eds), *Social determinants of health*. Oxford: Oxford University Press, 64–80.

Blas, E., & Kurup, A.S. (2010). *Equity, social determinants and public health programs*. Geneva: WHO Press. <http://whqlibdoc.who.int/publications/2010/9789241563970_eng.pdf>.

Blaxter, M. (2004). *Health*. Cambridge: Polity Press.

Booth, M.L., Chey, T., Wake, M., Norton, K., Hesketh, K., Dollman, J., & Robertson, I. (2003). Change in the prevalence of overweight and obesity among young Australians, 1969–1997. *American Journal of Clinical Nutrition*, 77, 29–36.

Borowski, A., & Encel, S.O.E. (2007). *Longevity and social change in Australia*. Sydney: UNSW Press.

Bortz, W.M. (2005). Biological basis of determinants of health. *American Journal of Public Health*, 95(3), 389–92.

Bourhis, R.Y., Roth, S., & MacQueen, G. (2002). Communication in the hospital setting: A survey of medical and everyday language use among patients, nurses, and doctors. *Social Science and Medicine*, 28(4), 339–46.

Bowes, J., & Grace, R. (2009). *Children, families and communities: Contexts and consequences*, 3rd edn. Melbourne: Oxford University Press.

Bowling, A. (1997). *Measuring health: A review of quality of life measurement scales*, 2nd edn. Buckingham, UK: Open University Press.

Bowling, A. (2005). *Ageing well: Quality of life in old age*. Berkshire: Open University Press.

Bowling, A., & Dieppe, P. (2005). What is successful ageing and who should define it? *British Medical Journal*, 331, 1458–551.

Boyle, P., Ariyaratne, Y., Barrington, R., Bartelink, H., Bartsch, G., Berns, A., et al. (2006). Tobacco: Deadly in any form or disguise. *Lancet*, 367(9524), 1710–12.

Boynton-Jarrett, R., Thomas, T., Peterson, R., Wiecha, J., Sobol, A., & Gortmaker, S. (2003). Impact of television viewing patterns on fruit and vegetable consumption among children and adolescents. *Pediatrics*, 112(6), 1321–6.

Braveman, P. (2010). Social conditions, health equity, and human rights. *Health and Human Rights*, 12(2), 31–48.

Braveman, P., & Gruskin, S. (2003). Defining equity in health. *Journal of Epidemiology and Community Health*, 57, 254–58.

Breslow, L. (1999). From disease prevention to health promotion. *Journal of the American Medical Association*, 281(11), 1030–3.

Bronfenbrenner, U. (1979). *The ecology of human development: Experiments by nature and design*. Cambridge, MA: Harvard University Press.

Brooks, M.V. (2008). Health-related hardiness in individuals with chronic illnesses. *Clinical Nursing Research*, 17(2), 98–117.

Broom, D. (1991). *Damned if we do: Contradictions in women's health care*. Sydney: Allen & Unwin.

Broom, D. (2009). Gender and health. In J. Germov (ed.), *Second opinion: An introduction to health sociology*, 4th edn. Melbourne: Oxford University Press, 130–55.

Brown, G., Price, R., & Anstey, N. (2010). Malaria. In A. Yung, D. Spelman, A. Street, J. McCormack, T. Sorrell, & P. Johnson (eds), *Infectious diseases: A clinical approach*, 3rd edn. Melbourne: IP Communications, 350–65.

Brown, L., Macintyre, K., & Trujillo, L. (2003). Interventions to reduce HIV/AIDS stigma: What have we learned? *AIDS Education and Prevention*, 15, 49–69.

Brown, P. (1995). Naming and framing: The social construction of diagnosis and illness. *Journal of Health and Social Behavior*, 35(Extra Issue), 34–52.

Brown, V. (2001). Monitoring changing environments in environmental health. *Environmental Health*, 1(1), 25–34.

Brownie, S. (2006). Why are elderly individuals at risk of nutritional deficiency? *International Journal of Nursing Practice*, 12(2), 110–18.

Browning, C., & Kendig, H. (2003). *Healthy ageing: A new focus on older people's health and wellbeing*. In P. Liamputtong & H. Gardner (eds), *Health, social change and communities*. Melbourne: Oxford University Press, 182–205.

Browning, C., & Kendig, H. (2004). Maximising health and well-being in older people. In R. Moodie & A. Hulme (eds), *Hands on health promotion*. Melbourne: IP Communications, 374–88.

Browning, C., & Thomas, S. (2007). *Definition and predictors of successful ageing and related concepts. Final report prepared for the Department of Human Services*. Melbourne: Department of Human Services.

Brundtland, G.H. (2005). The UDHR: Fifty years of synergy between health and human rights. In S. Gruskin, M. Grodin, S. Marks, & G. Annas (eds), *Perspectives on health and human rights*. New York: Routledge, 59–62.

Brundtland, G.H. (2011). *Opinion, climate change: 3 pieces of policy advice*. ABC Environment, Online, 21 February 2011. Article courtesy of the World Resources Institute.

Buckner-Brown, J., Tucker, P., Rivera, M., Cosgrove, S., Coleman, J.L., Penson, A., et al. (2011). Racial and ethnic approaches to community health: Reducing health disparities by addressing social determinants of health. *Family and Community Health*, 34(S1), S12–S22.

Buettner, D. (2010). *The Blue Zones: Lessons for living longer from the people who've lived the longest*. Washington, DC: National Geographic.

Bunton, R., & Petersen, A. (eds) (2005). Genetics and governance: An introduction. In *Genetic governance: Health, risk and ethics in the biotech era*. London: Routledge, 1–27.

Burge, P.J. (2004). Sick building syndrome. *Occupational and Environmental Medicine*, 61, 185–91.

Burgess, C.P., Johnston, F.H., & Bailie, R. (2007). Healthy country: Healthy people. Superior Indigenous health outcomes are associated with 'Caring for Country'. EcoHealth Conference, Deakin University, Melbourne.

Burke, V., Zhao, Y., Lee, A., Hunter, F., Spargo, R.M., Gracey, M., et al. (2007). Predictors of Type 2 diabetes and diabetes-related hospitalisation in an Australian Aboriginal cohort. *Diabetes Research and Clinical Practice*, 78(3), 360–8.

Caan, W. (2010). Editorial. *Journal of Public Mental Health*, 9(2), 2–3.

Cabal, L., Roa, M., & Sepúlveda-Oliva, L. (2003). What role can international litigation play in the promotion and advancement of reproductive rights in Latin America? *Health and Human Rights*, 7(1), 51–88.

Cameron, A.J., Welborn, T.A., Zimmet, P.Z., Dunstan, D.W., Owen, N., Salmon, J., et al. (2003). Overweight and obesity in Australia: The 1999–2000 Australian Diabetes, Obesity, and Lifestyle Study (AusDiab). *Medical Journal of Australia*, 178, 427–32.

Cancer Council Western Australia (2008). *The progress of tobacco control in Western Australia: Achievements, challenges and hopes for the future*. Perth: Cancer Council Western Australia. <www.cancerwa.asn.au/resources/2010-07-07-Tobacco-Control-Monograph.pdf>.

Canino, G., & Alegria, M. (2008). Psychiatric diagnosis: Is it universal or relative to culture? *Journal of Child Psychology and Psychiatry*, 49(3), 237–50.

Carlisle, C. (2001). HIV and AIDS. In T. Mason, C. Carlisle, C. Watkins, & E. Whitehead (eds), *Stigma and social exclusion in health care*. London: Routledge, 117–25.

Carter, O. (2008). Changes in the attitudes and beliefs of West Australian smokers, 1984–2007. In *The progress of tobacco control in Western Australia: Achievements, challenges and hopes for the future*. Perth: Cancer Council Western Australia, 23–9. <www.cancerwa.asn.au/resources/2010-07-07-Tobacco-Control-Monograph.pdf>.

Carter, R., & Moodie, M. (2005). The cost-effectiveness of obesity prevention. In D. Crawford & R.W. Jeffery (eds), *Obesity prevention and public health*. Oxford: Oxford University Press, 165–204.

Cashmore, J. (2001). Family, early development and the life course: Common risk and protective factors in pathways to prevention. In R. Eckersley, J. Dixon, & B. Douglas (eds), *The social origins of health and wellbeing*. Cambridge: Cambridge University Press, 216–24.

Castro, C.M., Wilson, C., Wang, F., & Schillinger, D. (2007). Babel babble: Physicians' use of unclarified medical jargon with patients. *American Journal of Health Behavior*, 31, S85–S95.

CDH&AC (Commonwealth Department of Health and Aged Care) (1999). *National environmental health strategy*. Canberra: Australian Government Publishing Service.

Center for Health Communication, Harvard School of Public Health (2011). *Harvard Alcohol Project*. <www.hsph.harvard.edu/research/chc/harvard-alcohol-project/index.html>.

Centre for Health Education, Training and Nutrition Awareness (2011). *Commitment to women*. <www.chetnaindia.org>.

CGE (Centre for Genetics Education) (2007a). *Fact Sheet #24: The human genetic code—The Human Genome Project and beyond*. <www.genetics.com.au/pdf/factsheets/fs24.pdf>.

CGE (2007b). *Fact Sheet #11: Environmental and genetic interactions—Complex patterns of inheritance 1*. <www.genetics.com.au/pdf/factsheets/fs11.pdf>.

CGE (2007c). *Fact Sheet #1: Genes and chromosomes*. <www.genetics.com.au/pdf/factsheets/fs01.pdf>.

CGE (2007d). *Fact Sheet #4: Changes to the genetic code*. <www.genetics.com.au/pdf/factsheets/fs04.pdf>.

CGE (2007e). *Fact Sheet #10: X-linked inheritance—Traditional patterns of inheritance 3*. <www.genetics.com.au/pdf/factsheets/fs10.pdf>.

CGE (2007f). *Fact Sheet #9: Autosomal dominant inheritance—Traditional patterns of inheritance 2*. <www.genetics.com.au/pdf/factsheets/fs09.pdf>.

CGE (2007g). *Fact Sheet #8*: Autosomal recessive inheritance—Traditional patterns of inheritance 1. <www.genetics.com.au/pdf/factsheets/fs08.pdf>.

CGE (2007h). *Fact Sheet #3: Genetic counselling*. <www.genetics.com.au/pdf/factsheets/fs03.pdf>.

CGE (2007i). *Fact Sheet #2: Genetic conditions—Overview*. <www.genetics.com.au/pdf/factsheets/fs02.pdf>.

CGE (2007j). *Fact Sheet #47: Cancer, genes and inherited predisposition overview—Cancer genetics 1*. <www.genetics.com.au/pdf/factsheets/fs47.pdf>.

CGE (2007k). *Fact Sheet #21: DNA genetic testing—Screening for genetic conditions and genetic susceptibility*. <www.genetics.com.au/pdf/factsheets/fs21.pdf>.

CGE (2007l). *Fact Sheet #48: Breast and ovarian cancer and inherited predisposition—Cancer genetics 2*. <www.genetics.com.au/pdf/factsheets/fs48.pdf>.

CGE (2007m). *Fact Sheet #23a: Life insurance products and genetic testing in Australia*. <www.genetics.com.au/pdf/factsheets/fs23a.pdf>.

Cha, D. (2003). *Hmong American concepts of health, healing and conventional medicine*. New York: Routledge.

Chang, H.C., Kung, Y-Y., Hsich, C-F., Hsiung, L.H-Y., Chang, S., & Chen, T.H-H. (2008). Biological risk factors relevant to chronic disease in three ethnic groups in Taiwan: Results from Li-Shin outreaching neighborhood screening (Lions A1). *Ethnicity and Disease*, 18, 228–34.

Chang, P.H., & Fortier, J.P. (1998). Language barriers to health care: An overview. *Journal of Health Care for the Poor and Underserved*, 9, S5–S20.

Chapman, A.R. (2010). The social determinants of health, health equity, and human rights. *Health and Human Rights*, 12(2), 17–30.

Chapman, J. (1990). Violence against women as a violation of human rights. *Social Justice*, 17(2), 54–70.

Chapman, K., Nicholas, P., & Supramaniam, R. (2006). How much food advertising is on the Australian television? *Health Promotion International*, 21(3), 172–80.

Chapman, S. (2004a). Advocacy for public health: A primer. *Journal of Epidemiology and Community Health*, 58, 361–5.

Chapman, S. (2004b). Public health advocacy. In R. Moodie & A. Hulme (eds), *Hands on health promotion*. Melbourne: IP Communications.

Chapman, S., & Freeman, B. (2008). Markers of the denormalisation of smoking and the tobacco industry. *Tobacco Control*, 17(1), 25–31.

Chapman, S., & Wakefield, M. (2001). Tobacco control advocacy in Australia: Reflections on 30 years of progress. *Health Education & Behavior*, 28(3), 274–89.

Charles, N., & Walters, V. (2008). Men are leavers-alone and women are worriers: Gender differences in discourses of health. *Health, Risk & Society*, 10(2), 117–32.

Charmaz, K. (1991). *Good days, bad days: The self in chronic illness and time*. New Brunswick, NJ: Rutgers University Press.

Chief Health Officer, Victoria, Australia (2011). *Pertussis epidemic*. <www.health.vic.gov.au/chiefhealthofficer/alerts/alert-2011-01-pertussis.htm>.

Choi, H., Schmidbauer, N., Sundell, J., Hasselgren, M., Spengler, J., Bornehag, C-G., et al. (2010). Common household chemicals and allergy risks in school-age children. *PLoS One*, 5(10), e13423.

Chopra, M., & Ford, N. (2005). Scaling up health promotion interventions in the era of HIV/AIDS: Challenges for a rights-based approach. *Health Promotion International*, 20(4), 383–90.

Chowell, G., Bertozzi, S.M., Colchero, M.A., Lopez-Gatell, H., Alpuche-Aranda, C., Hernandez, M., & Miller, M.A. (2009). Severe respiratory disease concurrent with the circulation of H1N1 influenza. *New England Journal of Medicine*, 361, 674–9.

Chronic Illness Alliance (2010). *Peak body for chronic illness organizations*. <www.chronicillness.org.au>.

City of Greater Geelong (2009). *Geelong health and wellbeing plan 2009–2013, A collaborative approach: The way forward*. <www.geelongaustralia.com.au/common/Public/Documents/8cc89d5225acc58-Geelong%20Health%20and%20Wellbeing%20Plan.pdf>.

Clarke, P.J., & Nieuwenhuijsen, E.R. (2009). Environments for healthy ageing: A critical review. *Maturitas*, 64(1), 9–14.

Clegg, G.A., & Richards, J.P. (2007). Chemicals in household products: Problems with solutions. *Environmental Management*, 40, 889–901.

Climate Change (2009). *Global Risks, Challenges and Decisions*, University of Copenhagan Climate Portal. <http://climatecongress.ku.dk/newsroom/congress_key_messages>.

Clinard, M.B., & Meier, R.F. (2008). *Sociology of deviance*, 13th edn. Belmont, CA: Thomson Wadsworth.

Coburn, D. (2000). Income inequality, social cohesion and the health status of populations: The role of neoliberalism. *Social Science and Medicine*, 51, 135–46.

Cockerham, W.C. (2007). *Social causes of health and disease*. Cambridge: Polity Press.

Cohen, A.K. (1974). *The elasticity of evil: Changes in the social definition of deviance*. Oxford: Blackwell.

Cohen, D. (2001). Advocacy: Its many faces and a common understanding. In D. Cohen, R. De la Vega, & G. Watson (eds), *Advocacy for social justice: A global action and reflection guide*. Bloomfield, CT: Kumarian Press, 7–10.

Coker, R. (2001). Just coercion? Detention of nonadherent tuberculosis patients. *Annals of the New York Academy of Sciences*, 953, 216–23.

Cole, E., & Buckle, P. (2004). Developing community resilience as a foundation for effective disaster recovery. *Australian Journal of Emergency Management*, 19(4), 6–15.

Colebunders, R., & Lambert, L. (2002). Management of co-infection with HIV and TB. *British Medical Journal*, 324, 802–3.

Collins Purdue, W., Stone, L.A., & Gostin, L.O. (2003). The built environment and its relationship to the public's health: The legal framework. *American Journal of Public Health*, 93(9), 1390–4.

Commonwealth Department of Health and Ageing (2006). *The annual cost of foodborne illness in Australia*. Canberra: Australian Government Publishing Service.

Commonwealth of Australia (1993). *Agreement between the Commonwealth of Australia and the State of South Australia in relation to the provision of public hospital services and other health services, from 1 July 1993 to June 1998 under Section 24 of the Health Insurance Act 1973 (CTH)*. Canberra: Australian Government Solicitor.

Commonwealth of Australia (2008). *2007 Australian National Children's Nutrition and Physical Activity Survey: Main findings*. Canberra: Commonwealth of Australia. <www.health.gov. au/internet/main/publishing.nsf/Content/health-pubhlth-strateg-food-monitoring. htm#07survey>.

Community Indicators Victoria (2007). *Swan Hill wellbeing report. Health Services Research*, 37, 85–101. <www.communityindicators.net.au/wellbeing_reports/swan_hill>.

Congress for the New Urbanism (2004). *Codifying new urbanism: How to reform municipal land development regulations*. Washington, DC: American Planning Association.

Connell, R. (2002). *Gender*. Cambridge: Polity Press.

Cook, R., Dickens, B., & Fathalla, M. (2003). *Reproductive health and human rights: Integrating medicine, ethics and law*. Oxford: Clarendon Press.

Coon, K.A., & Tucker, K.L. (2002). Television and children's consumption patterns. A review of the literature. *Minerva Pediatrica*, 54(5), 423–36.

Coon, K.A., Goldberg, J., Rogers, B.L., & Tucker, K.L. (2001). Relationship between use of television during meals and children's food consumption patterns. *Pediatrics*, 107(1), e7.

Cooper, H., Booth, K., & Gill, G. (2008). A trial of empowerment-based education in type 2 diabetes—global rather than glycaemic benefits. *Diabetes Research and Clinical Practice*, 82(20), 165–71.

Corbett, E.L., Watt, C.J., Walker, N., Maher, D., Williams, B.G., Raviglione, M.C., et al. (2003). The growing burden of tuberculosis: Global trends and interactions with the HIV epidemic. *Archives of Internal Medicine*, 163, 1009–21.

Corcoran, J., Faggian, A., & McCann, P. (2010). Human capital in remote and rural Australia: The role of graduate migration. *Growth and Change*, 41(2), 192–220.

Corrigan, P.W., & Lundin, R. (2001). *Don't call me nuts!: Coping with the stigma of mental illness*. Tinley Park, IL: Recovery Press.

Corrigan, P.W., & Penn, D.L. (1999). Lessons from social psychology on discrediting psychiatric stigma. *American Psychologist*, 54, 765–76.

Corrigan, P.W., Markowitz, F.E., Watson, A., Rowan, D., & Kubiak, M.A. (2003a). An attribution model of public discrimination towards persons with mental illness. *Journal of Health and Social Behavior*, 44, 162–79.

Corrigan, P.W., Rowan, D., Green, A., Lundin, R., River, L.P., Uphoff-Wasowski, K., White, K., & Kubiak, M.A. (2002). Challenging two mental illness stigmas: Personal responsibility and dangerousness. *Schizophrenia Bulletin*, 28, 293–309.

Corrigan, P.W., Thompson, V., Lambert, D., Sangster, Y., Noel, J.G., & Campbell, J. (2003b). Perceptions of discrimination among persons with serious mental illness. *Psychiatric Services*, 54, 1105–10.

Couture, S.M., & Penn, D.L. (2003). Interpersonal contact and the stigma of mental illness: A review of the literature. *Journal of Mental Health*, 12, 291–305.

Couzos, S., & Thiele, D.D. (2007). The ICESCR and the right to health: Is Australia meeting its obligations to Aboriginal peoples? *Medical Journal of Australia*, 186(10), 522–4.

Cox, N.J., & Bender, C.A. (1995). The molecular epidemiology of influenza viruses. *Seminars in Virology*, 6(6), 359–70.

Cox, N.J., & Subbarao, K. (2000). Global epidemiology of influenza: Past and present. *Annual Review of Medicine*, 51, 407–21.

Cox, S.M., & McKellin, W. (1999) 'There's this thing in our family': Predictive testing and the construction of risk for Huntington Disease. *Sociology of Health and Illness*, 21(5), 622–46.

Crocker, J., Major, B., & Steele, C. (1998). Social stigma. In D. Gilbert, S. Fiske, & G. Lindzey (eds), *Handbook of social psychology*, vol. 2, 4th edn. Boston: McGraw-Hill, 504–53.

Cromar, N., Cameron, S., & Fallowfield, H. (eds) (2004). *Environmental health in Australia and New Zealand*. Melbourne: Oxford University Press.

Cronan, K. (1998). Foundations of emergency management. *Australian Journal of Emergency Management*, Autumn, 20–23.

Crondstedt, M. (2001). Prevention, preparedness, response, recovery: An outdated concept. *Australian Journal of Emergency Management*, Autumn, 10–13.

Crosby, R., & Noar, S.M. (2010). Theory development in health promotion: Are we there yet? *Journal of Behavioural Medicine*, 33, 259–63.

Crystal, D. (1997). *The Cambridge encyclopedia of language*. Cambridge: Cambridge University Press.

Culhane-Pera, K.A., Cha, D., & Kunstadter, P. (2004). Hmong in Laos and the United States. In C.R. Ember & M. Ember (eds), *Encyclopedia of medical anthropology: Health and illness in the world's cultures*. New York: Kluwer Academic/Plenum, 729–43.

Cullinane, J. (2007). The domestication of AIDS: Stigma, gender, and the body politic in Japan. *Medical Anthropology*, 26(3), 255–92.

Cwikel, J. (2006). *Social epidemiology: Strategies for public health activities*. New York: Columbia University Press.

Dahlgren, G., & Whitehead, M. (1991). *Policies and strategies to promote social equity in health*. Stockholm: Institute of Futures Studies.

Dalton, C.B., Gregory, J., Kirk, M.D., Stafford, R.J., Kraa, E., & Gould D. (2004). Foodborne disease outbreaks in Australia, 1995 to 2000. *Communicable Diseases Intelligence*, 28(2), 211–24.

Danesi, M., & Perron, P. (1999). *Analyzing cultures: An introduction and handbook*. Bloomington and Indianapolis: University of Indiana Press.

Daniel, H., & Parker, R.G. (1993). *Sexuality, politics and AIDS in Brazil*. London: Falmer Press.

Daniel, T.M., Bates, J.H., & Downes, K.A. (1994). History of tuberculosis. In B.R. Bloom (ed.), *Tuberculosis: Pathogenesis, protection and control*. Washington, DC: American Society for Microbiology, 13–24.

Dart, J. (2008). The internet as a source of health information in three disparate communities. *Australian Health Review*, 32(3), 559–69.

Daube, M., & Walker, N. (2008). Advocating for tobacco control in Western Australia, 1971 to the present. In Cancer Council Western Australia, *The progress of tobacco control in Western Australia: Achievements, challenges and hopes for the future*. Perth: Cancer Council Western Australia, 55–70. <www.cancerwa.asn.au/resources/2010-07-07-Tobacco-Control-Monograph. pdf>.

Davidson, N., Skull, S., Calache, H., Murray, S., & Chalmers, J. (2006). Holes a plenty: Oral health status a major issue for newly arrived refugees in Australia. *Australian Dental Journal*, 51(4), 306–11.

Davis, K., Schoen, C., & Stemikis, K. (2010). *Mirror, mirror on the wall: How the performance of the U.S. health system compares internationally*. The Commonwealth Fund. Report No. 1400. <www.commonwealthfund.org/Content/Publications/Fund-Reports/2010/Jun/Mirror-Mirror-Update.aspx?page=all>.

Day, L.M. (1996). *Dairy farm injury in Victoria*. MUARC Accident Reports No 96. Melbourne: Monash University.

De Fossard, E. (2008). Using edu-tainment for distance education in community work. In *Communication for Behavior Change*, vol. 3. New Delhi: Sage Publications.

De Snoo, F.A., Riedijk, S.R., van Mil, A.M., Bergman, W., ter Huume, J.A.C., Timman, R., Bertina, W., & Tibben, A. (2008). Genetic testing in familial melanoma: Uptake and implications. *Psycho-Oncology*, 17(8), 790–6.

Delfin Lend Lease (n.d.). *Mawson Lakes: Fast facts*. <www.mawsonlakes.com.au/llweb/ mawsonlakes/main.nsf/all/ml_fastfacts>.

Delisle, H. (2002). *Programming of chronic disease by impaired foetal nutrition: Evidence and implications for policy and intervention strategies*. Geneva: WHO.

Denenberg, R.V., & Braverman, M. (1999). *The violence-prone workplace: A new approach to dealing with hostile, threatening and uncivil behavior*. Ithaca, NY: Cornell University Press.

Deng, R., Li, J., Sringernyuang, L., & Zhang, K. (2007). Drug abuse, HIV/AIDS and stigmatization in a Dai community in Yunnan, China. *Social Science and Medicine*, 64, 1560–71.

Denton, M., Prus, S., & Wallers, V. (2004). Gender differences in health: A Canadian study of the psychosocial, structural and behavioral determinants of health. *Social Science and Medicine*, 58(12), 2585–600.

Department of Foreign Affairs and Trade (2008). *Australia: A culturally diverse society*. Canberra: DFAT. <www.dfat.gov.au/facts/culturally_diverse.html>.

Department of Health and Ageing (2009). *Australian health management plan for pandemic influenza*. Canberra: Australian Government, Department of Health and Ageing.

Department of Health and Human Services (2009). *The Genetic Information Nondiscrimination Act of 2008: Information for researchers and health care professionals*. <www.genome.gov/Pages/ PolicyEthics/GeneticDiscrimination/GINAInfoDoc.pdf>.

Depp, C., & Jeste, D. (2006). Definitions and predictors of successful ageing: A comprehensive review of larger quantitative studies. *American Journal of Geriatric Psychiatry*, 14, 6–20.

Diamond, J. (2004). *Collapse: How societies choose to fail or succeed*. New York: Viking Press.

Dirven, R., & Verspoor, M. (2004). *Cognitive exploration of language and linguistics*. Amsterdam and Philadelphia: John Benjamins.

Docteur, E., & Oxley, H. (2003). *Health-care systems: Lessons from the reform experience*. Paris: OECD. <www.oecd.org/dataoecd/5/53/22364122.pdf>.

Dohrenwend, B.P., & Dohrenwend, B.S. (1974). Psychiatric disorders in urban settings. In G. Caplan (ed.), *Child and adolescent psychiatry: Sociocultural and community psychiatry*. New York: Basic Books, 424–49.

Doley, A., Sibly, C., Wigg, C., Crawford, P., Cowper, L., Barker. C., & Gale, P. (2008). Doctor on campus: A general practice initiative for detection and early intervention of mental health problems in a rural Australian secondary school. *Health Sociology Review*, 17(1), 11–16.

Doll, R., & Hill, A. (1950). Smoking and carcinoma of the lung. *British Medical Journal*, ii (4682), 739–48.

Doll, R., & Hill, A. (1954). The mortality of doctors in relation to their smoking habits: A preliminary report. *British Medical Journal*, i, 1451–5.

Doll, R., & Peto, R. (1976). Mortality in relation to smoking 20 years' observations on male British doctors. *British Medical Journal*, 2, 1525–36.

Doll, R., Gray, R., Hafner, B., & Peto, R. (1980). Mortality in relation to smoking 22 years' observations on female British doctors. *British Medical Journal*, 280, 967–71.

Doll, R., Peto, R., Boreham, J., & Sutherland, L. (2004). Mortality in relation to smoking 50 years' observations on male British doctors. *British Medical Journal*, 328, 1519–28.

Doll, R., Peto, R., Wheatley, K., Gray, R., & Sutherland, L. (1994). Mortality in relation to smoking 40 years' observations on male British doctors. *British Medical Journal*, 309, 901–11.

Donovan, R., & Henley, N. (2010). *Principles and practice of social marketing: An international perspective*, 2nd edn. Melbourne: IP Communications.

Dorozynski, A. (1994). British Government looks at effects of wealth on health. *British Medical Journal*, 308, 1257–8.

Dover, S. (2004). Sustainability and disaster management. *Australian Emergency Management Journal*, 19(1), 21–5.

Dover, V. (1999). Streets and squares should be safe, comfortable, and interesting to the pedestrian. Properly configured, they encourage walking and enable neighbors to know each other and protect their communities. In M. Leccese & K. McCormick (eds), *Charter of the new urbanism*. New York: McGraw-Hill, 147–51.

Dover, V., & King, J. (2008). Neighbourhood definition. In D. Farr (ed.), *Sustainable urbanism: Urban design with nature*. New Jersey: John Wiley & Sons, 127–31.

Doyle, J. (2004). The Cochrane Collaboration. In R. Moodie & A. Hulme (eds), *Hands on health promotion*. Melbourne: IP Communications, 13–15.

Draper, G., Turrell, G., & Oldenburg, B. (2004). *Health inequalities in Australia: Mortality. Health inequalities monitoring Series No. 1*. AIHW Cat. No. PHE 55. Canberra: Queensland University of Technology and AIHW.

Drewnowski, A., & Spencer, S.E. (2004). Poverty and obesity: The role of energy density and energy costs. *American Journal of Clinical Nutrition 79*, 6–16.

Drummond, M.F., Sculpher, M.J., Torrance, G.W., O'Brien, B.J., & Stoddart, G.L. (2007). *Methods for the economic evaluation of health care programmes*, 3rd edn. Oxford: Oxford University Press.

Duany, A., Plater-Zyberk, E., & Speck, J. (2000). *Suburban nation: The rise of sprawl and the decline of the American dream*. New York: North Point Press.

Dubos, R., & Dubos, J. (1952). *The white plague*. Boston: Little Brown & Co.

Duckett, S.J. (2000). *The Australian health care system*. Melbourne: Oxford University Press.

Duclos, P., & Hatcher, J. (1993). Epidemiology of influenza vaccination in Canada. *Canadian Journal of Public Health*, 84(5), 311–15.

Dunne, W.M. Jr, & Ledeboer, N.A. (2009). Mechanisms of infectious disease. In C.M. Porth & G.M. Wolters (eds), *Pathophysiology: Concepts of altered health states*, 8th edn. Philadelphia, PA: Lippincott Williams & Wilkins, 324–46.

Durie, M. (2005). *Nga tai matatu: Tides of Maori endurance*. Melbourne: Oxford University Press.

Durie, M., Milroy, H., & Hunter, E. (2009). Mental health and the Indigenous peoples of Australia and New Zealand. In L.J. Kirmayer & G.G. Valaskakis (eds), *Healing traditions: The mental health of Aboriginal peoples in Canada*. Vancouver: University of British Columbia Press, 36–55.

Durkheim, E. (1895/1982). *The rules of sociological method*. New York: Free Press.

Durrant, J. (2008). Physical punishment, culture, and rights: Current issues for professionals. *Journal of Developmental and Behavioral Pediatrics*, 29(1), 55–66.

Dushoff, J., Plotkin, J.B., Viboud, C., Earn, D.J.D., & Simonsen, L. (2005). Mortality due to influenza in the United States: An annualized regression approach using multiple-cause mortality data. *American Journal of Epidemiology*, 163(2), 181–7.

Dwyer, D. (2010). *Influenza*. In A. Yung, D. Spelman, A. Street, J. McCormack, T. Sorrell & P. Johnson (eds), *Infectious diseases: A clinical approach*, 3rd edn. Melbourne: IP Communications, 342–9.

Earle, S. (2000). Why some women do not breast feed: Bottle feeding and father's role. *Midwifery*, 16, 323–30.

Earle, S., & Letherby, G. (2008). Thinking sociologically about health and healthcare. In S. Earle & G. Letherby (eds), *The sociology of healthcare: A reader for health professionals*. New York: Palgrave Macmillan, xiv–xvii.

Ebden, M., & Townsend, M. (2007). Feeling blue? Then touch green. The benefits of conservation groups. EcoHealth Conference, Deakin University, Melbourne.

Ebi, K.L., & Semenza, J.C. (2008). Community-based adaptation to health impacts of climate change. *American Journal Preventive Medicine*, 35(5), 501–7.

Eckersley, R. (2001). Culture, health and wellbeing. In R. Eckersley, J. Dixon & B. Douglas (eds), *The social origins of health and wellbeing*. Cambridge: Cambridge University Press, 51–70.

Editors (1994). Gay rights victory at UN—I. *Human Rights Defender*. <www.austlii.edu.au/au/journals/HRD/1994/1.html>.

Edvardsson, B., Stenberg, B., Bergdahl, J., Erikson, N., Linden, G. & Widman, L. (2007). Medical and social prognoses of non-specific building-related symptoms (Sick Building Syndrome): A follow-up study of people previously referred to hospital. *International Archives of Occupational and Environmental Health*, 81, 805–12.

Eggleston, G., & Koob, P. (2004). The role of LGA in agricultural emergencies. *Australian Journal of Emergency Management*, 19(3), 29–31.

Eisenberg, J.N.S., Desai, M.A., Levy, K., Bates, S.J., Liang, S., & Naumoff, K. (2007). Environmental determinants of infectious diseases: A framework for tracking causal links and guiding public health research. *Environmental Health Perspectives*, 115(8), 1216–23.

Eisenbruch, M., Yeoa, S., Meiser, B., Goldstein, D., Tucker, K., & Barlow-Stewart, K. (2004). Optimising clinical practice in cancer genetics with cultural competence: Lessons to be learned from ethnographic research with Chinese-Australians. *Social Science and Medicine*, 59(2), 235–48.

Elder, G.J. (1974). *Children of the Great Depression*. Chicago: University of Chicago Press.

Elder, G.J. (1985). *Life course dynamics: Trajectories and transitions, 1968-1980*. Ithaca, NY: Cornell University Press.

Elder, G.J. (1994). Time, human agency, and social change: Perspectives on the life course. *Social Psychology Quarterly*, 57(1), 4-15.

EMA (Emergency Management Australia) (1996). *Australian emergency management arrangements*, 5th edn. Canberra: Australian Government Publishing Service.

EMA (2001). *Value your volunteers or lose them: The report on a national summit for volunteer leaders/managers*, Canberra, 11-12 October 2001. <www.ema.gov.au/www/emaweb/emaweb.nsf/Page/Home>.

Epstein, S. (1996). *Impure science: AIDS, activism and the politics of knowledge*. Berkeley: University California Press.

Erikson, E. (1968). *Identity: Youth and crisis*. New York: Norton.

Evans, G.S., Cadogan, D., Flueckigen, A., Hennes, C. & Kimber, I. (2008). Chemical pollution, respiratory allergy and asthma: A perspective. *Journal of Applied Toxicology*, 28(1), 1-5.

Evers-Kiebooms, G., Welkenhuysen, M., Claes, E., Decruyenaere, M., & Denayer, L. (2000). The psychological complexity of predictive testing for late onset neuro-genetic diseases and hereditary cancers: Implications for multidisciplinary counseling and for genetic education. *Social Science and Medicine*, 51(6), 831-41.

Evert, J., Lawler, E., Bogan, H., & Perls, T. (2003). Morbidity profiles of centenarians: Survivors, delayers, and escapers. *Journal of Gerontology, Medical Sciences*, 58A, 232-7.

Fadiman, A. (1997). *The spirit catches you and you fall down: A Hmong child, her American doctors, and the collision of two cultures*. New York: Farrar, Straus & Giroux.

Falk, G. (2001). *Stigma: How we treat outsiders*. Amherst, NY: Prometheus Books.

Falk, P. (1985). Corporeality and its fates in history. *Acta Sociologica*, 28(2), 115-36.

Farrow, A. (2008). Environmental pollutants and pediatric asthma. *Pediatric Health*, 2(3), 255-8.

Feldstein, P.J. (2005). *Health care economics*, 6th edn. New York: Delmar Cengage Learning.

Ferrucci, L., Izmirlian, G., Leveille, S., Phillips, C.L., Corti, M.C., & Brock, D.B. (1999). Smoking, physical activity, and active life expectancy. *American Journal of Epidemiology*, 149(7), 645-53.

Finney Lamb, C.E., Whelan, C.E., Klinken, A., & Michaels, C. (2009). Refugees and oral health: Lessons learned from stories of Hazara Health. *Australian Health Review*, 33(4), 618-27.

Fishback, P.V., & Kantor, S.E. (1998). The adoption of workers' compensation in the United States, 1900-1930. *Journal of Law and Economics*, 41(2), 305-42.

Fishback, P.V., & Kantor, S.E. (2006). *A prelude to the welfare state: The origins of workers' compensation*. Chicago: University of Chicago Press.

Flohr, C., Pascoe, D., & Williams, H. (2005). Atopic dermatitis and the 'Hygiene Hypothesis': Too clean to be true? *British Journal of Dermatology*, 152(2), 202-16.

Folland, S., Goodman, A.C., & Stano, M. (2010). *The economics of health and health care*, 6th edn. New Jersey: Prentice Hall.

Food Standards Australia and New Zealand (2011). *Antibiotics and food*. <www.foodstandards.gov.au/consumerinformation/antibioticsandfood.cfm>.

Ford, A.B., Haug, M.R., Stange, K.C., Gaines, A.D., Noelker, L.S., & Jones, P.K. (2000). Sustained personal autonomy: A measure of successful aging. *Journal of Aging and Health*, 12(4), 470-89.

Ford, L.R. (1992). Reading the skylines of American cities. *Geographical Review*, 82(2), 180-200.

Ford, N., Calmy, A., & Hurst, S. (2010). When to start antiretroviral therapy in resource-limited settings: A human rights analysis. *BMC International Health and Human Rights*, 10(1), 6-14.

Forster, C. (2009). *Australian cities: Continuity and change*, 3rd edn. Melbourne: Oxford University Press.

Foucault, M. (1973). *The birth of the clinic*. London: Tavistock.

Foucault, M. (1980). The politics of health in the eighteenth century. In C. Gordon (ed.), *Power/knowledge: Selected interviews and other writings, 1972-1977*. Brighton, USA: Harvest Press, 166-82.

Foucault, M. (1981). *The history of sexuality: An introduction*, trans. Harmondsworth: Penguin.

Fox, B.J. (2005). Framing tobacco control efforts within an ethical context. *Tobacco Control*, 14(Suppl. II), ii38-ii44.

Fox-Rushby, J., & Cairns, J. (2005). *Economic evaluation*. New York: Open University Press.

Frankenberg, E. (1995). The effects of access to health care on infant mortality in Indonesia: A fixed effects approach to evaluating health services. *Health Transitions Review*, 5(2), 143-62.

Freestone, R. (2010). *Urban nation: Australia's planning heritage*. Melbourne: CSIRO Publishing.

Freilich, R.H. (1998). The land use implications of transit oriented development: Controlling the demand side of transportation congestion and urban sprawl. *The Urban Lawyer*, 30(3), 547-72.

Freund, A.M., & Baltes, P.B. (1998). Selection, optimizing, and compensation as strategies of life management: Correlations with subjective indicators of successful aging. *Psychology and Aging*, 13(4), 531-43.

Fries, J. (1980). Aging, natural death, and the compression of morbidity. *New England Journal of Medicine*, 303(3), 130-5.

Fries, J. (1989). The compression of morbidity: Near or far? *Milbank Quarterly*, 67(2), 208-32.

Fries, J. (2002). Successful aging: An emerging paradigm of gerontology. *Clinics in Geriatric Medicine*, 18, 371-82.

Frumkin, H. (2002). Urban sprawl and public health. *Public Health Reports*, 117, 201-16.

Frumkin, H. (ed.) (2010). *Environmental health: From global to local*. San Francisco: John Wiley & Sons.

Fry, C.L., Treloar, C., & Maher, L. (2005). Ethical challenges and responses in harm reduction research: Promoting applied communitarian ethics. *Drug and Alcohol Review*, 24, 449-59.

FSANZ (Food Standards Australia New Zealand) (2001). *Australia and New Zealand Food Standards Code*. Melbourne: Anstat Legislation.

Furnass, B. (1996). Introduction. In B. Furnass, J. Whyte, J. Harris, & A. Baker (eds), *Survival, health and wellbeing into the twenty first century: Proceedings of a conference held at the Australian National University, November 30–December 1, 1995*.

Gaff, C., Cowan, R., Mesier, B., & Lindeman, G. (2006). Genetic services for men: The preferences of men with a family history of prostate cancer. *Genetics in Medicine*, 8(12), 771-8.

Galvao, J. (2005). Brazil and access to HIV/AIDS drugs: A question of human rights and public health. *American Journal of Public Health*, 95(7), 1110-16.

Ganapati, S. (2008). Critical appraisal of three ideas for community development in the United States. *Journal of Planning Education and Research*, 227, 382-99.

Gandy, M., & Zumia, A. (2002). The resurgence of disease: Social and historical perspectives on the new tuberculosis. *Social Science and Medicine*, 55(3), 385-96.

García-Moreno, G., Jansen, H.A.F.M., Ellsberg, M., Heise, L., & Watts, C. (2005). *WHO multi-country study on women's health and domestic violence against women*. Geneva: WHO.

Garn, H., & Renz, H. (2007). Epidemiological and immunological evidence for the Hygiene Hypothesis. *Immunobiology*, 212(6), 441-52.

Garnaut, R. (2008). *The Garnaut climate change review: Final report.* Commonwealth of Australia. Cambridge: Cambridge University Press.

Geithner, C.A., & McKenney, D.R. (2010). Strategies for aging well. *Strength and Conditioning Journal*, 32(5), 36–52.

Genat, B., & Cripps, K. (2009). Understanding the determinants of Aboriginal health. In H. Keleher & C. MacDougall (eds), *Understanding health: A determinants approach*, 2nd edn. Melbourne: Oxford University Press, 87–100.

Germov, J. (2005). *Second opinion: An introduction to health sociology*, 3rd edn. Melbourne: Oxford University Press.

Germov, J. (2009). The class origins of health inequality. In J. Germov (ed.), *Second opinion: An introduction to health sociology*, 4th edn. Melbourne: Oxford University Press, 85–110.

Germov, J., & Freij, M. (2009). Media and health: Moral panics, sinners, and saviours. In J. Germov (ed.), *Second opinion: An introduction to health sociology*, 4th edn. Melbourne: Oxford University Press, 348–63.

Giammattei, J., Blix, G., Marshak, H.H., Wollitzer, A.O., & Pettitt, D.J. (2003). Television watching and soft drink consumption: Associations with obesity in 11 to 13 year old children. *Archives of Pediatrics and Adolescent Medicine*, 157(9), 822–43.

Gifford, R. (2007). The consequences of living in high-rise buildings. *Architectural Science Review*, 50(1), 2–17.

Gilmore, N., & Somerville, M.A. (1994). Stigmatisation, scapegoating and discrimination in sexually transmitted diseases: Overcoming 'them' and 'us'. *Social Science and Medicine*, 39(9), 1339–58.

Gindroz, R. (1999). The revitalization of urban places depends on safety and security. The design of streets and buildings should reinforce safe environments, but not at the expense of accessibility and openness. In M. Leccese & K. McCormick (eds), *Charter of the new urbanism*. New York: McGraw-Hill, 133–7.

Ginsburg, Y., & Churchman, A. (1985). The pattern and meaning of neighbor relations in high-rise housing in Israel. *Human Ecology*, 13(4), 467–84.

Girling, C., & Kellet, R. (2005). *Skinny streets and green neighbourhoods: Design for environment and community*. New York: Island Press.

Glasgow, R.E., Warner, E.H., Kaplan, R.M., Vinicor, F., Smith, L., & Norman, J. (1999). If diabetes is a public health problem, why not treat it as one? A population based approach to chronic illness. *Annals of Behavioral Medicine*, 21(2), 159–70.

Glass, T.A. (2003). Assessing the success of successful aging. *Annals of Internal Medicine*, 139(5), 382–3.

Glover, J.D., Hetzel, D.M.S., & Tennant, S.K. (2004). The socioeconomic gradient and chronic illness and associated risk factors in Australia. *Australia and New Zealand Health Policy*, 1(8), 1–8.

Gochfield, M., & Goldstein, B.D. (1999). Lessons in environmental health in the twentieth century. *Annual Review of Public Health*, 20, 35–53.

Goffman, E. (1963). *Stigma: On the management of spoiled identity*. Englewood Cliffs, NJ: Prentice-Hall.

Goffman, E. (1990). *Stigma: Notes on the management of spoiled identity*. Harmondsworth: Penguin.

Goldhaber, M.D. (2007). *A people's history of the European Court of Human Rights*. New Brunswick, NJ: Rutgers University Press.

Goldman, L.R. (2004). Environmental health practice. In R. Detels, J. McEwen, R. Beaglehole & H. Tanaka (eds), *Oxford textbook of public health*, 4th edn. Oxford: Oxford University Press.

Goldsworthy, D., Jirojwong, S., & Liamputtong, P. (2009). Emerging population health issues and health promotion. In S. Jirojwong & P. Liamputtong (eds), *Population health, communities and health promotion: Assessment, planning, implementation and evaluation.* Melbourne: Oxford University Press, 92–103.

Goris, J.M., Peterssen, S., Stamatakis, E., & Veerman, J.L. (2010). Television food advertising and the prevalence of childhood overweight and obesity: A multicountry comparison. *Public Health Nutrition*, 13(7), 1003–12.

Gorski, J.A., Slifer, K.J., Kelly-Suttka, J., & Lowery, K. (2004). Behavioral interventions for pediatric patients' acute pain and anxiety: Improving health regimen compliance and outcomes. *Children's Health Care*, 33(1), 1–20.

Gostin, L.O., & Lazzarini, Z. (1997). Prevention of HIV/AIDS among injection drug users: The theory and science of public health and criminal justice approaches to disease prevention. *Emory Law Journal*, 46(2), 587–696.

Gostin, L., Mann, J., & Gostin, L. (1994). Towards the development of a human rights impact assessment for the formulation and evaluation of health policies. *Health and Human Rights* 1(1), 58–80.

Gottlieb, T., Hoy, J., & McDonald, M. (2010). *Fever: Mechanisms and symptomatic treatment.* In A. Yung, D. Spelman, A. Street, J. McCormack, T. Sorrell & P. Johnson (eds), *Infectious diseases: A clinical approach*, 3rd edn. Melbourne: IP Communications, 18–26.

Gracey, M., & King, M. (2009). Indigenous health Part 1: Determinants and disease patterns. *The Lancet*, 374, 65–75.

Gray, D., & Saggers, S. (2009). Indigenous health: The perpetuation of inequality. In J. Germov (ed.), *Second opinion: An introduction to health sociology*, 4th edn. Oxford University Press: Melbourne, 156–74.

Grayson, L., & Howden, B. (2010). *Antibacterial agents.* In A. Yung, D. Spelman, A. Street, J. McCormack, T. Sorrell & P. Johnson (eds), *Infectious diseases: A clinical approach*, 3rd edn. Melbourne: IP Communications, 585–608.

Grayson, R. (1995). *Evaluating Sydney's community gardens.* Australian City Farms and Community Gardens Network. <http://communitygarden.org.au/evaluation>.

Grbich, C. (ed.) (1999). *Health in Australia: Sociological concepts and issues.* Melbourne: Longman/ Prentice Hall.

Green, J. (2010). The WHO Commission on the Social Determinants of Health. *Critical Public Health*, 20(1), 1–4.

Green, J., & Tones, K. (2010). *Health promotion: Planning and strategies*, 2nd edn. London: Sage Publications.

Griffin, D.E. (2007). Mealses virus. In D.E. Knipe & P.M. Holey (eds), *Fields virology*, 5th edn. Philadelphia: Lippincott Williams & Wilkins, 1551–86.

Griffith, C.H., Wilson, J.F., Langen, S., & Haist, S.A. (2003). House staff nonverbal communication skills and standardized patient satisfaction. *Journal of General Internal Medicine*, 18(3), 170–4.

Griffith, L., Raina, P., Wu, H., Zhu, B., & Stathokostas, L. (2010). Population attributable risk for functional disability associated with chronic conditions in Canadian older adults. *Age and Ageing*, 39(6), 738–45.

Griffiths, J., Rao, M., Adshead, F., & Thorpe, A. (eds) (2009). *The health practitioner's guide to climate change: Diagnosis and cure*. London: Earthscan.

Groake, A., Curtis, R., Couglin, R., & Gsel, A. (2005). The impact of illness representations and disease activity on adjustment in women with rheumatoid arthritis: A longitudinal study. *Psychology and Health*, 20(5), 597–613.

Gruskin, S., & Tarantola, D. (2005). Health and human rights. In S. Gruskin, M. Grodin, S. Marks & G. Annas (eds), *Perspectives on health and human rights*. New York: Routledge, 3–57.

Gruskin, S., Mills, E.J., & Tarantola, D. (2007). History, principles and practice of health and human rights. *The Lancet*, 370, 449–55.

Guralnik, J., & Kaplan, G. (1989). Predictors of healthy aging: Prospective evidence from the Alameda County Study. *American Journal of Public Health*, 79, 703–8.

Guttman, N., & Zimmerman, D.R. (2000). Low-income mothers' views on breastfeeding. *Social Science and Medicine*, 50(10), 1457–73.

Habibis, D. (2009). The illness experience: Lay perspectives, disability, and chronic illness. In J. Germov (ed.), *Second opinion: An introduction to health sociology*, 4th edn. Melbourne: Oxford University Press, 288–306.

Hadlow, J., & Pitts, M. (1991). The understanding of common health terms by doctors, nurses, and patients. *Social Science and Medicine*, 32(2), 193–6.

Haines, A. (2009). Introduction. In J. Griffiths, M. Rao, F. Adshead, & A. Thorpe (eds), *The health practitioner's guide to climate change. Diagnosis and cure* (p. xx). London: Earthscan.

Haines, L., Wan, K.C., Lynn, R., Barrett, T.G., & Shield, J.P.H. (2007). Rising incidence of Type 2 diabetes in children in the UK. *Diabetes Care*, 30(5), 1097–101.

Halford, J.C.G., Boyland, E.J., Brown, V., Highes, G.M., Stacey, L., McKean, S., & Dovey, T.M. (2007). Beyond-brand effect of television food advertisements on food choice in children: The effects of weight status. *Public Health Nutrition*, 11(9), 897–904.

Hall, J.A., Epstein, A.M., & McNeil, B.J. (1989). Multidimensionality of health status in an elderly population: Construct validity of a measurement battery. *Medical Care*, 27(3), S168–S177.

Hall, K.B., & Porterfield, G.A. (2001). *Community by design: New urbanism for suburbs and small communities*. New York: McGraw-Hill.

Hall, W.D., Morley, K.I., & Lucke, J.C. (2004). The prediction of disease risk in genomic medicine: Scientific prospects and implications for public policy and ethics. *EMBO Reports European Molecular Biology Organisation* Special Issue, S22–S26.

Hancock, T. (1985). The mandala of health: A model of the human ecosystem. *Family and Community Health*, 8Z(3), 1–10.

Hancock, T. (1993). Health, human development and the community ecosystem: Three ecological models. *Health Promotion International*, 8(1), 41–7.

Hancock, T. (1994). Sustainability, equity, peace and the (green) politics of health. In C. Chu & R. Simpson (eds), *Ecological public health: From vision to practice*. Griffith and Toronto: Institute of Applied Environmental Research and Centre for Health Promotion, 36–46.

Hancock, T., & Perkins, F. (1985). The mandala of health: A conceptual model and teaching tool. *Health Education*, Summer, 8–10.

Hanlon, P., Walsh, D., & Whyte, B. (2006). *Let Glasgow flourish*. Glasgow: Glasgow Centre for Population Health.

Hardey, M. (1998). *The social context of health*. Buckingham, PA: Open University Press.

Harrigan, J.A., Oxman, T.E., & Rosenthal, R. (1985). Rapport expressed through nonverbal behavior. *Journal of Nonverbal Behavior*, 9(2), 95–110.

Harris, E., Nutbeam, D., & Sainsbury, P. (2001). Does our limited analysis of the dimensions of poverty limit the way we seek solutions? In R. Eckersley, J. Dixon, & B. Douglas (eds), *The social origins of health and wellbeing*. Cambridge: Cambridge University Press, 259–68.

Harris, E., Wise, M., Hawe, P., Finlay, P., & Nutbeam, D. (1995). *Working together: Intersectoral action for health*. Canberra: Australian Government.

Harris, P., Nagy, S., & Vardaxis, N. (2010). *Mosby's dictionary of medicine, nursing and allied health professions*, 2nd edn. Sydney: Mosby Elsevier.

Harrison, M., Coyne, R., Lee, A.J., Leonard, D., Lowson, S., Groos, A., & Ashton, B.A. (2007). The increasing cost of basic foods required to promote health in Queensland. *Medical Journal of Australia*, 186(1), 9–14.

Hart, J.T. (2006). *The political economy of health care: A clinical perspective*. Bristol: Policy Press.

Hartog, J., & Hartog, E.A. (1983). Cultural aspects of health and illness behavior in hospitals. *Western Journal of Medicine*, 139, 910–16.

Harvey, P.W. (2006). Social determinants of health: Why we continue to ignore them in the search for improved population health outcomes. *Australian Health Review*, 30(4), 419–24.

Hassan, R., Scholes, R., & Ash, N. (eds) (2005). *Ecosystems and human well-being: Current state and trends*. Washington, DC: Millennium Ecosystem Assessment.

Havemen-Nies, A., De Groot, L., & Van Staveren, W.A. (2003). Dietary quality, lifestyle factors, and healthy ageing in Europe: The SENECA study. *Age and Ageing*, 32(4), 427–34.

Hawe, P. (2009). The social determinants of health: How can a radical agenda be mainstreamed? *Canadian Journal of Public Health*, 100(4), 291–4.

Hayden, M.R. (2003). Predictive testing for Huntington's disease: A universal model? *The Lancet Neurology*, 2, 141–2.

Hayflick, L. (2007). Biological aging is no longer an unsolved problem. *Annals of New York Academy of Sciences*, 1100, 1–13.

Health and Development Africa (2007). *Soul City, it's real: Evaluation report, Series 7*. <www.soulcity.org.za/research/evaluations/soul-city-its-real-evaluation-report-2007/evaluation-report-2007/view>.

Health-Canada (2001). Workshop on healthy aging. <www.hc-sc.gc.ca/seniors-aines/pubs/healthy_aging/intro_e.htm>.

Heggenhougan, H.K., & Shore, L. (1986). Cultural components of behavioural epidemiology: Implications for primary health care. *Social Science and Medicine*, 22(11), 1235–45.

Heijnders, M., & Van Der Meij, S. (2006). The fight against stigma: An overview of stigma-reduction strategies and interventions. *Psychology, Health, and Medicine*, 11, 353–63.

Heikkinen, E. (1999). *Determinants of healthy ageing: Implications for research policy*. Jyvaskyla, Finland: University of Jyvaskyla.

Helman, C.G. (2007). *Culture, health and illness*, 5th edn. London: Hodder Arnold.

Henderson-Wilson, C. (2009). Inner city high-rise living: A catalyst for social exclusion and social connectedness? In A.Taket, B.R. Crisp, A. Nevill, G. Lamaro, M. Graham, & S. Barter-Godfrey (eds), *Theorising social exclusion*. London: Routledge, 68–77.

Henderson-Wilson, C. (2010). Sustainable highrise developments: Factors impacting on residents' health and wellbeing. In M.K. Tolba, A. Abdel-Hadi, & S. Soliman (eds), *Environment, health, and sustainable development: Advances in people-environment studies*, vol. 1. Cambridge: Hogrefe Ltd, 59–72.

Hendryx, M., Ahern, A., Lovrich, N., & McCurdy, A. (2002). Access to health care and community social capital. *Health Services Research*, 37, 85–101.

Henson, C., Chapman, S., McLeod, L., Johnson, N., McGeechan, K., & Hickie, I. (2009). More us than them: Positive depictions of mental illness on Australian television news. *Australian and New Zealand Journal of Psychiatry*, 43, 554–60.

Herek, G.M. (2002). Thinking about AIDS and stigma: A psychologist's perspective. *Journal of Law, Medicine, and Ethics*, 30, 594–607.

Herek, G.M., & Glunt, E.K. (1993). Public reactions to AIDS in the United States: A second decade of stigma. *American Journal of Public Health*, 83(4), 573–7.

Hertzman, C. (2000). The case for an early childhood development strategy. *Isuma: Canadian Journal of Policy Research*, 1(4), 10–18.

Hertzman, C., & Power, C. (2004). Child development as a determinant of health across the life course. *Current Paediatrics*, 14(5), 438–43.

Hill, E.K., Alpi, K.M., & Auerbach, M. (2010). Evidence-based practice in health education and promotion: A review and introduction to resources. *Health Promotion Practice*, 11(3), 358–66.

Hill, J., & Radimer, K. (1997). A content analysis of food advertisements in television for Australian children. *Australian Journal of Nutrition and Dietetics*, 54(4), 174–82.

Hitchings, E., and Moynihan, P.J. (1998). The relationship between television food advertisements recalled and actual foods consumed by children. *Journal of Human Nutrition and Dietetics*, 11(6), 511–17.

Hoey, L.M., Ieropoli, S.C, White, V.M., & Jefford, M. (2008). Systematic review of peer-support programs for people with cancer. *Patient Education and Counseling*, 70, 315–37.

Hogerzeil, H.V., Samson, M., Casanovas, J.V., & Rahmani-Ocora, L. (2006). Is access to essential medicines as part of the fulfilment of the right to health enforceable through the courts? *The Lancet*, 368, 305–11.

Holstein, M.B., & Minkler, M. (2003). Self, society and the 'New Gerontology'. *The Gerontologist*, 43(6), 787–96.

Honari, M. (1993). Advancing health ecology: Where to from here? In N. Newman (ed.), *Health and ecology: A nursing perspective*. Proceedings of the First National Nursing the Environment Conference, Australian Nursing Federation, Melbourne.

Horsley, A., Cunningham, S., & Innes, A. (2009). *Cystic fibrosis*. Oxford Respiratory Medicine Library. New York: Oxford University Press.

Horton, G., & McMichael, A. (2008). Climate change health check 2020. The Climate Institute, <www.climateinstitute.org.au>.

Howard, C.M., & Mathews, W.K. (2006). *On deadline: Managing media relations*, 4th edn. Long Grove, IL: Waveland Press.

Hoy, J., & Richmond J. (2008). Standard precautions and infection control. In D. Bradford, J. Hoy, & G. Matthews (eds), *HIV, viral hepatitis and STIs: A guide for primary care*. Sydney: Australasian Society for HIV Medicine, 146–51.

Hughes, C.C. (1996). The culture bound syndromes and psychiatric diagnosis. In J.E. Mezzich, A. Kleinman, H. Fabrega, & D.L. Parron (eds), *Culture and psychiatric diagnosis: A DSM-IV perspective*. Washington, DC: APA, 289–308.

Hulme, A. (1998). An analysis of collaboration in the Municipal Public Health Plan process in a number of Victoria municipalities. Unpublished Honours thesis, Deakin University, Melbourne.

Human Diseases and Conditions (2010). *Chronic illness.* <www.humanillnesses.com/Behavioral-Health-Br-Fe/Chronic-Illness.html>.

Human Genetics Society of Australasia (2008). *Genetic testing and life insurance in Australia.* <www.hgsa.org.au/website/wp-content/uploads/2009/12/2008-PS01.pdf>.

Human Genetics Society of Australasia (2010). *Policy: Testing and screening.* <www.hgsa.org.au/category/documents/docs-policy-testing-and-screening>.

Human Rights Commission (2011). *Disability Discrimination Act 1992.* <www.hreoc.gov.au/disability_rights/index.html>.

Hunt, P. (2009). Missed opportunities: Human rights and the Commission on Social Determinants of Health. *Global Health Promotion*, 16 (Suppl 1), 36–41.

Hurlimann, A.C., & Mackay, J.M. (2006). What attributes of recycled water make it fit for residential purposes? The Mawson Lakes Experience. *Desalination*, 187, 167–77.

Hurst, J., & Siciliani, L. (2003). *Tackling excessive waiting times for elective surgery: A comparison of policies in twelve OECD countries.* OECD Health Working papers, No. 6. Paris: OECD. <www.oecd.org/dataoecd/24/32/5162353.pdf>.

Hutchison, E. (2005). The life course perspective: A promising approach for bridging the micro and macro worlds for social workers. *Families in Society*, 86(1), 143–52.

Hutchison, E. (2010). A life course perspective. In E. Hutchison (ed.), *Dimensions of human behavior: The changing life course.* London: Sage Publications, 3–38.

IACHR (Inter-American Commission on Human Rights) (2011). *Annual report of the Inter-American Commission on Human Rights 2010.* Washington, DC: IACHR.

INDEPTH Network (2007). *Measuring health equity in small areas: Findings from demographic surveillance systems.* INDEPTH Network. Hampshire, England: Ashgate. <www.indepth-network.org>.

Institute of Medicine (2001). *Crossing the quality chasm: A new health system for the twenty-first century.* Washington, DC: National Academies Press.

Intergenerational Report (2010). <www.population.org.au/index.php/publications/spa-articles/aging/464-the-2010-intergenerational-report>.

Irwin, A., & Scali, E. (2007). Action on the social determinants of health: A historical perspective. *Global Public Health*, 2(3), 235–56.

Ishay, M.R. (2008). *The history of human rights: From ancient times to the globalization era*, 2nd edn. Berkeley, CA: University of California Press.

Itzin, C., Taket, A., & Barter-Godfrey, S. (2010). *Domestic and sexual violence and abuse: Tackling the health and mental health effects.* London: Routledge.

Izumi, Y., Amaya, F., Hosokawa, K., Ueno, H., Hosokawa, T., Hashimoto, S., & Tanaka, Y. (2010). Five-day pain management regimen using patient-controlled analgesia facilitates early ambulation after cardiac surgery. *Journal of Anesthesia*, 24(2), 187–91.

Jaakkola, M.S., Yang, L., Leromnimon, A., & Jaakkola, J.J.K. (2007). Office work exposure and respiratory and sick building syndrome symptoms. *Occupational and Environmental Medicine*, 64(3), 178–84.

Jacobs, G. (2011). 'Take control or lean back?': Barriers to practicing empowerment in health promotion. *Health Promotion Practice*, 12(1), 94–101.

Jacobs, P. (1997). *The economics of health and medical care*, 4th edn. Frederick, MA: Aspen Publications.

Jacobson, P.D., & Banerjee, A. (2005). Social movements and human rights rhetoric in tobacco control. *Tobacco Control*, 14(Suppl. II), ii45–ii49.

Janus, S.S., & Janus, C.L. (1993). *The Janus report on sexual behaviour.* New York: John Wiley & Sons.

Jirojwong, S., & Liamputtong, P. (2009). An introduction: Population health and health promotion. In S. Jirojwong & P. Liamputtong (eds), *Population health, communities and health promotion: Assessment, planning, implementation and evaluation.* Melbourne: Oxford University Press, 3–25.

Jones, E.E., Farina, A., Hastort, A.H., Markus, H., Miller, D.T., et al. (1984). *Social stigma: The psychology of marked relationships.* New York: W.H. Freeman and Company.

Jones, K., & Creedy, D. (2008). *Health and human behaviour,* 2nd edn. Melbourne: Oxford University Press.

Jonsson, U. (2003). *Human rights approach to development programming.* Nairobi: UNICEF.

Judd, M. (2004). Trauma in the city of Kerma: Ancient versus modern injury patterns. *International Journal of Osteoarchaeology*, 14(1), 34–51.

Julian, R. (2009). Ethnicity, health, and multiculturalism. In J. Germov (ed.), *Second opinion: An introduction to health sociology*, 4th edn. Oxford University Press: Melbourne, 175–96.

Karasek, R., Baker, D., Marxer, F., Ahlbom, A., & Theorell, T. (1981). Job decision latitude, job demands and cardiovascular disease: A prospective study of Swedish men. *American Journal of Public Health*, 71(7), 694–705.

Katz, I. (1981). *Stigma: A social psychological analysis.* Hillsdale, NJ: Erlbaum.

Kausikan, B. (1996). Asia's different standard. In H.J. Steiner & P. Alston (eds), *International human rights in context.* Oxford: Clarendon Press, 226–33.

Kawachi, I., Kennedy, B.P., & Glass, R. (1999). Social capital and self-rated health: A contextual analysis. *American Journal of Public Health*, 89(8), 1187–93.

Kawachi, I., Subramanian, S., & Almeida-Filho, N. (2002). A glossary for health inequalities. *Journal of Epidemiology and Community Health* (Glossary), 56(9), 647–52.

Kazi, A., Falmi, Z., Hatcher, J., Kadir, M.M., Niaz, U., & Wasserman, G.A. (2006). Social environment and depression amongst pregnant women in urban areas of Pakistan: Importance of social relations, *Social Science and Medicine*, 63(6), 1466–76.

Keane, H. (2003). Critiques of harm reduction, morality and the promise of human rights. *International Journal of Drug Policy*, 14, 227–32.

Kelaher, M., Paul, S., Lambert, H., Ahmed, W., & Davey-Smith, G. (2008). The impact of different measures of socioeconomic position on the relationship between ethnicity and health. *Annuals of Epidemiology*, 18, 351–6.

Kelbaugh, D. (1999). Architecture and landscape design should grow from local climate: Topography, history, and building practice. In M. Leccese & K. McCormick (eds), *Charter of the new urbanism.* New York: McGraw-Hill, 155–60.

Keleher, H., & Joss, N. (2009). Determinants of healthy ageing. In H. Keleher & C. MacDougall (eds), *Understanding health: A determinants approach*, 2nd edn. Melbourne: Oxford University Press, 367–78.

Keleher, H. & MacDougall, C. (2009). Understanding health. In H. Keleher & C. MacDougall (eds), *Understanding health: A determinants approach*, 2nd edn. Melbourne: Oxford University Press, 3–16.

Keleher, H., & Murphy, B. (2004). Understanding health: An introduction. In H. Keleher & B. Murphy (eds), *Understanding health: A determinants approach.* Melbourne: Oxford University Press, 1–8.

Keller, V.F., & Carroll, J.G. (1994). A new model for physician–patient communication. *Patient Education and Counseling*, 23, 131–40.

Kelly, B., Smith, B., King, L., Flood, V., & Bauman, A. (2007). Television food advertising to children: The extent and nature of exposure. *Public Health Nutrition*, 10(11), 1234–40.

Kelly, B.P., & Chau, J.Y. (2007). Children's television sub-standards: A call for significant amendments. *Medical Journal of Australia*, 186(1), 18.

Kelly, M.P., Morgan, A., Bonnefoy, J., Butt, J., & Bergman, V. (2007). *The social determinants of health: Developing an evidence base for political action*. Final Report to WHO Commission on Social Determinants of Health. London: National Institutes for Health and Clinical Excellence.

Kendig, H., & Browning, C. (2010). A social view on healthy ageing: Multi-disciplinary perspectives and Australian evidence. In C. Phillipson & D. Dannefer (eds), *The Sage handbook of social gerontology*. Los Angeles: Sage Publications, 459–71.

Kennedy, D., Stocker, L., & Burke, G. (2010). Australian local government action on climate change adaptation: Some critical reflections to assist decision-making. *Local Environment*, 15(9–10), 805–16.

Kenneway, E., & Kenneway, N. (1947). A further study into the incidence of cancer of the lung and larynx. *British Journal of Cancer*, 1, 260–98.

Kenneway, N., & Kenneway, E. (1936). A study of the incidence of cancer of the lung and larynx. *Journal of Hygiene*, 36, 236–67.

Kenny, A. (2004). Medical dominance and power: A rural perspective. *Health Sociological Review*, 13, 158–65.

Kernick, D. (2002). *Getting health economics into practice*. Oxford: Radcliffe Medical Press.

Khoury, M.J., Burke, W., & Thomson, E.J. (eds) (2000). *Genetics and public health in the 21st century: Using genetic information to improve health and prevent disease*. New York: Oxford University Press.

Kickbusch, I. (2007). The move towards a new public health. *IUHPE—Promotion and Education Supplement*, 2, 9.

Kickbusch, I., & O'Byrne, D. (1995). Community as the focus for health and health changes. *Promotion and Education*, 2, 17–20.

King, H., Aubert, R., & Herman, W. (1998). Global burden of diabetes, 1995–2025: Prevalence, numerical estimates and projections. *Diabetes Care* 21, 1414–31.

King, M., Smith, A., & Gracey, M. (2009). Indigenous health Part 2: The underlying causes of the health gap. *The Lancet*, 374, 76–85.

Kirmayer, L.J., & Sartorius, N. (2007). Cultural models and somatic syndromes. *Psychosomatic Medicine*, 69, 832–40.

Kitagawa, T., Owada, M., Urakami, T., & Yamauchi, K. (1998). Increased incidence of non-insulin dependent Diabetes Mellitus among Japanese school children correlates with an increased intake of animal protein and fat. *Clinical Pediatrics*, 37, 111–16.

Kitchener, S., Leggat, P.A., Brennan, L., & McCall, B. (2002). Importation of dengue by soldiers returning from East Timor to North Queensland, Australia. *Journal of Travel Medicine*, 9(4), 180–3.

Kizer, K.W. (2000). Lessons learned in public health emergency management: Personal reflections. *Journal of Prehospital and Disaster Medicine*, 15(4), 209–14.

Kleinman, A., Eisenberg, L., & Good, B. (1978). Culture, illness, and care: Clinical lessons from anthropologic and cross-cultural research. *Annals of Internal Medicine*, 88(2), 251–8.

Klin, A., & Lemish, D. (2008). Mental disorders stigma in the media: Review of studies on production, content, and influences. *Journal of Communication*, 13(5), 434–49.

Kotler, P., Adam, S., Denize, S., & Armstrong, G. (2009). *Principles of marketing*, 4th edn. Sydney: Pearson Education Australia.

Kramsch, C. (1998). *Language and culture*. Oxford and New York: Oxford University Press.

Krieger, N. (2003). Genders, sexes and health: What are the connections—and why does it matter? *International Journal of Epidemiology*, 32, 652–7.

Krimm, R.W. (1998). Making mitigation a realty. *Australian Journal of Emergency Management*, Autumn, 60–3.

Krolewski, A., Warram, J.H., Rand, L.I., & Kahn, R. (1987). Epidemiologic approach to the etiology of Type I Diabetes Mellitus and its complications. *New England Journal of Medicine*, 317, 1390–8.

Krug, E.G., Dahlberg, L.L., Mercy, J.A., Zwi, A.B., & Lozano, R. (eds) (2002). *World report on violence and health*. Geneva: WHO.

Labonte, R. (1997). *Power participation and partnerships for health promotion*. Melbourne: VicHealth.

LaDeau, S.L., Kilpatrick, A.M., & Marra, P.P. (2007). West Nile emergence and large-scale declines of North American bird populations. *Nature*, 447, 710–14.

Lamb, K.L., Brodie, D.A., & Roberts, K. (1988). Physical fitness and health-related fitness as indicators of a positive health state. *Health Promotion*, 3, 171–82.

Laris, P., Gleeson, S., & Alperstein, G. (2008). *Social determinants of health: Areas for action*. Australian Health Promotion Association, NSW Branch.

Larsen, K.M., & Smith, C.K. (1991). Assessment of non-verbal communication in the physician-patient interview. *Journal of Family Practice*, 12(3), 481–8.

Laverack, G. (2007). *Health promotion practice: Building empowered communities*. London: Open University Press.

Lawless, S., Kippax, S., & Crawford, J. (1996). Dirty, diseased and undeserving: The positioning of HIV positive women. *Social Science and Medicine*, 43(9), 1371–7.

Lawn, S. (2008). 'The needs of strangers': Understanding social determinants of mental illness. *Social Alternatives*, 27(4), 36–41.

Lawrence, R.J. (2003). Human ecology and its applications. *Landscape and Urban Planning*, 65, 31–40.

LeBel, T.P. (2008). Perceptions of and responses to stigma. *Sociology Compass*, 2(2), 409–32.

LeBlanc, M.M., & Kelloway, E.K. (2003). Predictors and outcomes of workplace violence and aggression. *Journal of Applied Psychology*, 87(3), 444–53.

Lee, A.M., & Lee, S. (1996). Disordered eating and its psychosocial correlates among Chinese adolescent females in Hong Kong. *International Journal of Eating Disorders*, 20(2), 177–83.

Lee, K. (2010). How do we move forward on the social determinants of health: The global governance challenges. *Critical Public Health*, 20(1), 5–14.

Lee, W.R. (1973). Emergence of occupational medicine in Victorian times. *British Journal of Industrial Medicine*, 30, 118–24.

Leeder, S. (1999). *Healthy medicine: Challenges facing Australia's health services*. Sydney: Allen & Unwin.

Leeder, S. (2007). The scope, mission and method of contemporary public health. *Australian and New Zealand Journal of Public Health*, 31(6), 505–8.

Leggett, B.A. (2009). Family-based screening for colorectal cancer: The Australian perspective. *Journal of Gastroenterololy & Hepatology*, 24, Supplement 3, S29–S32.

Leroux-Roels, I., & Leroux-Roels, G. (2009). Current status and progress of prepandemic and pandemic influenza vaccine development. *Expert Review of Vaccines*, 8(4), 401–23.

Letteney, S., & LaPorte, H.H. (2004). Deconstructing stigma: Perceptions of HIV-seropositive mothers and their disclosure to children. *Social Work in Health Care*, 38, 105–23.

Leveille, S.G., Guralnik, J.M., Ferrucci, L., & Langlois, J.A. (1999). Aging successfully until death in old age: Opportunities for increasing active life expectancy. *American Journal of Epidemiology*, 149(7), 654–64.

Levin, B.W., & Browner, C.H. (2005). The social construction of health: Critical contributions from evolutionary, biological and cultural anthropology. *Social Science and Medicine*, 61(4), 745–50.

Levitas, R., Pantazis, C., Fahmy, E., Gordon, D., Llyod, E., & Patsios, D. (2007). *The multidimensional analysis of social exclusion*: Bristol Institute for Public Affairs, University of Bristol. <www.cabinetoffice.gov.uk/social_exclusion_task_force/publications/multidimensional.aspx>.

Levy, B.R. (2000). Handwriting as a reflection of aging self-stereotypes. *Journal of Geriatric Psychiatry*, 33, 81–94.

Levy, B.R. (2003). Mind matters: Cognitive and physical effects of aging self-stereotypes. *Journal of Gerontology*, 58B(4), 203–11.

Levy, B.R. (2009). Stereotype embodiment: A psychosocial approach to ageing. *Current directions in psychological science*, 18, 332–6.

Liamputtong Rice, P. (2000). *Hmong woman and reproduction*. Westport, CT: Bergin & Garvey.

Liamputtong Rice, P., Ly, B., & Lumley, J. (1994). Soul loss and childbirth: The case of a Hmong woman. *Medical Journal of Australia*, 160, 577–8.

Liamputtong, P. (2006). Motherhood and 'moral career': Discourses of good motherhood among Southeast Asian immigrant women in Australia. *Qualitative Sociology*, 29(1), 25–53.

Liamputtong, P. (2007). *The journey of becoming a mother amongst women in northern Thailand*. Lanham, MD: Lexington Books.

Liamputtong, P. (2009a). Treating the afflicted body: Perceptions of infertility and ethnomedicine among fertile Hmong women in Australia. In L. Culley, N. Hudson, & F. van Rooij (eds), *Marginalized reproduction: Ethnicity, infertility and reproductive technologies*. Oxford: Earthscan Publisher, 151–64.

Liamputtong, P. (2009b). *Qualitative research methods*, 3rd edn. Melbourne: Oxford University Press.

Liamputtong, P. (2010a). *Performing qualitative cross-cultural research*. Cambridge: Cambridge University Press.

Liamputtong, P. (2010b). The science of words and the science of numbers: Research methods as foundations for evidence-based practice in health. In P. Liamputtong (ed.), *Research methods in health: Foundations for evidence-based practice*. Melbourne: Oxford University Press, 3–26.

Liamputtong, P., & Kitisriworapan, S. (2011). Good mother, infant feeding and social change in northern Thailand. In P. Liamputtong (ed.), *Infant feeding practices: A cross-cultural perspective*. Springer: New York, 141–59.

Liamputtong, P., Haritavorn, N., & Kiatying-Angsulee, N. (2009). HIV and AIDS, stigma and AIDS support groups: Perspectives from women living with HIV and AIDS in central Thailand. *Social Science and Medicine*, special issue on Women, Motherhood and AIDS Care in Resource Poor Settings, 69(6), 862–8.

Liggins, F. (2009). Greenhouse gas emissions: The hard facts. In J. Griffiths, M. Rao, F. Adshead, & A. Thorpe (eds) (2009). *The health practitioner's guide to climate change: Diagnosis and cure*. London: Earthscan.

Lin, V., Smith, J., & Fawkes, S. (2007). *Public health practice in Australia: The organised effort*. Sydney: Allen & Unwin.

Link, B.G., & Phelan, J.C. (2001). Conceptualizing stigma. *Annual Review of Sociology*, 27, 363–85.

Link, B.G., Struening, E.L., Neese-Todd, S., Asmussen, S., & Phelan, J.C. (2002). On describing and seeking to change the experience of stigma. *Psychiatric Rehabilitation Skills*, 6, 201–31.

Link, K. (2007). *Understanding new, resurgent and resistant diseases: How man and globalization create and spread illness*. Westport, CT: Praeger.

Littlewood, R. (1996). Cultural comments on culture bound syndromes. In J.E. Mezzich, A. Kleinman, H. Fabrega, & D.L. Parron (eds), *Culture and psychiatric diagnosis: A DSM-IV perspective*. Washington, DC: APA, 309–12.

Littlewood, R., & Lipsedge, M. (1985). Culture bound syndromes. In K. Granville-Grossman (ed.), *Recent advances in clinical psychiatry*. Edinburgh: Churchill Livingstone, 105–42.

Liu, S., Jones, R.N., & Glymour, M.M. (2010). Implications of lifecourse epidemiology for research on determinants of adult disease. *Public Health Reviews*, 32. <www.publichealthreviews.eu/upload/pdf_files/8/Glymour_for_website.pdf>.

Lorentz, C., Wieben, E., Tefferi, A., Whiteman, D., & Dewald, G. (2002). Primer on medical genomics, part I: History of genetics and sequencing of the human genome. *Mayo Clinical Proceedings*, 77, 773–82.

Lorig, K., Sobel, D., Gonzalez, V., & Minor, M. (2006). *Living a healthy life with chronic conditions*, 3rd edn. Boulder, CO: Bull Publishing Company.

Lovell, N.C. (1997). Trauma analysis in paleopathology. *Yearbook of Physical Anthropology*, 40, 139–70.

Lowry, R., Wechsler, H., Galuska, D.A., Fulton, J.E., & Kann, L. (2002). Television viewing and its associations with overweight, sedentary lifestyle, and insufficient consumption of fruits and vegetables among US high school students: Differences by race, ethnicity, and gender. *Journal of School Health*, 72(10), 413–21.

Lundberg, P.C., & Kerdonfag, P. (2010). Spiritual care provided by Thai nurses in intensive care units. *Journal of Clinical Nursing*, 19, 1121–8.

Lupien, S., & Wan, N. (2004). Successful ageing: From cell to self. *Philosophical Transactions of the Royal Society of London*, 359, 1413–26.

Luszcz, M.A., Paull, I., & Fitzgerald, K.M. (1985). Knowledge of ageing: An intergenerational comparison. *Australasian Journal on Ageing*, 4(3), 9–14.

Lynch, J., & Smith, G.D. (2005). A life course approach to chronic disease epidemiology. *Annual Review of Public health*, 26, 1–35.

Lyttleton, C. (2000). *Endangered relations: Negotiating sex and AIDS in Thailand*. Amsterdam: Harwood Academic Press.

Lyttleton, C. (2004). Fleeing the fire: Transformation and gendered belonging in Thai HIV/AIDS support groups. *Medical Anthropology*, 23, 1–40.

Lyttleton, C., Beesey, A., & Sitthikriengkrai, M. (2007). Expanding community through ARV provision in Thailand. *AIDS Care*, 19(Supplement 1), S44–S53.

MacArthur, I. (2002). *Local environmental health planning: Guidance for local and national authorities*. WHO Regional Publications, European Series, No. 95. Copenhagen: World Health Organization.

MacDonald, J.J. (2010). Health equity and the social determinants of health in Australia. *Social Alternatives*, 29(2), 34–40.

Macintyre, S., & Ellaway, A. (2000). Ecological approaches: Rediscovering the role of the physical and social environment. In L.F. Berkman & I. Kawachi (eds), *Social epidemiology*. New York: Oxford University Press, 332–48.

Mackenzie, E.R., Taylor, L., Bloom, B.S., Hufford, D.J., & Johnson, J.C. (2003). Ethnic minority use of complementary and alternative medicine (CAM): A national probability survey of CAM utilizers. *Alternative Therapies in Health and Medicine*, 9(4), 50–6.

Macklin, J. (1992). *Enough to make you sick: How income and environment affect health*. Research Paper No, 1, National Health Strategy, Canberra.

MacLachlan, M. (2006). *Culture and health: A critical perspective towards global health*. Chicester, UK: John Wiley & Sons.

Macmillan, R., & Elliason, S.R. (2004). Characterising the life course as role configurations and pathways: A latent structure approach. In J.T. Mortimer & M.J. Shananhan (eds), *Handbook of the life course*. New York: Springer, 529–54.

Madsen, K.L., Hviid, A., Vestergard, M., Schendel, D., Wohlfahrt, J., Thorsen, J., & Melbye, M. (2002). A population based study of measles, mumps and rubella vaccination and autism. *New England Journal of Medicine*, 347(19), 1477–82.

Magarey, A.M., Daniels, M., & Boulton, T.J. (2001). Prevalence of overweight and obesity in Australian children and adolescents: Reassessment of 1985 and 1995 data against new standard definitions. *Medical Journal of Australia*, 174, 561–5.

Mahnken, J.E. (2001). Rural nursing and health care reforms: Building a social model of health. *Journal of Rural and Remote Health Research, Education, Policy and Practice*. <www.rrh.org.au/publishedarticles/article_print_104.pdf>.

Maier, R.M., Palmer, M.W., Anderson, G.L., Halonen, M.J., Josephson, K.C., Maier, R.S., et al. (2010). Environmental determinants of and impact on childhood asthma by the bacterial community in household dust. *Applied and Environmental Microbiology*, 76(8), 2663–7.

Major, B., & O'Brien, L.T. (2005). The social psychology of stigma. *Annual Review of Psychology*, 56, 393–421.

Major, B., Quinton, W.J., McCoy, S.K., & Schmader, T. (2000). Reducing prejudice: The target's perspective. In S. Oskamp (ed.), *Reducing prejudice and discrimination*. Mahwah, NJ: Lawrence Erlbaum Associates, 211–37.

Maneesriwongul, W., Panutat, S., Putwatana, P., Srirapo-ngam, Y., Ounprasertpong, L., & Williams, A.B. (2004). Educational needs of family caregivers of persons living with HIV/AIDS in Thailand. *Journal of the Association of Nurses in AIDS Care*, 15(3), 27–36.

Mann, J., & Tarantola, D. (1998). Responding to HIV/AIDS: A historical perspective. *Health and Human Rights: An International Journal*, 2(4), 5–8.

Marieb, E.N., & Hoehn, K. (2010). *Human anatomy and physiology*, 8th edn. San Francisco: Pearson Education Inc.

Marijuana Linked to Salmonellosis (1982). *The New York Times*, 27 May. <www.nytimes.com/1982/05/27/us/marijuana-linked-to-salmonellosis.html>.

Markowitz, F.E. (2005). Sociological models of mental illness stigma. In P.W. Corrigan (ed.), *On the stigma of mental illness: Practical strategies for research and social change*. Washington, DC: APA, 129-44.

Marmot, M. (2000). Social determinants of health: From observation to policy. *Medical Journal of Australia*, 172(8), 379-82.

Marmot, M. (2003). Understanding inequalities in health. *Perspectives in Biology and Medicine*, 46(3), S9-S23.

Marmot, M. (2004). *Status syndrome: How your social standing directly affects your health and life expectancy*. London: Bloomsbury Press.

Marmot, M. (2010). *Fair society, healthy lives: The Marmot review*. London: University College London.

Marmot, M., & Wilkinson, R.G. (eds) (1999). *Social determinants of health*. Oxford: Oxford University Press.

Marmot, M., & Wilkinson, R.G. (eds) (2006). *Social determinants of health*, 2nd edn. Oxford: Oxford University Press.

Marmot, M., Stansfeld, S., Patel, C., North, F., Head, J., White, I., Brunner, E., Feeney, A., & Davey Smith, G. (1991). Health inequities amongst British civil servants: The Whitehall II study. *The Lancet*, 237(8754), 1387-93.

Marrickville Council (2007). *Community gardens policy directions*. Sydney: Marrickville Council Publication.

Marshall, W.A., & Tanner, J.M. (1969). Variations in pattern of pubertal changes in girls. *Archives of Diseases in Childhood*, 44(235), 291-303.

Marshall, W.A., & Tanner, J.M. (1970). Variations in the pattern of pubertal changes in boys. *Archives of Diseases in Childhood*, 45(239), 13-23.

Marteau, T.M., & Croyle, R.T. (1998). Psychological responses to genetic testing. *British Medical Journal*, 316(7132), 693-6.

Marteau, T., & Richards, M. (eds) (1995). *The troubled helix: Social and psychological implications of the new human genetics*. Cambridge: Cambridge University Press.

Martin, C.M., & Peterson, C. (2010). The social construction of chronicity: A key to understanding chronic care transformations. *Journal of Evaluation in Clinincal Practice*, 15, 579-85.

Martin, J., Rogers, M., & Winter, C. (eds) (2009). *Climate change in regional Australia: Social learning and adaptation*. Ballarat, Vic.: VUURN Press.

Mason, P. (2008). *Tourism impacts, planning, and management*. Oxford, UK: Butterworth-Heinemenn.

Mason, T., Carlisle, C., Watkins, C., & Whitehead, E. (2001). Introduction. In T. Mason, C. Carlisle, C. Watkins, & E. Whitehead (eds), *Stigma and social exclusion in health care*. London: Routledge, 1-13.

Mathers, C., Penm, R., Carter, R., & Stevenson, C. (1998). *Health system cost of diseases and injury in Australia, 1993-94: An analysis of costs, service use and mortality for major disease and injury groups*. Canberra: AIHW.

Mathers, C., Stevenson, C., Carter, R., & Penm, R. (1998). *Disease costing methodology used in the Disease Cost and Impacts Study, 1993-94*. Canberra: AIHW.

Mathur, S., Moon, L., & Leigh, S. (2006). Aboriginal and Torres Strait Islander people with coronary heart disease: Further perspectives on health status and treatment. Canberra: AIHW. <www.aihw.gov.au/publications/index.cfm/title/10266>.

Matthews, K.A., & Haynes, S.G. (1986). Type A behavior pattern and coronary disease risk: Update and critical evaluation. *American Journal of Epidemiology*, 123(6), 923-60.

Mausner, J.S., & Kramer, S. (1985). *Epidemiology: An introductory text*. Philadelphia, PA: W.B. Saunders Company.

Mayer, K.U. (2009). New directions in life course research. *Annual Review of Sociology*, 35, 413–33.

McCally, M., Haines, A., Fein, O., Addington, W., Lawrence, R., Cassel, J., & Blankenship, E. (2008). Poverty and ill health. In P. Brown (ed.), *Perspectives in medical sociology*. Long Grove, IL: Waveland Inc., 5–23.

McCarthy, A.J., & Goodman, S.J. (2010). Reassessing conflicting evolutionary histories of the paramyxoviridae and the origins of respiroviruses with Bayesian Multigene Phylogenies. *Infection, Genetics and Evolution*, 10(1), 97–107.

McCurdy, S.A., & Carroll, D.J. (2000). Agricultural injury. *American Journal of Industrial Medicine*, 38(4), 463–80.

McHugh, P. (1970). A commonsense conception of deviance. In J.D. Douglas (ed.), *Deviance and responsibility: The social construction of moral meanings*. New York: Basic Books, 61–88.

McLaren, L., & Hawe, P. (2005). Ecological perspectives in health research. *Journal of Epidemiology and Community Health*, 59, 6–14.

McMichael, A., Campbell-Lendrum, H., Corvalen, C., Ebi, K., Githeko, A.K., Schwraga, J.D., & Woodward, A. (eds) (2003). *Climate change and human health: Risks and responses*. Geneva: WHO.

McMichael, A.J. (1993). *Planetary overload*. Cambridge: Cambridge University Press.

McMichael, A.J. (2000). The urban environment and health in a world of increasing globalization: Issues for developing countries. *Bulletin of the World Health Organization*, 78, 1117–26.

McMichael, A.J. (2001). *Human frontiers, environments and disease: Past patterns, uncertain futures*. Cambridge: Cambridge University Press.

McNamara, B., & Rosenwax, L. (2007). The mismanagement of dying. *Health Sociology Review*, 16(5), 373–83.

McNeil, W. (1976). *Plagues and peoples*. New York: Anchor Press/Doubleday.

McPake, B., & Normand C. (2008). *Health economics: An international perspective*, 2nd edn. London: Routledge.

Mechanic, D. (1974). Social structure and personal adaptation: Some neglected dimensions. In G.V. Coelho, D.A. Hamburg, & J.E. Adams (eds), *Coping and adaptation*. New York: Basic Books, 32–44.

Mechanic, D. (1995). Sociological dimensions of illness behavior. *Social Science and Medicine*, 41, 1207–16.

Medicare Australia (2011). *How does the Medicare Safety Net work?* <www.publichealth.gov.au/interactive_graphics/australia_2010/sa/private_health.html>.

Mendes de Leon, C.F., Glass, T.A., Beckett, L.A., Seeman, T.E., Evans, D.A., & Berkman, L.F. (1999). Social networks and disability transitions across eight intervals of yearly data in the new haven EPESE. *The Journals of Gerontology, Social Sciences*, 54B(3), S162–S172.

Menec, V. (2003). The relation between everyday activities and successful aging: A six-year longitudinal study. *Journal of Gerontology Psychological Sciences and Social Sciences*, 53B, S74–S82.

Merrill, R.M. (2010). *Introduction to epidemiology*. Sudbury, MA: Jones & Bartlett.

Merzel, C., & D'Afflitti, J. (2003). Reconsidering community-based health promotion: Promise, performance, and potential. *American Journal of Public Health*, 93(4), 557–74.

Metcalf, B., Hosking, J., Jeffery, A., Voss, L., Henley, W., & Wilkin, T. (2010). Fatness leads to inactivity, but inactivity does not lead to fatness: A longitudinal study in children. *Archives of Disease in Children*, 95(6), 1–6.

Metcalfe, S.A., Bittles, A.H., O'Leary, P., & Emery, J. (2009). Australia: Public Health Genomics. *Public Health Genomics*, 12, 121–8.

Metz, B., Davidson, O.R., Bosch, P.R., Dave, R., & Meye, L.A. (eds) (2007). *Contribution of Working Group III to the Fourth Assessment Report of the Intergovernmental Panel on Climate Change*. Cambridge: Cambridge University Press.

Metzler, M. (2007). Editorial. Social determinants of health: What, how, why and now. *Preventing Chronic Disease*, 4(4), 1–4.

Miller, C.A. (2009). *Nursing for wellness in older adults*, 5th edn. Philadelphia, PA: Wolters Kluwer/ Lippincott Williams & Wilkins.

Ministry of Health (New Zealand) (2010). *Tatau kahukura: Maori health chart book 2010*, 2nd edn. Wellington: Ministry of Health.

Ministry of Maori Development (New Zealand) (2009a). *Maori health*. Wellington: Te Puni Kokiri. <www.tpk.govt.nz/en/in-print/our-publications/fact-sheets/maori-health/download/ tpk-maorihealth-2009-en.pdf>.

Ministry of Maori Development (New Zealand) (2009b). Statement of intent 2009–2012. Wellington: Te Puni Kokiri. <www.tpk.govt.nz/en/in-print/our-publications/corporate- documents/statement-of-intent-2009-12/page/1>.

Minkler, M., & Fadem, P. (2002). 'Successful aging': A disability perspective. *Journal of Disability Policy Studies*, 12(4), 229–35.

Molster, C., Charles, T., Samanek, A., & O'Leary, P. (2009). Australian study on public knowledge of human genetics and health. *Public Health Genomics*, 12, 84–91.

Montia, G. (2008). Genetic testing moratorium extended to 2014. *Insurance Daily* 16 June 2008. <www.insurancedaily.co.uk/2008/06/16/genetic-testing-moratorium-extended-to-2014>.

Monto, A.S. (2008). Epidemiology of influenza. *Vaccine*, 26 (Supplement 4), D45–D48.

Moodie, M., & Carter, R. (2010). Economic evaluation of obesity interventions. In E. Waters, B. Swinburn, J. Seidell, & R. Uauy (eds), *Preventing childhood obesity: Evidence policy and practice*. West Sussex: Wiley-Blackwell, 167–74.

Moon, G., & Gillespie, R. (1995). *Society and health: An introduction to social science for health professionals*. London: Routledge.

Mooney, G., & Scotton R. (1999). *Economics and Australian health policy*. Sydney: Allen & Unwin.

Morabia, A. (2006). *A History of epidemiologic methods and concepts*. Basel: Birkhauser.

Morgan, R.E., & David, S. (2002). Human rights: A new language for aging advocacy. *Gerontologist*, 42(4), 436–42.

Morley, B., Chapman, K., Mehta, K., King, L., Swinburn, B., & Wakefield, M. (2008). Parental awareness and attitudes about food advertising to children in Australian television. *Australian and New Zealand Journal of Public Health*, 32(4), 341–7.

Morris, S., Devlin, N., & Parkin, D. (2007). *Economic analysis in health care*. West Sussex: John Wiley & Sons.

Mortimer, J.T., & Shananhan, M.J. (2004). *Handbook of the life course*. New York: Springer.

Mowbray, M. for the WHO Commission on Social Determinants of Health (2007). Social determinants and Indigenous health: The international experience and its policy implications. International Symposium on the Social Determinants of Indigenous Health, Adelaide, April 2007. Geneva: WHO. <www.who.int/social_determinants/resources/indigenous_health_ adelaide_report_07.pdf>.

Moyn, S. (2010). *The last utopia: Human rights in history*. Cambridge, MA: Harvard University Press.

Muecke, M. (1979). An explanation of 'wind illness' in northern Thailand. *Culture, Medicine and Psychiatry*, 3, 267–300.

Municipal Association of Victoria (2007). *Human services: Municipal public health planning*. <www.mav.asn.au/CA256C2B000B597A/ListMaker?ReadForm&1=10-None~&2=0-PP+-+HS+-+Public+Health+-+Municipal+Public+Health+Planning+-+TOC~&3=~&V=Listing~&K=TOC+MPHP~&REFUNID=7CBB7163636D5FCECA25726500023FC9~>.

Muntaner, C., Sridharan, S., Solar, O., & Benach, J. (2009). Commentary: Against unjust global distribution of power and money: The report of the WHO commission on the social determinants of health: Global inequality and the future of public health policy. *Journal of Public Health Policy*, 30(2), 163–75.

Murphy, E. (1999). 'Breast is best': Infant feeding decisions and maternal deviance. *Sociology of Health & Illness*, 21, 187–208.

Murray, C.J.L., & Lopez, A.D. (1997a). Global mortality, disability and the contribution of risk factors: Global Burden of Disease Study. *The Lancet*, 349, 1436–42.

Murray C.J.L., & Lopez A.D. (1997b). Mortality by cause for eight regions of the world: Global burden of disease study. *The Lancet*, 349, 1269–76.

Nadesan, M.H., & Sotirin, P. (1998). The romance and science of 'breast is best': Discursive contradictions and contexts of breast-feeding choices. *Text and Performance Quarterly*, 18, 217–32.

Nagengast, C. (1997). Women, minorities, and indigenous peoples: Universalism and cultural relativity. *Journal of Anthropological Research*, 53(3), 349–69.

Naidoo, J., & Wills, J. (2009). *Foundations for health promotion: Public health and health promotion practice*, 3rd edn. Edinburgh: Bailliere Tindall.

Najman, J. (2001). A general model of the social origins of health and well-being. In R. Eckersley, J. Dixon, & B. Dixon (eds), *The social origins of health and well-being*. Cambridge: Cambridge University Press, 73–83.

Nash, D., Mostashari, F., Fine, A., Miller, J., O'Leary, D., Murray, K., et al. (2001). The outbreak of the West Nile virus infection in the New York City area in 1999. *New England Journal of Medicine*, 344, 1807–14.

National Audit Office (2008). *End of life: Report by the Comptroller and Auditor-General*. London: The Stationery Office.

National Cancer Institute (2002). *Making health communication programs work*. Bethesda, MD: National Institutes of Health, US Department of Health and Human Services. <www.cancer.gov/pinkbook>.

National End of Life Intelligence Network (2010). *Variations in place of death in England: Inequalities or appropriate consequence of age, gender and cause of death?* <www.endoflifecare-intelligence.org.uk/resources/publications.aspx#neolcin>.

National Health Priority Action Council (2006). *National chronic disease strategy*. Canberra: Australian Government Department of Health and Ageing. <www.health.gov.au/internet/main/publishing.nsf/content/7E7E9140A3D3A3BCCA257140007AB32B/$File/stratal3.pdf>.

National Health Survey (2008). <www.abs.gov.au/AUSSTATS/abs@.nsf/DetailsPage/4364.02007-2008%20(Reissue)?OpenDocument>.

National Public Health Partnership (2001). *Preventing chronic disease: A strategic framework*. <www.dhs.vic.gov.au/nphp/publications/strategies/chrondis-bgpaper.pdf>.

National Public Health Partnership (2002). *The role of local government in public health regulation*. Melbourne: NPHP Publication.

Navarro, V. (2007). *Neoliberalism, globalization and inequities: Consequences for health and quality of life*. Amityville, NY: Baywood Publishers.

NCRVWC (National Council to Reduce Violence against Women and their Children) (2009). *Time for action: The national council's plan for Australia to reduce violence against women and their children, 2009-2021*. Canberra: Commonwealth of Australia.

Ndinda, C., Chimbwete, C., McGrath, N., Pool, R., & MDP GROUP (2007). Community attitudes towards individuals living with HIV in rural Kwa-Zulu Natan, South Africa. *AIDS Care*, 19(1), 92–101.

Nelkin, D., & Lindee, M.S. (1995). *The DNA mystique: The gene as a cultural icon*. New York: W.H. Freeman & Company.

Nettleton, C., Napolitano, D.A., & Stephens, C. (2007). An overview of current knowledge of the social determinants of Indigenous health. Symposium on the Social Determinants of Indigenous Health, Adelaide, April 2007. Geneva: WHO. <http://som.flinders.edu.au/FUSA/SACHRU/Symposium/Social%20Determinants%20of%20Indigenous%20Health.pdf>.

Neville, L., Thomas, M., & Bauman, A. (2005). Food advertising on Australian television: The extent of children's exposure. *Health Promotion International*, 20(2), 105–12.

Newman, A., Arnold, A., Naydeck, B., Fried, L.P., Burke, G.L., Enright, P. et al. (2003). 'Successful aging': Effect of subclinical cardiovascular disease. *Archives of Internal Medicine*, 163(19), 2315–22.

Newman, J.E., Sorenson, J.R., DeVellis, B.M., & Cheuvront, B. (2002). Gender differences in psychosocial reactions to cystic fibrosis carrier testing. *American Journal of Medical Genetics*, 113(2), 151–7.

Newman, J.H., & Baron, R.A. (1998). Workplace violence and workplace aggression: Evidence concerning specific forms, potential causes, and preferred targets. *Journal of Management*, 24(3), 391–419.

Newton-John, H., & Eisen, D. (2010). *Tetanus*. In A. Yung, D. Spelman, A. Street, J. McCormack, T. Sorrell, & P. Johnson (eds), *Infectious diseases: A clinical approach*, 3rd edn. Melbourne: IP Communications, 366–73.

NHHRC (National Health and Hospital Reform Commission) (2009a). *Final report*. <www.health.gov.au/internet/nhhrc/publishing.nsf/Content/nhhrc-report>.

NHHRC (2009b). *A healthier future for all Australians: Interim report December 2008*. Canberra: Commonwealth of Australia.

NHHRC (2009c). *A healthier future for all Australians: Final report May 2009*. Canberra: Commonwealth of Australia.

NHMRC (National Health and Medical Research Council) (2005). *Cultural competency in health: A guide for policy, partnerships and participation*. Canberra: NHMRC.

Nicholson, K.G. (2009). Influenza and vaccine development: A continuing battle. *Expert Review of Vaccines*, 8(4), 373–4.

Nicholson, R., & Stephenson, P. (2004). Environmental determinants of health. In H. Keleher & B. Murphy (eds), *Understanding health: A determinants approach*. Melbourne: Oxford University Press, 23–9.

Nicholson, R., & Stephenson, P. (2009). Natural environments as a determinant of health. In H. Keleher & C. MacDougall (eds), *Understanding health: A determinants approach*, 2nd edn. Melbourne: Oxford University Press, 112–33.

Nunn, A., Da Fonesca, E., & Gruskin, S. (2009). Changing global essential medicines norms to improve access to AIDS treatment: Lessons from Brazil. *Global Public Health*, 4, 131–49.

Nussbaum, M. (2001). Symposium on Amartya Sen's philosophy: 5 adaptive preferences and women's options. *Economics and Philosophy*, 17, 67–88.

Nussbaum, M. (2005). *Women and human development: The capabilities approach*. Cambridge: Cambridge University Press.

O'Brien, S.J., Elson, R., Gillespie, I.A., Adak, G.K., & Cowden, J.M. (2002). Surveillance of foodborne outbreaks of infectious intestinal disease in England and Wales 1992–1999: Contributing to evidence-based food policy? *Public Health*, 116, 75–80.

O'Connor-Fleming, M.L., & Parker, E. (2001). *Health promotion: Principles and practice in the Australian context*, 2nd edn. Sydney: Allen & Unwin.

Office of Women's Policy (2009). *A right to respect: Victoria's plan to prevent violence against women 2010–2020*. Melbourne: Department of Planning and Community Development, Victorian Government.

O'Flaherty, M., & Ulrich, G. (2010). The professionalization of human rights field work. *Journal of Human Rights Practice*, 2(1), 1–27.

OHCHR/WHO (Office of the United Nations High Commissioner for Human Rights and World Health Organization) (2008). The Right to Health, Fact sheet No. 31. <www.who.int/hhr/activities/factsheets/en/index.html>.

Oldenburg, R. (1999). *The great good place: Cafes, coffee shops, bookstores, bars, hair salons, and other hangouts at the heart of a community*. Cambridge, MA: Da Capo Press.

Oldmeadow, L.B., Edwards, E.R., Kimmel, L.A., Kipen, E., Robertson, V.J., & Bailey, M.J. (2006). No rest for the wounded: Early ambulation after hip surgery accelerates recovery. *ANZ Journal of Surgery*, 76(7), 607–11.

Olsen, J.A. (2009). *Principles in health economics and policy*. New York: Oxford University Press.

Omran, A. (1971). *The epidemiologic transition: A theory of the epidemiology of population change*. <www.milbank.org/quarterly/830418omran.pdf>.

O'Shaughnessy, M., & Stadler, J.M. (2008). *Media and society*, 4th edn. Melbourne: Oxford University Press.

Pagram, R. (1999). Shifts in emergency management service provision: A case for new innovative leadership. *Australian Journal of Emergency Management*, Autumn, 28–30.

Palmer, G.R., & Short, S.D. (2000). *Health care & public policy*, 3rd edn. Melbourne: Macmillan Publishers.

Palmore, E. (1977). Facts on aging: A short quiz. *The Gerontologist*, 17, 315–20.

Parfrey, P., & Barrett, B. (2009). *Clinical epidemiology: Practice and methods*. Totowa, NJ: Humana; London: Springer.

Parker, R., & Aggleton, P. (2003). HIV and AIDS-related stigma and discrimination: A conceptual framework and implications for action. *Social Science and Medicine*, 57(1), 13–24.

Parker, R.G. (1996). *Empowerment, community mobilization, and social change in the face of HIV/ AIDS*. AIDS 10(Supplement 3), S27–S31.

Parkes, T. (2000). Good practice in emergency management. *Australian Journal of Emergency Management*, Autumn, 1.

Parry, M.L., Canziani, O.F., Palutikof, J.P., van der Linden, P.J., & Hanson, C.E. (eds) (2007). *Climate Change 2007: Impacts, adaptation and vulnerability: Contribution of Working Group II to the Fourth Assessment Report of the Intergovernmental Panel on Climate Change*. Cambridge: Cambridge University Press.

Parry, Y.K. (2009). *The social determinants of health*. Poster for the Australian Health Promotion Association National Conference. Adelaide Hindmarsh Education Centre, 31 August 2009.

Parry, Y.K. (2011). The impact of social determinants of health on paediatric emergency department use: A mixed methods analysis. Unpublished PhD thesis, Social Health Sciences, Flinders University, Adelaide.

Parsons, T. (1951). *The social role*. Glencoe, IL: Free Press.

Paynter, N., Chasman, D., Paré, G., Buring, J., Cook, N., Miletich, J., & Ridker, P. (2010). Association between a literature-based genetic risk score and cardiovascular events in women. *Journal of the American Medical Association*, 303(7), 631–7.

People's Health Movement (2011). *People's charter for health*. <www.phmovement.org/files/ phm-pch-english.pdf>.

Perry, L., Steinbeck, K.S., Dunbabin, J.S., & Lowe, J.M. (2010). Lost in transition? Access to and uptake of adult health services and outcomes for young people with type 1 diabetes in regional New South Wales. *Medical Journal of Australia*, 193(8), 444–9.

Pescosolido, B.A., Martin, J.K., Lang, A., & Olafsdottir, S. (2008). Rethinking theoretical approaches to stigma: A framework integrating normative influences on stigma (FINIS). *Social Science and Medicine*, 67(3), 431–40.

Petersen, A., & Bunton, R. (2002). *The new genetics and the public's health*. London: Routledge Press.

Peterson, C.L. (1999). *Stress at work: A sociological perspective*. Amityville, NY: Baywood Publishers.

Peterson, C.L., & Murphy, G. (2010). Transition from the labor market: Older workers and retirement. *International Journal of Health Services*, 40(4), 609–27.

Pfefferbaum, B., Doughty, D.E., Reddy, C., Patel, N., Gurwitch, R.H., Nixon, S.J., & Tivis, R.D. (2002). Exposure and peritraumatic response as predictors of posttraumatic stress in children following the 1995 Oklahoma City Bombing. *Journal of Urban Health*, 79(3), 354–63.

Phelps, C.E. (2010). *Health economics*, 4th edn. New York: Addison Wesley.

PHIDU (Primary Health Care Research & Information Service) (2006). *Use of services by statistical local area, SA (including health region)*. <www.publichealth.gov.au>.

PHIDU (2010). *Monitoring inequality in Australia, private health insurance rates in Adelaide by quintile*. <www.publichealth.gov.au/interactive_graphics/australia_2010/sa/private_ health.html>.

Phillips, R., & Kingsley, J. (2007). Healthy country, healthy people: An Indigenous Victorian EcoHealth Conference, December, Deakin University, Melbourne.

Phillipson, C., & Dannefer, D. (2010). *The Sage handbook of social gerontology*. Los Angeles: Sage Publications.

Picard, M. (2005). *Principles into practice: Learning from innovative rights-based programmes*. London: CARE International UK.

Pickett, K., & Wilkinson, R. (eds) (2009). *Health and human inequality: Major themes in health and social welfare*, vols 1–4. London: Routledge.

Pinhas-Hamiel, O., & Zeitler P. (2005). The global spread of Type 2 Diabetes Mellitus in children and adolescents. *Journal of Pediatrics*, 146, 693–700.

Piotrow, P.T., & De Fossard, E. (2004). Entertainment-education as a public health intervention. In A. Singhal, M.J. Cody, E.M. Rogers, & M. Sabido (eds), *Entertainment-education and social change: History, research, and practice*. Mahwah, NJ: Lawrence Erlbaum Associates, 39–60.

Pirkis, J.E., Burgess, P.M., Francis, C., Blood, R.W., & Jolley, D.J. (2006). The relationship between media reporting of suicide and actual suicide in Australia. *Social Science & Medicine*, 62, 2874–86.

Pollack, A. (2010). The genome at 10; awaiting the genome payoff. *New York Times*, 15 June, A15.

Pollard, C.M., Daly, A.M., & Binns, C.W. (2009b). Consumer perceptions of fruit and vegetables serving sizes. *Public Health Nutrition*, 12(5), 637–43.

Pollard, C.M., Lewis, J.M., & Binns, C.W. (2008b). Selecting interventions to promote fruit and vegetable consumption: From policy to action, a planning framework case study in Western Australia. *Australia and New Zealand Health Policy*, 5(27), 7 pages. <www.anzhealthpolicy.com/content/5/1/27>.

Pollard, C.M., Miller, M., Daly, A.M., Crouchley, K.E., O'Donoghue, K.J., Lang, A.J., & Binns, C.W. (2008a). Increasing fruit and vegetable consumption: Success of the Western Australian Go for 2&5® campaign. *Public Health Nutrition*, 11(3), 314–20.

Pollard, C.M., Miller, M., Woodman, R.J., Meng, R., & Binns, C.W. (2009a). Changes in knowledge, beliefs, and behaviors related to fruit and vegetable consumption among Western Australian adults from 1995 to 2004. *American Journal of Public Health*, 99(2), 355–61.

Ponce, N.A., Afable-Munsuz, A., & Nordyke, R.J. (2007). Conceptualising the impact of genetic testing on cancer disparities in the USA. *International Journal of Healthcare Technology Management*, 8, 536–48.

Poticha, S. (2008). The integration of transportation, land use, and technology. In D. Farr (ed.), *Sustainable urbanism: Urban design with nature*. New Jersey: John Wiley & Sons, 114–19.

Pour-Jafari, H., & Pourjafari, B. (2009). Lost in translation: Limitations of a universal approach in genetic counseling. *Journal of Genetic Counseling*, 19(1), 5–6.

Power, C., Manor, O., & Matthews, S. (1999). The duration and timing of exposure: Effects of socio-economic environment on adult health. *American Journal of Public Health*, 89(7), 1059–66.

Productivity Commission (2011). *Caring for older Australians*. Draft Inquiry Report, Canberra.

Puhl, R., & Brownell, K.D. (2003). Ways of coping with obesity stigma: Review and conceptual analysis. *Eating Behaviors*, 4, 53–78.

Queensland Government, Department of Emergency Services (2005). *Queensland disaster management planning guidelines: For local government*. Kedron, Qld: Department of Emergency Services.

Queensland Health (2001). *Social determinants of health: The role of the Public Health Services Act*. Brisbane: Queensland Government.

Queensland Health (2010). *Hydatid disease*. <http://access.health.qld.gov.au/hid/InfectionsandParasites/Parasites/hydatidDisease_fs.asp>.

Ragland, D.R., & Brand, R.J. (1988). Type A behavior and mortality from coronary heart disease. *New England Journal of Medicine*, 318, 65–9.

Rambaut, A., Pybus, O.G., Nelson, M.I., Viboud, C., Taubenberger, K., & Holmes, E.C. (2008). The genomic and epidemiological dynamics of human influenza A virus. *Nature*, 453(7195), 615–19.

Raphael, D. (2000). The question of evidence in health promotion. *Health Promotion International*, 15(4), 355–67.

Rasanathan, K., Norenhag, J., & Valentine, N. (2010). Realizing human rights-based approaches for action on the social determinants of health. *Health and Human Rights*, 12(2), 49–59.

Rawls, J. (1971). *A theory of justice*. Oxford: Oxford University Press.

Reed, D., Foley, D., White, L., Heimovitz, H., Burchfiel, C.M., & Masaki, K. (1998). Predictors of healthy aging in men with high life experiences. *American Journal of Public Health*, 88, 1463–8.

Rees, S. (2004). Human rights and the significance of psychosocial and cultural issues in domestic violence policy and intervention for refugee women. *Australian Journal of Human Rights*, 10(2). <www.austlii.edu.au/au/journals/AJHR/2004/19.html>.

Rees, W., & Wackernagel, M. (1994). Ecological footprints and appropriated carrying capacity: Measuring the natural capital requirements of the human economy. In A-M. Jansson, M. Hammer, C. Folke, & R. Costanza (eds), *Investing in natural capital: The ecological economics approach to sustainability*. Washington: Island Press, 362–90.

Reidpath, D.D. (2004). Social determinants of health. In H. Keleher & B. Murphy (eds), *Understanding health: A determinants approach*. Melbourne: Oxford University Press, 9–22.

Reidpath, D.D., & Chan, K.Y.A. (2005). A method for the quantitative analysis of the layering of HIV-related stigma. *AIDS Care*, 17(4), 425–32.

Reingold, A. (1998). Outbreak investigation: A perspective. *Emerging Infectious Diseases*, 4(1), 21–7.

Reynaert, C.C., & Gelman, S.A. (2007). The influence of language forms and conventional wording on judgments of illness. *Journal of Psycholinguistic Research*, 36(4), 273–95.

Rice, T. (2003). *The economics of health reconsidered*, 2nd edn. Washington, DC: Academy Press.

Richards, M. (1995). Families, kinship and genes. In T. Marteau & M. Richards (eds), *The troubled helix: Social and psychological implications of the new human genetics*. Cambridge: Cambridge University Press, 249–73.

Richards, M., & Ponder, M. (1996). Lay understanding of genetics: A test of a hypothesis. *Journal of Medical Genetics*, 33(12), 1032–6.

Riso, L.P., Mivatake, R.K., & Thase, M.E. (2002). The search for determinants of chronic depression: A review of six factors. *Journal of Affective Disorders*, 70(2), 103–15.

Ritter, L.A., & Hoffman, N.A. (2010). *Multicultural health*. Sudbury, MA: Jones & Bartlett.

Roach Anleu, S.L. (2006). *Deviance, conformity and control*, 4th edn. Sydney: Pearson Education Australia.

Roach Anleu, S.L. (2009). The medicalisation of deviance. In J. Germov (ed.), *Second opinion: An introduction to health sociology*, 4th edn. Melbourne: Oxford University Press, 242–68.

Roberts, C.A. (2005). The study of paleopathology. In C. Roberts & K. Manchester (eds), *Archaeology of disease*. Stroud, NSW: Sutton Publishing, 1–21.

Robertson, S. (2007). *Understanding men and health: Masculinities, identity and well-being*. Berkshire: Open University Press/McGraw Hill.

Robinson, T.N. (2001). Television viewing and childhood obesity. *Pediatric Clinics of North America*, 48, 1017–25.

Roos, N., & Havens, B. (1991). Predictors of successful aging: A twelve-year study of Manitoba elderly. *American Journal of Public Health*, 81, 63–8.

Rosen, G. (1993). *History of public health*. Baltimore, MD: Johns Hopkins University Press.

Rosen, G. (1998). *A history of public health*, 2nd edn. Baltimore, MD: Johns Hopkins University Press.

Rosner, D., & Markowitz, G.E. (1987). *Dying for work: Workers' safety and health in twentieth century America*. Bloomington, IN: Indiana University Press.

Rouche, B. (1984). Annals of medicine: A contemporary touch. *The New Yorker*, 13 August, 76–85.

Rowe, J., & Kahn, R.L. (1997). Successful ageing. *The Gerontologist*, 37(4), 433–40.

Rowe, R., & Thomas, A. (2008). *Climate change adaptation: A framework for local action*. Policy Signpost #3. Melbourne: McCaughey Centre: VicHealth Centre for the Promotion of Mental Health and Community Wellbeing, University of Melbourne.

Roy, R., Symonds, R.P., Kumar, D.M., Ibrahim, K., Mitchell, A., & Fallowfield, L. (2005). The use of denial in an ethnically diverse British cancer population: A cross-sectional study. *British Journal of Cancer*, 92, 1393–7.

Rudlin, D., & Falk, N. (2009). *Sustainable urban neighbourhood: Building the 21st century home*. Oxford: Architectural Press.

Rutter, N. (1996). Transitions and turning points in developmental psychopathology: As applied to the age span between childhood and mid adulthood. *International Journal of Behavioral Development*, 6(3), 603–26.

Saggers, S., Walter, M., & Gray, D. (2011). Culture, history and health. In R. Thackrah & K. Scott (eds), *Indigenous Australian health and cultures: An introduction for health professionals*. Sydney: Pearson, 1–21.

Salmon, J., Campbell, K., & Crawford, D. (2006). Television viewing habits associated with obesity risk factors: A survey of Melbourne school children. *Medical Journal of Australia*, 184(2), 64–7.

Salter, J. (1998). Risk management in the emergency management context. *Australian Journal of Emergency Management*, 12(4), 22–7.

Samson, C. (1999). Biomedicine and the body. In C. Samson (ed.), *Health studies: A critical and cross-cultural reader*. Oxford: Blackwell, 3–21.

Sandiford, P., Cassel, J., Montenegro, M., & Sanchez, G. (1995). The impact of women's literacy on child health and its interaction with access to health services. *Population Studies*, 49, 5–17.

Santrock, J.W. (2004). *Child development*, 10th edn. Boston: McGraw Hill.

Sarafino, E.P. (2006). *Health psychology: Biopsychosocial interactions*. New York: Wiley Publishers.

Satariano, W.A. (2006). *Epidemiology of aging: An ecological approach*. Sudbury, MA: Jones & Bartlett.

Sayce, L. (2000). *From psychiatric patient to citizen: Overcoming discrimination and social exclusion*. New York: St Martin's Press Inc.

Saylor, C.F., Cowart, B.L., Lipovsky, J.A., Jackson, C., & Finch, A.J. (2003). Media exposure to September 11: Elementary school students' experiences and posttraumatic symptoms. *The American Behavioral Scientist*, 46(12), 1622–42.

Scambler, G. (2003). Deviance, sick role and stigma. In G. Scambler (ed.), *Sociology as applied to medicine*. Edinburgh: Saunders, 192–202.

Scambler, G. (2009). Health-related stigma. *Sociology of health and illness*, 31(3), 441–55.

Scheff, T. (1966). *Being mentally ill: A sociological theory*. Chicago: Aldine Publishing.

Schneiderman, N., Ironson, G., & Seigel, S.D. (2005) Stress and health: Psychological, behavioral and biological determinants. *Annual Review of Clinical Psychology*, 1, 607–28.

Schrader, T. (2004). Poverty and health in Australia. *New Doctor*, 80, 17–19.

Seeman, T.E., & Crimmins, E. (2001). Social environment effects on health and aging: Integrated epidemiologic and demographic approaches and perspectives. *Annals New York Academy of Sciences*, 954, 88–117.

Seeman, T.E., Berkman, L.F., Charpentier, P.A., & Blazer, D.G. (1995). Behavioural and psychosocial predictors of physical performance: MacArthur studies of successful aging. *Journals of Gerontology, Medical Sciences*, 50, M177–M183.

Seeman, T.E., Charpentier, P.A., Berkman, L.F., Tinetti, M.E., Guralnik, J.M., & Albert, M., et al. (1994). Predicting changes in physical performance in a high-functioning elderly cohort: MacArthur studies of successful aging. *Journals of Gerontology, Medical Sciences*, 49(3), M97–M108.

Selye, H. (1956). *The stress of life*. New York: McGraw Hill.

Sen, A. (1984). *Resources, values, and development*. Oxford: Blackwell.

Sen, A. (2009). *The idea of justice*. London: Penguin.

Settersten, R.A.J., & Mayer, K.U. (1997). The measurement of age, age structuring and the life course. *Annual Review of Sociology*, 23, 233–61.

Shaw, M., Dorling, D., & Davey Smith, G. (2006). Poverty, social exclusion, and minorities. In M. Marmot & R. Wilkinson (eds), *Social determinants of health*. Oxford: Oxford University Press, 196–223.

Sherman, P. (2007). *Stigma, mental illness, and culture*. <www.scribd.com/doc/11731670/The-Stigma-of-Mental-Illness>.

Shih, M. (2004). Positive stigma: Examining resilience and empowerment in overcoming stigma. *ANNALS of the American Academy of Political and Social Science*, 591(1), 175–85.

Shiloh, S. (1996). Decision-making in the context of genetic risk. In T. Marteau & M. Richards (eds), *The troubled helix: Social and psychological implications of the new human genetics*. Cambridge: Cambridge University Press, 82–103.

Shisana, O. (2010). *The social and environmental determinants of nutrition*. <www.doh.gov.za/docs/sp/2010/sp0315.html>.

Shoaf, K.I., & Rottman, S.J. (2000). The role of public health in disasters preparedness, mitigation, response and recovery. *Journal of Prehospital and Disaster Medicine*, 15(4), 18–20.

Simbayi, L.C., Kalichman, S., Strebel, A., Cloete, A., Henda, N., & Mqeketo, A. (2007). Internalized stigma, discrimination, and depression among men and women living with HIV/AIDS in Cape Town, South Africa. *Social Science and Medicine*, 64(9), 1823–31.

Simonsen, L., Clarke, M.J., Schonberger, L.B., Arden, L.B., Cox, N.J., & Fukuda, K. (1998). Pandemic versus epidemic influenza mortality: A pattern of changing age distribution. *Journal of Infectious Diseases*, 178, 53–60.

Simonsen, L., Reichert, T.A., Viboud, C., Blackwelder, W.C., Taylor, R.J. & Miller, M.A. (2005). Impact of influenza vaccination on seasonal mortality in the US elderly population. *Archives of Internal Medicine*, 165, 265–72.

Singer, M., & Baer, H. (2007). *Introducing medical anthropology: A discipline in action*. Lanham, MD: AltaMira Press.

Singh, J.A., Govender, M., & Mills, E.J. (2007). Do human rights matter to health? *The Lancet*, 370, 521–7.

Singhal, A., & Rogers, E.M. (2003). *Combating AIDS: Communication strategies in action*. New Delhi: Sage Publications.

Singhal, A., & Rogers, E.M. (2004). The status of entertainment-education worldwide. In A. Singhal, M.J. Cody, E.M. Rogers, & M. Sabido (eds), *Entertainment-education and social change: History, research, and practice*. Mahwah, NJ: Lawrence Erlbaum Associates, 3–20.

Slavin, M., Chen, S., & Morrissey, O. (2010). Systemic fungal infections. In A. Yung, D. Spelman, A. Street, J. McCormack, T. Sorrell, & P. Johnson (eds), *Infectious diseases: A clinical approach*, 3rd edn. Melbourne: IP Communications, 399–411.

Smedley, B.D., Sith, A.Y., & Nelson, A.R. (eds) (2002). *Unequal treatment: Confronting racial and ethnic disparities in health care*. Washington, DC: National Academies Press.

Snowdon, D. (2002). *Aging with grace: What the Nun Study teaches us about leading longer, healthier, and more meaningful lives*. New York: Bantam Books.

Social Inclusion Unit, Department of the Prime Minister and Cabinet (2009). *The Australian Public Service Social Inclusion policy design and delivery toolkit*. Canberra: Commonwealth of Australia.

Solar, O., & Irwin, A. (2007). *A conceptual framework for action on the social determinants of health*. Draft discussion paper for the Commission on Social Determinants of Health. Geneva: WHO.

Solomon, S., Qin, D., Manning, M., Chen, Z., Marquis, M., Averyt, K.B., Tignor, M., & Miller, H.L. (eds) (2007). *Contribution of Working Group I to the Fourth Assessment Report of the Intergovernmental Panel on Climate Change*. Cambridge: Cambridge University Press.

Sontag, S. (1991). *Illness as metaphor: AIDS and its metaphors*. London: Penguin Books.

Sparks, M. (2010). A health promotion approach to addressing health equity. *Global Health Promotion*, 17(1), 77–82.

Spector, R.E. (2009). *Cultural diversity in health and illness*, 7th edn. Upper Saddle River, NJ: Pearson Prentice Hall.

Sringernyuang, L., Thaweesit, S., & Nakapiew, S. (2005). A situational analysis of HIV/AIDS-related discrimination in Bangkok, Thailand. *AIDS Care*, 17(Supplement 2), S165–S174.

Stacey, M. (1995). The new genetics: A feminist view. In T. Marteau & M. Richards (eds), *The troubled helix: Social and psychological implications of the new human genetics*. Cambridge: Cambridge University Press, 331–49.

Stack, S. (2003). Media coverage as a risk factor in suicide. *Journal of Epidemiology and Community Health*, 57, 238–40.

Stafford, J., Mitchell, H., Stoneham, M., & Daube, M. (2009). *Advocacy in action: A toolkit for public health professionals*, 2nd edn. Perth: Public Health Advocacy Institute of Western Australia. <www.phaiwa.org.au/index.php/component/attachments/download/35>.

State of Victoria (2009). *January 2009: Heatwave in Victoria. An assessment of health impacts*. Melbourne: Victorian Department of Human Services.

Steuteville, R., & Langdon, P. (2003). *New urbanism: Comprehensive report and best practices guide*. New York: New Urban Publications.

Stewart, M., Brown, J.B., Boon, H., Galajda, J., Meredith, L., & Sangster, M. (1999). Evidence on patient–doctor communication. *Cancer Prevention and Control*, 3(1), 25–30.

Stoneham, M. (2003). Developing an environmental health research framework. *Environmental Health*, 3(3), 37–42.

Stoppard, M. (2010). We must start to prepare for our ageing population. *Daily Mirror*, London, 23 November, 34.

Story, M. (2003). Television and food advertising: An international threat to children? *Nutrition & Dietetics*, 60(2), 72–3.

Strasburger, V.C., Wilson, B.J., & Jordan, A.B. (2009). *Children, adolescents, and the media*. 2nd edn. Los Angeles, CA: Sage Publications.

Strategic Review of Health Inequalities in England post-2010 (2010). *Fair society, healthy lives: The Marmot Review*. <www.marmotreview.org>.

Strawbridge, W., Cohen, R., Shema, S., & Kaplan, G. (1996). Successful aging: Predictors and associated activities. *American Journal of Epidemiology*, 144, 135–41.

Stuber, J., Galea, S., & Link, B.G. (2008). Smoking and the emergence of a stigmatized social status. *Social Science and Medicine*, 67, 420–30.

Sudak, H.S., & Sudak, D.M. (2005). The media and suicide. *Academic Psychiatry*, 29(5), 495–9.

Sullivan, M. (2003). The new subjective medicine: Taking the patient's point of view on health care and health. *Social Science and Medicine*, 56, 1595–604.

Susser, M., & Stein, Z. (2009). *Eras in epidemiology: The evolution of ideas*. New York: Oxford University Press.

Suwankhong, D. (2011). Traditional healers (*mor pheun baan*) in southern Thailand: A contribution towards Thai health. Unpublished PhD thesis, School of Public Health, La Trobe University, Melbourne.

Swan Hill Rural City Council (2006). Food for all. <www.swanhill.vic.gov.au>.

Swinburn, B., & Cameron-Smith, D. (2009). Biological determinants of health. In H. Keleher & C. MacDougall (eds), *Understanding health: A determinants approach*, 2nd edn. Melbourne: Oxford University Press, 248–69.

Syme, S.L. (2004). Social determinants of health: The community as an empowered partner. *Preventing Chronic Disease*, 1(1), 1–5.

Symonds, P.V. (2004). *Gender and the cycle of life: Calling in the soul in a Hmong village*. Seattle: University of Washington Press.

Taket, A. (2012). *Health equity, social justice and human rights*. London: Routledge.

Talbot, L., & Verrinder, G. (2009). *Promoting health: The primary health care approach*. Sydney: Elsevier Australia.

Tamlyn, J.A. (2003). Costs of chronic illness in rural and regional Victoria. *Health Issues Journal*, 74, 23–5.

Tannahill, A. (2008a). Health promotion: The Tannahill model revisited. *Public Health*, 122, 1387–91.

Tannahill, A. (2008b). Beyond evidence—to ethics: A decision-making framework for health promotion, public health and health improvement. *Health Promotion International*, 23(4), 380–90.

Taylor, B. (2001). HIV, stigma and health: Integration of theoretical concepts and the lived experiences of individuals. *Journal of Advanced Nursing*, 35(5), 792–8.

Taylor, D., & Bury, M. (2007). Chronic illness, expert patients and care transition. *Sociology of Health and Illness*, 29(1), 27–45.

Taylor, D.N., Wachsmuth, I.K., Shangkuan, Y., Schmidt, E.V., Barrett, T.J., Schrader, J.S., et al. (1982). Salmonellosis associated with marijuana: A multistate outbreak traced by plasmid fingerprinting. *New England Journal of Medicine*, 306(21), 1249–53.

Taylor, S.D. (2004). Predictive genetic test decisions for Huntington's disease: Context, appraisal and new moral imperatives. *Social Science and Medicine*, 58(1), 137–49.

Taylor, S.D. (2008a). The concept of health. In S. Taylor, M. Foster, & J. Fleming (eds), *Health care practice in Australia*. Melbourne: Oxford University Press, 3–21.

Taylor, S.D. (2008b). Gender and genetic risk: Exploring conceptualisation and interface within health care. Full refereed paper, Complete Conference Proceedings of the Australian Sociological Association (TASA), Melbourne.

Taylor, S.D. (2012). A population-based survey in Australia of men's and women's perceptions of genetic risk and predictive genetic testing and implications for primary care. *Public Health Genomics*. <www.ornl.gov/sci/techresources/Human_Genome/home.shtml>.

Taylor, S.D., Foster, M., & Fleming, J. (eds) (2008a). *Health care practice in Australia: Policy, context and innovation*. Melbourne: Oxford University Press.

Taylor, S.D., Treloar, S., Barlow-Stewart, K., Stranger, M., & Otlowski, M. (2008b). Investigating genetic discrimination in Australia: A large-scale survey of clinical genetics clients. *Clinical Genetics*, 74(1), 20–30.

Temple-Smith, M., Stoove, M., Smith, A., O'Brien, M., Mitchell, D., Banwell, C., Bammer, G., Jolley, D., & Gifford, S. (2007). Gender differences in seeking care for hepatitis C in Australia. *Journal of Substance Use*, 12(1), 59–70.

Thackrah, R., & Scott, K. (eds) (2011). *Indigenous Australian health and cultures: An introduction for health professionals*. Sydney: Pearson.

Thomas, F. (2006). Stigma, fatigue and social breakdown: Exploring the impacts of HIV/AIDS on patient and carer well-being in the Caprivi Region, Namibia. *Social Science and Medicine*, 63(12), 3174–87.

Thompson, S., Corkery, L., & Judd, B. (2007). The role of community gardens in sustaining healthy communities. Unpublished paper, Faculty of the Built Environment, University of New South Wales, Sydney.

Tilley, J.J. (2000). Cultural relativism. *Human Rights Quarterly*, 22(2), 501–47.

Tong, S., Dale, P., Nicholls, N., Mackenzie, J.S., Wolff, R., & McMichael, A.J. (2008). Climate variability, social and environmental factors, and Ross River virus transmission: Research development and future research needs. *Environmental Health Perspectives*, 116, 1591–7.

Townsend, M., & Mahoney, M. (2004). Ecology, people, place and health. In H. Keleher & B. Murphy (eds), *Understanding health: A determinants approach*. Melbourne: Oxford University Press, 269–75.

Treasury (Australia) (2007). *Intergenerational report*. Canberra: Commonwealth of Australia.

Trewin, D. (2001). *Measuring wellbeing: Frameworks for Australian social statistics*. Canberra: ABS.

Trowbridge, M.J., Gurka, M.J., & O'Connor, R.E. (2009). Urban sprawl and delayed ambulance arrival in the U.S. *American Journal of Preventive Medicine*, 37(5), 428–32.

UNAIDS (Joint United Nations Programme on HIV/AIDS) (2005). *Getting the message across: The mass media and the response to HIV/AIDS*. UNAIDS Best Practice Collection (UNAIDS Catalogue No. UNAIDS/05.29E). Geneva: UNAIDS. <http://data.unaids.org/Publications/IRC-pub06/jc1094-mediasa-bp_en.pdf>.

UNFPA and Harvard School of Public Health (2010). A human rights-based approach to programming: Practical information and training materials. <www.unfpa.org/public/publications/pid/4919>.

Unger, J.B., McAvay, G.J., Bruce, M.L., Berkman, L.F., & Seeman, T.E. (1999). Variation in the impact of social network characteristics on physical functioning in elderly persons: MacArthur studies of successful aging. *Journals of Gerontology, Social Sciences*, 54B(5), S245–S251.

United Nations (1945). Charter of the United Nations and Statute of the International Court of Justice. Geneva: United Nations. <www.un.org/en/documents/charter>.

United Nations (1948). Universal Declaration of Human Rights. Geneva: United Nations <www.un.org/en/documents/udhr>.

United Nations (2009). World Population Prospects: The 2008 Revision. New York: UN, Department of Economic and Social Affairs, Population Division (advanced Excel tables). <http://data.un.org/Data.aspx?d=PopDiv&f=variableID%3A14>.

Unwin, N., Whiting, D., & Roglic, G. (2010). Social determinants of diabetes and challenges of prevention. *The Lancet*, 375(9733), 2204–5.

US Department of Energy (2008). *Genetic disease information*. <www.ornl.gov/sci/techresources/Human_Genome/medicine/assist.shtml>.

US Department of Energy (2009). Potential benefits of Human Genome Project research. <www.ornl.gov/sci/techresources/Human_Genome/project/benefits.shtml>.

US Department of Energy (2010). *Human Genome Project Information*. <www.ornl.gov/sci/techresources/Human_Genome/home.shtml>.

US Department of Health and Human Services National Institute of Health (2011). *ARRA investments in environmental determinants of cardiovascular disease*. <http://report.nih.gov/recovery/investmentreports/ViewARRAInvRpt.aspx?csid=139>.

Usdin, S., Singhal, A., Shongwe, T., Goldstein, S., & Shabalala, A. (2004). No short cuts in entertainment-education: Designing Soul City step-by-step. In A. Singhal, M.J. Cody, E.M. Rogers, & M. Sabido (eds), *Entertainment-education and social change: History, research, and practice*. Mahwah, NJ: Lawrence Erlbaum Associates, 153–75.

Vaillant, G.E., & Mukamal, K. (2001). Successful aging. *American Journal of Psychiatry*, 158(6), 839–47.

VanLandingham, M., Im-em, W., & Saengtienchai, C. (2005). Community reaction to persons with HIV/AIDS and their parents: An analysis of recent evidence from Thailand. *Journal of Health and Social Behavior*, 46, 392–410.

Vaughan, C. (2009). Vulnerability and globalisation. In H. Keleher & C. MacDougall (eds), *Understanding health: A determinants approach*, 2nd edn. Melbourne: Oxford University Press, 170–84.

Vaughan, J., & Harvy, B. (2009). Health care firms scraps bulk billing. *Adelaide now*. <www.news.com.au/adelaidenow>.

Venkatapuram, S., Bell, R., & Marmot, M. (2010). The right to sutures: Social epidemiology, human rights, and social justice. *Health and Human Rights*, 12(2), 3–16.

Verrinder, A. (2000). *Human ecology and health*. Bendigo, Vic.: La Trobe University.

Verrinder, G.K. (2011). Health and quality of life. In T. Fitzpatrick (eds), *Understanding environmental and social policy*. London: Policy Press.

VicHealth (1999). *Mental health promotion plan. Foundation document: 1990–2002*. Melbourne: VicHealth.

VicHealth (2004). *The health costs of violence: Measuring the burden of disease caused by intimate partner violence. A summary of findings*. Melbourne: Department of Human Services.

VicHealth (2010a). *Food security*. <www.vichealth.vic.gov.au/Programs-and-Projects/Healthy-Eating/Food-Security.aspx>.

VicHealth (2010b). Ten ways local government can act on food security. *VicHealth Online*. <www.vichealth.vic.gov.au>.

VicHealth (2010c). Growing food locally: Supporting residents to grow and harvest food. Information sheet series. *VicHealth Online*. <www.vichealth.vic.gov.au>.

Vickery, K. (2010). Widening the psychiatric gaze: Reflections on PsychoDoctor, depression and recent transitions in Japanese mental health care. *Transcultural Psychiatry*, 47(3), 363–91.

Victorian Department of Health (2010). *Using policy to promote mental health and wellbeing: An introduction for policy makers*. <www.health.vic.gov.au>.

Victorian Department of Human Services (1999). *The Victorian burden of disease study: Mortality*. Melbourne: DHS.

Victorian Department of Human Services (2009). *Heatwave planning guide: Development of heatwave plans in local councils in Victoria*. Melbourne: Environmental Health Unit Publication.

Victorian Government Department of Human Services (2003). *Integrated health promotion resource kit*. Melbourne: Rural and Regional Health and Aged Care Services Division, Victorian Government Department of Human Services.

Victorian Healthcare Association (2010). *Population health approaches to planning*. Position statement. Melbourne: VHA.

Vlahov, D., & Galea, S. (2004). Urbanization, urbanicity and health. *Journal of Urban Health: Bulletin of the New York Academy of Sciences*, 79(4), S1–S12.

Vlahov, D., Freudenberg, N., Proietti, F., Ompad, D., Quinn, A., Nandi, V., & Galea, S. (2007). Urban as a determinant of health. *Journal of Urban Health*, 84(Supplement 1), 16–26.

Vlassoff, C. (2007). Gender differences in determinants and consequences of health and illness. *Journal of Health Population and Nutrition*, 25(1), 47–61.

Vlassoff, C., & Ali, F. (2011). HIV-related stigma among South Asians in Toronto. *Ethnicity & Health*, 16(1), 25–42.

Von Mutius, E. (2007). Allergies, infection and the Hygiene Hypothesis: The epidemiological avenue. *Immunobiology*, 212(6), 433–9.

Vos, T. (2010). *Pamphlet A: The ACE-Prevention Project, ACE-prevention pamphlets*. Queensland: Centre for Burden of Disease and Cost-Effectiveness, University of Queensland.

Vos, T., Astbury, J., Piers, L.S., Magnus, A., Heenan, M., Stanley, L., Walker, L., & Webster, K. (2006). Measuring the impact of intimate partner violence on the health of women in Victoria, Australia. *Bulletin of the World Health Organization*, 84(9), 739–44.

Vos, T., Carter, R., Barendregt, J., Mihalopoulos, C., Veerman, L., Magnus, A., et al. (2010). *Assessing cost-effectiveness in prevention (ACE-Prevention)*. Melbourne: Centre for Burden of Disease and Cost-effectiveness, University of Queensland and Deakin Health Economics, Deakin University.

Vujovic, O., Hoy, J., & Mijch, A. (2010). HIV infection and AIDS. In A. Yung, D. Spelman, A. Street, J. McCormack, T. Sorrell, & P. Johnson (eds), *Infectious diseases: A clinical approach*, 3rd edn. Melbourne: IP Communications, 319–41.

Wade, N. (2010). A decade later, Genetic map yields few new cures. *New York Times*, 12 June, A16.

Wadsworth, M., & Butterworth, S. (2006). Early life. In M. Marmot & R. Wilkinson (eds), *Social determinants of health*. Oxford: Oxford University Press, 31–53.

Wahlqvist, M.L. (2002). Chronic disease prevention: A life cycle approach which takes account of the environmental impact and opportunities of food, nutrition and public health policies—the rationale for an eco-nutritional disease nomenclature. *Asia Pacific Journal of Clinical Nutrition*, 11(suppl), S759–S762.

Wake, M., Hesketh, K., & Waters, E. (2003). Television, computer use and body mass index in Australian primary school children. *Journal of Paediatrics and Child Health*, 39, 130–4.

Wakefield, A.J., Murch, S.H., Anthony, A., Linnell, J., Casson, D.M., Malik, M., Berelowitz, M., Dhillon, A.P., et al. (1998). Ileal-lymphoid-nodular hyperplasia, non-specific colitis, and pervasive developmental disorder in children. *The Lancet*, 351(9103), 637–41.

Waldron, I. (2005). Gender differences in mortality: Causes and variations in different societies. In P. Conrad (ed.), *The sociology of health and illness: Critical perspectives*, 7th edn. New York: Worth Publishers, 38–55.

Walker, A. (2002). A strategy for active ageing. *International Social Security Review*, 55, 121–39.

Walker, C., Peterson, C.L., Millen, N., & Martin, C. (eds) (2003). In *Chronic illness: New perspectives and new direction*. Croydon: Tertiary Press, 1–13.

Walker, R., Hassall, J., Chaplin, S., Congues, J., & Bajayo, R. (2011). A systematic review: The implications of climate change for health and community services. South East Healthy

Communities Partnership, School of Public Health, La Trobe University and South East Health Communities Partnership.

Wang, Z., Hoy, W.E., & Si, D. (2010). Incidence of Type 2 diabetes in Aboriginal Australians: An 11 year prospective cohort study. *BMC Public Health*, 10, 487–91.

Wardle, J., Carnell, S., Haworth, C., & Plomin, R. (2008). Evidence for a strong genetic influence on childhood adiposity despite the force of the obesogenic environment. *The American Journal of Clinical Nutrition*, 87(2), 398–404.

Washington, H., & Cook, J. (2011). *Climate change deniers: Heads in the sand.* UK: Earthscan.

Watters, E. (2010). *Crazy like us: The globalization of the American psyche.* New York: Free Press.

Webb, P., & Bain, C. (2011). *Essential epidemiology: An introduction for students and health professionals.* Cambridge: Cambridge University Press.

Webb, S.D. (1984). Rural-urban differences in mental health. In H. Freeman (ed.), *Mental health and the environment.* London: Churchill Livingston, 226–49.

Webber, R. (2009). *Communicable disease epidemiology and control: A global perspective.* Wallingford, UK and Cambridge, MA: Cabi.

Weil, J. (2000). *Psychosocial genetic counselling.* Oxford: Oxford University Press.

Weindling, P. (1985). *The social history of occupational health.* Beckenham, Kent: Croom Helm Ltd.

Weitz, R. (2010). *The sociology of health, illness, and health care: A critical approach,* 5th edn. Boston: Wadsworth Cengage Learning.

Werner, D. (1997). *Questioning the solution: The politics of primary health care and child survivial with an in-depth critique of oral rehydration therapy.* Palo Alto, CA: Health Wrights.

West, G.B., & Bergman, A. (2009). Toward a systems biology framework for understanding aging and health span. *Journal of Gerontology Series A: Biolocial Sciences and Medical Sciences*, 64A(2), 205–8.

Wheaton, B., & Gotlieb, I.H. (1997). Trajectories and turning points over the life course: Concepts and themes. In I.H. Gotlieb & B. Wheaton (eds), *Stress and adversity over the life course.* Cambridge: Cambridge University Press, 1–28.

White, K. (2001). What's happening in general practice: Capitalist monopolisation and a state bailing out. *Health Sociology Review*, 10, 5–18.

White, K. (2009). *An introduction to the sociology of health and illness,* 2nd edn. London: Sage Publications.

Whitehead, E., Carlisle, C., Watkins, C., & Mason, T. (2001a). Historical developments. In T. Mason, C. Carlisle, C. Watkins, & E. Whitehead (eds), *Stigma and social exclusion in health care.* London: Routledge, 11–28.

Whitehead, E., Mason, T., Carlisle, C., & Watkins, C. (2001b). The changing dynamic of stigma. In T. Mason, C. Carlisle, C. Watkins, & E. Whitehead (eds), *Stigma and social exclusion in health care.* London: Routledge, 29–39.

WHO (World Health Organization) (1952). Constitution of the World Health Organization. In WHO (ed.), *World Health Organization handbook of basic documents,* 5th edn. Geneva: WHO, 3–20.

WHO (1978). *Alma-Ata 1978: Primary health care.* Geneva: WHO.

WHO (1986). *Ottawa Charter for Health Promotion.* Geneva: WHO.

WHO (1997a). *Health and environment in sustainable development, five years after the Earth Summit.* Geneva: WHO.

WHO (1997b). *Violence against women: A health priority issue, FRH/WHD/97.8.* Geneva: WHO.

WHO (1998). *Health promotion glossary*. Geneva: WHO.

WHO (2002a). Active aging: A policy framework. <http://whqlibdoc.who.int/hq/2002/who_nmh_nph_02.8.pdf>.

WHO (2002b). 25 questions and answers on health and human rights. Geneva: WHO. <www.who.int/hhr/activities/publications/en>.

WHO (2005a). *Chronic diseases and their common risk factors*. Information sheet #1. Geneva: WHO.

WHO (2005b). *Ecosystems and human well-being: Health synthesis. Millennium ecosystem assessment*. <www.who.int/globalchange/publications/ecosystems05/en/index.html>.

WHO (2005c). The global burden of oral diseases and risks to oral health. *Bulletin of the World Health Organization*, 83(9). <www.scielosp.org/scielo.php?pid=S0042-96862005000900011&script=sci_arttext&tlng=en>.

WHO (2008). *The World Health Report 2008: Primary health care: Now more than ever*. http://www.who.int/whr/2008/en/index.html

WHO (2009a). *The Bangkok Charter for Health Promotion in a Globalized World*. In *Milestones in Health Promotion. Statements from Global Conferences*. Geneva: WHO.

WHO (2009b). *Protecting health from climate change. Connecting science policy and people*. <www.who.int/globalchange/publications/reports/9789241598880/en/index.html>.

WHO (2009c). *Milestones in health promotion: Statements from global conferences*. <www.who.int/healthpromotion/milestones/en>.

WHO (2010a). *Tetanus*. <www.who.int/immunization_monitoring/diseases/tetanus/en/index.html>.

WHO (2010b). *Global summary of the AIDS epidemic* 2009, 1–11. <www.who.int/hiv/data/2010_globalreport_core_en.ppt>.

WHO (2010c). Set of recommendations on the marketing of food and non-alcoholic beverages to children. Geneva, WHO. <http://whqlibdoc.who.int/publications/2010/9789241500210_eng.pdf>.

WHO (2010d). Urbanization and health. *Bulletin of the World Health Organization*, 88 (4). <www.who.int/bulletin/volumes/88/4/10-010410/en>.

WHO (2011a). *Bovine spongiform encephalopathy*. <www.who.int/topics/encephalopathy_bovine_spongiform/en>.

WHO (2011b). *Smallpox*. <www.who.int/mediacentre/factsheets/smallpox/en>.

WHO (2011c). *Chronic diseases and their common risk factors*. <www.who.int/chp/chronic_disease_report/media/Factsheet1.pdf>.

WHO (2011d). *Malaria*. <www.who.int/topics/malaria/en>.

WHO (2011e). *Infectious diseases*. Retrieved 13 March 2011 from: http://www.who.int/topics/infectious_diseases/en/

WHO CSDH (Commission on Social Determinants of Health) (2005). *Action on the social determinants of health: Learning from previous experiences*. Geneva: WHO.

WHO CSDH (2007). *A conceptual framework for action on the social determinants of health*. Geneva: WHO. <www.who.int/social_determinants/resources/csdh_framework_action_05_07.pdf>.

WHO CSDH (2008a). *Backgrounder 3*. http://www.who.int.social_determinants/tools/resources/en/index.html

WHO CSDH (2008b). *Closing the gap in a generation: Health equity through action on the social determinants of health*. Final Report of the Commission on Social Determinants of Health. Geneva: WHO.

Wilkinson, R.G. (1997a). Income, inequality and social cohesion. *American Journal of Public Health*, 87, 104–6.

Wilkinson, R.G. (1997b). Socioeconomic determinants of health: Health inequities: Relative or absolute material standards. *British Medical Journal*, 314, 591–4.

Wilkinson, R.G., & Marmot, M. (eds) (2003). *Social determinants of health: The solid facts*. Copenhagen: WHO Regional Office for Europe.

Wilkinson, R.G., & Pickett, K.E. (2006). Income inequality and population health: A review and explanation of the evidence. *Social Science and Medicine*, 62(7), 1768–84.

Wilkinson, R.G., & Pickett, K. (2009). *The spirit level: Why more equal societies almost always do better*. London: Allen-Lane (Penguin).

Williams, A. (1987). Health economics: The cheerful face of a dismal science. In A. Williams (ed.), *Health and economics*. London: Macmillan, 1–11.

Williams, D.R., & Rucker, T.D. (2000). Understanding and addressing racial disparities in health care. *Health Care Financing Review*, 21(4), 75–90.

Williams, D.R., Gonzalez, H.M., Williams, S., Mohammed, S.A., Moomal, H., & Stein, D.J. (2008). Perceived discrimination, race and health in South Africa. *Social Science and Medicine*, 67(3), 441–52.

Williamson, R.C. (1981). Adjustment to the high rise: Variables in a German sample. *Environment and Behavior*, 13(3), 289–310.

Willis, E. (1998). The 'new genetics' and the sociology of medical technology. *Journal of Sociology*, 34(2), 170–83.

Willis, E. (2004). *The sociological quest: An introduction to the study of social life*, 4th edn. Sydney: Allen & Unwin.

Willis, E. (2005). Public health and the 'new genetics': Balancing individual and collective outcomes. In R. Bunton & A. Petersen (eds), *Genetic governance: Health, risk and ethics in the biotech era*. London: Routledge, 155–69.

Willis, E. (2009a). The Australian health care system. In E. Willis, L. Reynolds, & H. Keleher (eds), *Understanding the Australian health care system*. Sydney: Elsevier Australia, 3–15.

Willis, E. (2009b). *Purgatorial time in hospitals*. Germany: LAP Lambert Academic.

Willis, E. (2009c). The human genome project: A sociology of medical technology. In J. Germov (ed.), *Second opinion: An introduction to health sociology*, 4th edn. Melbourne: Oxford University Press, 328–46.

Willis, E., Miller, R., & Wyn, J. (2001). Gendered embodiment and survival for young people with cystic fibrosis. *Social Science and Medicine*, 53(9), 1163–74.

Willis, K., & Elmer, S. (2007). *Society, culture and health: An introduction to sociology for nurses*. Melbourne: Oxford University Press.

Wilson, T. (2005). New United Nations world population projections. *People and Place*, 13(1), 14–22.

Winsten, J.A. (1994). Promoting designated drivers: The Harvard Alcohol Project. *American Journal of Preventative Medicine*, 10(3), S11–S14.

Winsten, J.A., & DeJong, W. (2001). The designated driver campaign. In R.E. Rice & C.K. Atkin (eds), *Public communication campaigns*, 3rd edn. Thousand Oaks, CA: Sage Publications, 290–4.

Women's Health West (2008). *Improving maternity services in Australia: Submission response to a discussion paper from the Australian Government.* <www.whwest.org.au>.

Wonderling, D., Gruen, R., & Black, B. (2005). *Introduction to health economics.* New York: Open University Press.

Wong, S., & Regan, S. (2009). Patient perspectives on primary health care in rural communities: Effects of geography on access, continuity and efficiency. *Rural and Remote Health*, 9, 1–12.

Woodward, D.R., Cumming, F.J., Ball, P.J., Williams, H.M., Hornsby, H., & Boon, J.A. (1997). Does television affect teenagers' food choices? *Journal of Human Nutrition and Dietetics*, 10, 229–35.

Worm, I. (2010). *Human rights and gender equality and health: Overview of impact assessment tools.* Health and Human Rights Working Paper Series No 7. Geneva: WHO. <www.who.int/hhr/information/papers/en/index.html>.

Yang, L.H., Kleinman, A., Link, B.G., Phelan, J.C., Lee, S., & Good, B. (2007). Culture and stigma: Adding moral experience to stigma theory. *Social Science and Medicine*, 64, 1524–35.

Yassi, A., Kjellstrom, T., de Kok, T., & Guidotti, T.L. (2001). *Basic environmental health.* New York: Oxford University Press.

Yeatman, H. (2007). *National survey of food and nutrition activities of Australian local governments: A snapshot of Victorian local governments.* Wollongong, NSW: VicHealth/University of Wollongong publication.

Yeatman, H. (2008). Action or inaction? Food and nutrition in Australian local governments. *Public Health Nutrition*, 12(9), 1399–407.

Yuill, C. (2010). The social model of health. In C. Yuill, I. Crinson, & E. Duncan (eds), *Key concepts in health studies.* Thousand Oaks, CA: Sage Publications, 11–14.

Yung, A., Spelman, D., Street, A., McCormack, J., Sorrell, T., & Johnson, P. (eds) (2010). *Infectious diseases: A clinical approach*, 3rd edn. Melbourne: IP Communications.

Zarcadoolas, C., Pleasant, A.F., & Green D.S. (2006). Defining health literacy. In C. Zarcadoolas, A.F. Pleasant & D.S. Green (eds), *Advancing health literacy: A framework for understanding and action.* San Francisco, CA: Jossey-Bass, John Wiley & Sons, 45–67.

Zhang P., Zhang, X., Brown, J., Vistisen, D., Sicree, R., Shaw, J., & Nichols, G. (2010). Global healthcare expenditure on diabetes for 2010 and 2030. *Diabetes Research and Clinical Practice*, 87(3), 293–301.

Zhou, Y.R. (2007). 'If you get AIDS... You have to endure it alone': Understanding the social constructions of HIV/AIDS in China. *Social Science and Medicine*, 65(2), 284–95.

Zimmet, P. (1999). Diabetes epidemiology as a trigger to diabetes research. *Diabetologia*, 42, 499–518.

Zimmet, P., Alberti, K.G.M.M., & Shaw, J. (2001). Global and societal implications of the diabetes epidemic. *Nature*, 414, 782–7.

Zuppa, J.A., Morton, H., & Mehta, K. (2003). Television food advertising: Counterproductive to children's health? A content analysis using the Australian Guide to Healthy Eating. *Nutrition and Dietetics*, 60(2), 78–84.

Index

access to health services   100, 200, 328, 330–41

ACE-Prevention study   318–19

Acquired Immune Deficiency
    Syndrome (AIDS)   29–30, 36, 133–4
    see also HIV/AIDS

Active Ageing Network   105

Active Ageing policy framework (WHO)   103–4

activities of daily living (ADLs)   96, 99, 101

Adams, J.   79

adapted social ecological model   207–10

adaptive or specific defences against
    infection   33–5

addiction   180, 247

adolescence   217

Advance Care Planning (ACP)   224–5

advertising   262–3
    food   263–4
    tobacco   261–2

age
    concepts of   221
    as health determinant   12, 77, 79, 93,
        142, 208
    human rights   289

aged care   103, 315–16

ageing
    active ageing   103–5
    biomedical model of health   94–6
    environmental determinants of health   96–7
    functional health   79, 96–7
    health policies   102–4
    'healthy ageing'   94, 97–8, 103–4
    homeostatic mechanisms   142
    individual ageing   97
    longevity   96
    mental health   102
    population ageing   77, 93
    positive ageing   98
    predictors of good outcomes   101–2
    productive ageing   98
    psychosocial models   96–7
    SOC model   97
    social determinant of health   96–7, 100–2
    social environment   97
    stereotyping   94, 98–100
    'successful ageing'   94–6, 98

Ageing Well Research Network   105

agency/structure debate   203–5, 223

Aggleton, P.   252, 254

agricultural adaptation   147–8

Airs, waters and places (Hippocrates)   45

alcohol use   10, 81, 101, 110–11,
    249, 270–1, 309, 321

alleles   61

allocative efficiency   303

allostatic load   100

Alma Ata Declaration (WHO)   88

Anderson, T.   286

Andreasen, A.   265

Angus, J.   98

anorexia nervosa   240

Anson, D.   87

anthropogenic change   125–35

antibiotics
    fed to animals   37, 42
    incorrect use   36

antibodies   35

antigens   35

antiretroviral drugs   29, 252, 295, 298

anti-tobacco
    campaigns   298
    media advocacy   268–9

arbovirus diseases   143, 149–50

Archive for Life Course Research   228

arthritis   78, 118

asbestos   158

Ashkenazi Jewish families   62

Asian flu   28

Association of British Insurers   73

asthma   78–9, 82, 85, 118,
    131–2, 309

attributable risk   50

Australian Bureau of Statistics   212, 308, 325

Australian Council for New Urbanism   173

Australian Council on Children and
    the Media   264

Australian Council on Smoking and
    Health (ACOSH)   269

Australian Immunisation Handbook
    (Department of Health and
    Ageing and NHMRC)   39, 42

Australian Institute of Health and
    Welfare (AIHW)   2, 9, 14, 75, 78, 80,
                90, 196, 308, 320, 324
Australian National Children's Nutrition
    and Physical Activity Survey   263
Australian Research Alliance for
    Children and Youth   124
Australian Social Inclusion Board   196
Australian Television Communications and
    Media Authority   264
autism and vaccination   40
autosomes   62

B lymphocytes   35
baby boomers   95, 183
bacteria   25-7
Baltes, M.   97
Baltes, P.B.   97
Banerjee, A.   298
Barker, K.   270
Barmah forest virus   144
Bartley, M.   217-18, 226
Baum, F.   82
Bauman, Z.   179
Beauchamp, D.   192
behaviour change communication   264
behavioural approach to health   3
behavioural determinants of health   81-2
behavioural genetics   85
behaviours, health related   68
beliefs, health related   68-9
Ben-Shlomo, Y.   79
Bernardi, G.   293
best practice   108, 115-16, 137, 184, 235,
            237, 241, 272, 304, 317-18
Better Health Channel (Victorian
    Government)   42
Bickenbach, J.E.   284
biofuels   146
biological determinants of health   11-12, 79
    see also genetics
biological model of health   3
biomedical model of health   3-4, 67, 198-200
    ageing   94-6
birth weight   215, 223
Bisaillon, L.M.   286
Bishop, B.   103
Black Balloon, The [film]   254
Black Report   87, 182

Blane, D.   215, 225
Blaxter, M.   4, 199
blood pressure   10, 81, 83, 85, 101, 188
bottle-feeding   245, 249
Bourdieu, Pierre   223
bovine spongiform
    encephalopathy (BSE)   22, 30, 43
Bowling, A.   97, 99
BRCA1 and BRCA2   63
breast cancer   62-4, 67-8, 78, 88,
            237, 309, 312-14
breastfeeding   245-6
Bristol Exclusion Matrix   190-1
Bronfenbrenner, U.   206-7
Brooks, M.V.   83
Broom, D.   198
Brownie, S.   79
Browning, C.   100
Brundtland, G.H.   145, 287
built environment   126
bulimia nervosa   239
bulk-billing   333
burden of disease
    Australia   309
    chronic illnesses   78
    diabetes   78
    lifestyle factors   320
    longevity effects   96
    prevalence   55
    studies   308, 310-14
Cabal, L.   298
Cameron-Smith, D.   11
cancer
    ageing   101
    immigrant rates of   237
    mortality   78
    non-communicable disease risk factors   118
    social gradient and   224
Candida albicans   24, 31
capabilities model   191-2
car-dependence   97, 155-6, 159-60
cardiovascular disease   78-82, 85, 97, 101, 118
CARE International   296-8
Caring for older Australians (Australian
    Productivity Commission)   103
Center for Communication Programs,
    Johns Hopkins Bloomberg School
    of Public Health   277

Center for Health Communication [US]   271
Center for Reproductive Rights   298
Centers for Disease Control and
    Prevention [US]   55, 106, 135, 276
Centre for Aboriginal Economic Policy
    and Research, Australian National
    University   228
Centre for Evidence-Based Medicine [UK]   324
Centre for Health and Society, University of
    Melbourne   212
Centre for Health Economics (CHE-UK)   324
Centre for Health Economics, Monash
    University   323
Centre for Health Economics Research and
    Evaluation, University of Technology,
    Sydney   323
Centre for Reviews and Dissemination [UK]   324
Chadwick, Edwin   87
Chang, H.C.   79
Chapman, K.   264
Chapman, S.   112–13, 268–9
Charmaz, K.   77
Chau, J.Y.   264
chicken pox   47
childcare facilities   210
Chinese-Australians   68
Chlamydia (C. trachomatis)
    HIV and   11
    notifiable disease   26
    prevalence   25
    sexual transmission   25
cholera   143
    causation   45–6
cholesterol   10, 60, 81, 83
Chopra, M.   297
chromosomes   60–1, 95
chronic illnesses   91
    definition   46
    determinants   78–87
    determinants of health   118
    genetics   84–90
    health promotion   119
    major diseases   78
    mortality   45, 77
    social gradient   225
    see also non-communicable
        diseases (NCDs)
chronic obstructive pulmonary disease   78, 309

circulatory diseases   80
Clarke, P.J.   97
climate change   136–52
    adaptation   147–9
    agricultural adaptation   147–8
    alternative power sources   146
    Australia   153
    carbon cycle   139
    climate change literacy   137
    definition   137
    deniers   139
    as environmental determinant
        of health   12, 82
    extreme cold   140–2, 149
    extreme weather events   82, 114, 140–1,
        143–4, 156–7
    food security   12, 114
    fossil fuels   138–9, 146
    greenhouse gas emissions   147
    health promotion approach   114–15
    health sector adaptation   148–9
    heatwaves   12, 149, 153, 156, 168
    impacts in Australia   13
    infectious disease vectors   12
    key messages   140
    mental health   144
    mitigation   145–7
    vulnerable populations   142
    see also global warming
Climate change adaptation: A framework for local
    action (Southern Grampians and
    Glenelg Primary Care Partnership)   114–15
Climate Change and Primary Healthcare
    Intervention Framework   151
Climate Institute of Australia   153
Clinard, M.B.   243, 246
cloning   58
Closing the gap (WHO)   192
Coalition on Food Advertising to Children   264
Cochrane Collaboration   115
Cohen, A.K.   245
cohorts   216
colorectal cancer   78, 309
Committee on Economic, Social and
    Cultural Rights: Australia   282
Committee on the Elimination of Racial
    Discrimination: Australia   283
communicable diseases see infectious diseases

Communicable Diseases Surveillance program 150
Communication for Social Change
        Consortium   277
Communication Initiative Network   276
Community Ecosystem Model   206
community enablement   120–1
community gardens   170–3
community health movement   183
complementary and alternative medicine   79
Compression of Morbidity hypothesis   96
Congress for the New Urbanism   173
contagious diseases see infectious diseases
Convention on Migrant Workers   292
Convention on the Rights of Persons with
        Disabilities   284
Convention on the Rights of the Child   291
Cook, R.   298
coronary heart disease   78, 81, 215, 223, 312–14
cost of illness studies   308, 310–15
cost-benefit analysis (CBA)   317
cost-utility analysis (CUA)   317
Council for Responsible Genetics   75
Cox, S.M.   70
Creedy, D.   5
Creutzfeld-Jakob disease (CJD)   30
Crick, Francis   58, 84
Crimmins, E.   97
Crocker, J.   248
CSIRO (Australian Commonwealth Scientific
        and Research Organisation)   144
cultural competency   232, 235–7, 241
cultural concepts of health   5–8, 68, 199, 230–41
cultural diversity   156
cultural relativism   284
culture
    definition   215, 230
    language and   230–4
culture-bound syndromes   238–40
cyclones   142
cystic fibrosis   62, 85, 87

Dalton, C.B.   158
DALY (Disability Adjusted Life Year)   309–13
Dart, J.   259
Daube, M.   269
David, S.   298
De Fossard, E.   269–70
De Mortibus Artificum Diatriba (Ramazzini)   45
Deakin Health Economics   323
decision rules in health economics   310

Delisle, H.   214–15
demand   304, 307
dementia   96, 309
dengue fever   131
dental health   127, 233, 316, 332, 340
Denton, M.   79
Depp, C.   100
depression   78, 81, 83, 222, 240, 249, 309, 321
description in health economics   308, 310
determinants of health   2–3, 8–16, 87, 109–11
    chronic illnesses   78–87, 89, 118
    see also behavioural determinants of health;
        biological determinants of health;
        environmental determinants of health;
        psychological determinants of health;
        psychosocial determinants of health;
        social determinants of health
deviance   243–56
diabetes   85, 88, 91, 101, 118, 200, 239
    epidemiology   52–3
    type 2   50, 52–3, 78–84, 309, 321
Dickens, Charles   217
difference   243
diphtheria   39
direct costs   310, 315
disability   209, 247
Disability Discrimination Act 1992   73
discrimination   247, 249–52, 254
disease, definition   4, 237
disease genetics   85
distributive efficiency   303
DNA   58, 60–1, 84
    'fingerprinting'   59
    genetic tests   63–6, 70
Docteur, E.   330
Doll, R.   184–5
domestic violence   128, 272, 298–9, 309
Donovan, R.   265–6
Draper, G.   320
Durkheim, Emile   223, 243
Durrant, J.   284
Earle, S.   246
early life as health determinant   180
Ebi, K.L.   148
Echinococcus granulosus, E. granulosus
    (hydatid tapeworms)   31–2
ecological models of health   206–10
economic rationalism   319
economics of health   302–22

education as health determinant   10, 69, 78,
        101–2, 110–12, 116–17, 150, 178, 202–4, 223,
                            259, 281–2, 289
edu-tainment   269–72
efficiency   303, 305–8, 322
Eisenbruch, M.   68
Elder, Glen   214–16, 218–20, 222–3
Elliason, S.R.   218
embedded energy   146
emergency management   156, 165–7
Emergency Management Australia   167
employment as health determinant   10, 80, 110,
                            180, 208–9, 288
encephalitis   143–4
endemic, definition   47
Enterobius vermicularis, E. vermicularis
            (pinworms)   31
entertainment-education   269–72
environmental determinants of health   154–72
    ageing   96–7
    biological factors   156
    chemical factors   156
    chronic illnesses   82
    definition   12
    extreme cold   140–2, 149
    global warming   12, 141
    heat-stroke   141, 149
    physical factors   156
    poverty and   13
    responses   157–9
    social factors   156
    vulnerable populations   142
    see also climate change; town planning
environmental health   155, 157–9
Environmental Health Practitioners   157–9
environmental sustainability   210
epidemics   45, 47
Epidemiologic Transition Theory   94
epidemiology   44–55
    definition   45
    diabetes   52–3
    history   45–6
    incidence   49
    influenza   51–2
    prevalence   49
    rates   48–9
    risk   50–1
    see also social epidemiology
Equality Trust, The   196

equity   116–19, 190, 279
    see also health equity; health inequality
Equity, social determinants and public health
        programmes (Blas & Kurup)   192
Erikson, Erik   217–18
Escherichia coli (E. coli)   24
ethics and predictive genomic testing   65–6
'ethnic cleansing'   248
ethnicity as health determinant   13–14
eugenics   59
eukaryotes   25
European Convention on Human Rights   294
European Court of Human Rights   294
evaluation in health economics   317–19
evidence base for health determinants   183–5
evidence-based health promotion   115–16, 184
evidence-based medicine   79–80, 184, 237
explanation in health economics   320–1
extreme weather events   82, 114, 140–1,
                            143–4, 156–7

    see also heatwaves

Fadem, P.   98
Fair society, healthy lives: The Marmot
        review (Marmot)   192, 196
Falk, G.   247
Falk, P.   67
Family Safety Net   338
Farming Zones   164
Flannery, Tim   153
floods   143, 156
Food Act 1984 (Vic.)   157–8
Food for All (VicHealth)   170–1
food security   114, 169–70, 173, 180
    vulnerable populations   143
Food Standards Australia and
        New Zealand   42
food-borne illnesses   158–9
Ford, N.   295, 297
fossil fuels   138–9, 146
Foucault, M.   253–4
Fox, B.J.   298
Freeman, B.   269
free-radical theory   95
Friedman, Milton   306
Fries, J.   96
Fry, C.L.   298
functional health   96–7
fungi   25, 30

gastroenteritis 158–9
Geithner, C.A. 79
gender
    burden of disease 309
    genes and 72
    as health determinant 12–14, 87, 202
    human rights 289
    obesity 312–14
    as 'tribal identity' 247
gene therapy 86
General Household Survey [UK] 225
general practitioners 330–1, 338–41
genes 60–1
    gender and 72
genetic 'carriers' 62
genetic conditions 61–2
genetic counselling 68
genetic determinism 59–60
genetic discrimination 73
Genetic Information Non-discrimination Act
    (GINA) of 2008 [USA] 73
genetic literacy 69
genetic markers 100
genetic mutations 61–2, 85
genetic reductionism 88
genetic risk 62
genetic tests 63–6, 70
geneticisation 67
genetics 57–74
    chronic illnesses 79, 84–90
    social context 87–9
genome 61
genotype 61
Germov, J. 198–9, 201, 203
Giardia 156
Glasgow, R.E. 84
Global Alert and Response Network (WHO) 131
Global Lawyers and Physicians—Working
    Together for Human Rights 301
global warming 139–41
Global warming and the political ecology
    of health (Baer & Singer) 143
Glover, J.D. 80
glucose levels 10, 53, 101
'Go for 2 & 5®' Campaign 265–7, 274
Goffman, E. 247–8, 251
Goldhaber, M.D. 294
Gostin, L. 284–6, 296
government failure 303, 308

GP Plus 340–1
GP Super Clinics 340–1
Gram staining 25
Graunt, John 45
Grayson, R. 170
Green Star—Healthcare v1 148
greenhouse gas emissions 147
Griffiths, J. 137
Groake, A. 79
Gruskin, S. 296

H1N1 influenza ('swine flu') 22, 28
Habermas, Jürgen 223
haemophilia 62
Haines, A. 137
HALCyon Healthy Ageing across the
    Life Course 106
Hall, J.A. 96
Hall, W.D. 65
Hancock, T. 206
Hanta virus 143
harm reduction 268, 298
Harvard Alcohol Project, The 270–1
Harvard School of Public Health 297
Harvey, P.W. 80
Hawaiians 68
hazardous waste 155–6
health
    as absence of disease 4
    behavioural approach 3
    biological model 3
    biomedical model 3–4
    as cultural construct 2–3, 5–8
    definitions 2–4, 198, 230
    health promotion approach 3
    Hmong concepts 6–8
    Indigenous Australians' concepts 5–6
    influence of location 3
    as social construct 2, 198–201
    social justice approaches 15
    Thai concepts 6
    see also determinants of health
Health and Human Rights 298
health communication 264, 273–5
health economics 302–22
Health Economics Research Group [UK] 324
health equity 279
    human rights 293–5
health expenditure projections 316–17

health iceberg model 185–6
health inequality 15, 79–81, 202–3, 234–5, 329
health inequities 279
health insurance 306, 308, 328–32, 334–8
Health Insurance Commission 308, 325
health literacy 259
health policy 200–1
health promotion 107–23
   advocacy 112–13, 122
   approach to health 3
   chronic illnesses 119
   collaboration 111–12, 121
   definition 108–9
   enabling 113, 120–1
   evidence-based 115–16
   history 183–5
   influenza 121–2
   local government 156, 168–72
   mass media and 264–75
   mediation 113
   see also Ottawa Charter for Health
      Promotion (WHO)
health services 290
   access to 100, 200, 328, 330–41
health sociology 201
healthcare system 326–42
   bulk-billing 333
   Family Safety Net 338
   market-based model 333
   Medicare 334–5, 338
   primary care 338–9
   private insurance model 331–2, 334
   public-contract service delivery model 330–1
   public-integrated model 330–1, 334
   role substitution 340
   as structural determinant of
      health 327, 329–30
   sustainability 315–16
   universal healthcare 328–30, 334–5
   user pays healthcare 328–31, 335, 337–8
   waiting times 328, 331–2, 336
   welfare-based model 330, 334
   see also health services
Health-Environment-Economy model 206
Healthier future for all Australians,
   A (NHHRC) 192
Healthy Cities program (WHO) 88
heat-stroke 141, 149

heatwaves 12, 149, 153, 156, 168
Heikkinen, E. 104
helminths 31–2
Henley, N. 265–6
hepatitis B 156
hepatitis C 202
Herek, G.M. 249
Herpes 36
Hertzman, C. 223–4
Hill, A. 184–5
Hippocrates 45
HIV/AIDS
   co-infection with tuberculosis 134
   human rights approach 280, 295–6
   morbidity 36
   overview 29–30
   rights limitations 285
   risk factors 11
   stigmatisation 247, 249–55
   virology 29–30, 36
   World Health Organization 43
Hmong health concepts 6–8
Hoehn, K. 34
Hogerzeil, H.V. 295
Holstein, M.B. 98
homosexuals/homosexuality 29, 244–5,
      251–3, 292–3
Hong Kong flu 28
household chemicals 130–1
household structure 209
housing 209, 288, 328
Howard, C.M. 267
Hulme Chambers, A. 149
Human Genetics Society of
   Australasia (HGSA) 75
Human Genome Project 59, 61, 67, 75, 84–5
human rights
   absolute and relative 284
   approach to health 280
   convenants, conventions and
      treaties 281–2, 291–2
   homosexuality 292–3
   inalienable 283
   Indigenous Australians 282–3
   justifiable limitations 284–6
   policy analysis 295–7
   public health practice 297–9
   right to health 286–7, 295

social determinants of health   287–91
social justice   279, 293–5
   see also Universal Declaration on Human
       Rights (United Nations)
Huntington's disease   62–3, 70–1, 73, 85
Hutchison, E.   215, 221
hydatid tapeworm (*Echinococcus granulosus*,
   E. granulosus)   31–2, 43
hypertension   79, 85, 312–14

illness behaviour   230, 237–9
illness, definition   4, 237
immunisation   38–41, 182
Immunise Australia Program   39, 41–2
incidence   49
income inequality   189–90, 202–3, 288
incremental cost-effectiveness ratio (ICER)   317
Indigenous Australians
   Closing the Gap Strategy   234, 241
   diabetes   53
   health concepts   5–6, 235
   health inequalities   234–5
   health status   15, 234–5
   human rights   282–3
   life expectancy at birth   15, 116, 202
   NGO advocacy   294
   social inclusion   235
indirect costs   310
Indonesian concepts of health   231, 238–9
infant mortality and morbidity   332
infectious diseases
   biology   22–5
   carriers   27
   defences against infection   33–4
   humoral immunity   35
   immunisation   38–41
   morbidity   36
   normal flora   24
   parasites   24, 31–3
   pathogens   23–31
   susceptibility factors   37
   vaccination   38–41
   World Health Organization   43
inflammatory bowel disease   85
influenza   28–9, 156
   epidemiology   51–2
   health promotion   121–2
   immunisation   39, 52
Institute for Life Course and Aging   227

intangible costs   311
Inter-American Commission on Human
   Rights (IACHR)   298–9
interest groups   327, 330
Intergenerational Report, The   77
Intergovernmental Panel on Climate
   Change   140, 153
intermediary determinants of
   health   327–8, 332–4
International Centre for Life Course Studies
   in Society and Health   228
International Covenant on Civil and
   Political Rights (ICCPR)   281, 289–90,
       292, 294
International Covenant on Economic,
   Social and Cultural
   Rights (ICESCR)   281, 284, 286–7,
       289–91, 294
International Network for Economic, Social
   and Cultural Rights   301
International Panel on Climate Change   144
internet
   advertising   262
   as health information provider   259
irrigation   147–8
Irwin, A.   183, 185, 327
ischaemic heart disease   78, 81, 83, 309, 312–14
Ishay, M.R.   281

Jacobson, P.D.   298
Japhet, Garth   271
Jeste, D.   100
Jones, E.E.   247
Jones, K.   5
Jonsson, U.   296
Joss, N.   12
Journal of Emergency Management   173

Kahn, R.L.   96, 98
Karasek, R.   81
karyotype   60
Kawachi, I.   15
Keane, H.   298
Keleher, H.   2–3, 12
Kelly, B.P.   264
Khoury, M.J.   63
kidney disease   78
Kitisriworapan, S.   245
Klin, A.   261

Koch, Robert   23
Kotler, P.   262
Kuh, D.   79
Kyoto Protocol   145

labelling theory   248
Lamb, K.L.   97
language
    culture and health   231–4
    medical   232–3
    non-verbal   232
Lawn, S.   13
Lazzarini, Z.   286
LeBel, T.P.   252–3
Legionnaire's Disease   132
Lemish, D.   261
Levy, B.R.   98
Liamputtong, P.   245, 252, 254
life course approach to health   213–26
    agency   223
    cohorts   216
    'life and historical times'   220
    life events   219
    'linked lives'   222
    outcome effects   223
    social gradient   223–5
    'timing of lives'   220–1
    trajectories   218
    transitions   216–18
    turning points   219
life events   219
life expectancy
    Australia   202
    at birth   15
    female   93
    income inequality   190
    Indigenous Australians   202
    influences   93
    international comparisons   116, 187–8
    male   93
    Maoris   234
    per capita income   192
    Preston Curve   192–3
    social class and   187
    socio-economic status   320
Lin, V.   68
Lindee, M.S.   67
linguistic relativity   231
living environment   155

local government
    community gardens   170–2
    emergency management   156, 165–7
    environmental health   157–9
    health promotion   156, 168–72
    Municipal Health and
        Well-being Plans   157, 168–9
    responsibilities   156
longevity   96
Longitudinal and Life Course Studies: An
    International Journal   228
lung cancer   78, 309
Lupien, S.   94
Lyme Disease   143
Lyttleton, C.   253

MacArthur, I.   157
MacDougall, C.   2–3
Macmillan, R.   218
macroparasites   24
'mad cow disease'   22, 30
Magic Mountain, The (Mann)   133
malaria
    mosquitoes   38
    overview   32–3
    parasite   36
    protozoa   24
    surveillance   150
    thalassaemia minor   61
    World Health Organization   43
managed care plans   331
Mandala of Health   206
Mann, J.   251, 280
Mann, Thomas   133
Maoris   234–5
Marieb, E.N.   34
market failure   303, 308
marketing   261–4
Marmot, M.   80, 180–1, 187–8, 199
Martin, C.M.   199
Marx, Karl   223
Mason, T.   247
mass media   257–76
    advocacy   267–9
    definition   258–9
    developing promotion materials   272–5
    globalisation   259
    health promotion and   264–75
    marketing   261–4

mental health and   261
  representations of health   259–61
  social marketing   264–72, 277
Mathews, W.K.   267
McKellin, W.   70
McKenny, D.R.   79
McMichael, A.   137
measles   126
measles, mumps, and Rubella (MMR)
  vaccination   40
media advocacy   267–9
Medicare   334–5, 338
Meier, R.F.   243, 246
melanoma   66, 82
mental health
  ageing   102
  'blemishes of individual character' 247
  climate change   144
  definitions   4
  health gradient   80
  mass media and   261
  stigma   248
  urban sprawl   160–1
merit goods   306, 308
metazoa   24–5
Metzler, M.   79–80
microparasites   24
Milestones in Health Promotion (WHO) 183
Millennium Development Goals (WHO) 192, 196
MindMatters program   295
Minkler, M.   98
Molster, C.   69
'moral career'   248
morbidity
  infectious diseases   36
  National Notifiable Diseases
    Surveillance System   56
  rates   49
Morbillivirus   126
Morgan, R.E.   298
mortality
  breast cancer   78
  cancer   78
  cardiovascular disease   78
  coronary heart disease   78
  male and female infants   45
  mental health   78
  rates   48–9
  social gradient   224
  stroke   78

mosquito-borne diseases   131, 149–50, 153, 156
  malaria   32–3, 38
Moyn, S.   281
multi-factorial disorders   62–3
multiple sclerosis   85
Municipal Health and Well-being
  Plans (MHWP)   157, 168–9
Muntaner, C.   279
Murphy, E.   245–6
Murphy, G.   77
Murray Valley encephalitis   144
Mycobacterium tuberculosis   133
Myriad Genetics   66

Nagengast, C.   284
National Aboriginal Community
  Controlled Health Organisations   294
National Cancer Institute [US]   272
National Chronic Disease Strategy of 2005 78
National Congress of Australia's First Peoples 283
National Food Safety Standards   158
National Health and Hospitals Reform
  Commission   224
National Health and Medical Research
  Council (NHMRC)
  cultural competency   236, 241
National Health Priority Areas   168
National Health Service [UK]   182–3
National Health Survey   320
National Institute of Health [USA]   83
National Notifiable Diseases
  Surveillance System   56, 150
National Public Health Partnership   78
National Stigma Clearinghouse   255
National Strategy for an Ageing
  Australia (NSAA) (Bishop)   103
Natural and political observation on the bills of
  mortality (Graunt)   45
natural environment, access to   209
Nelkin, D.   67
New Urbanism   155, 161–6, 173
  see also urbanisation
Nieuwenhuijsen, E.R.   97
non-communicable diseases (NCDs)   118–19
non-specific defences against infection 33–4
normal flora   24
normative economics   304, 306
nosocomial (hospital-acquired) infections 31
NSW Health Centre for Genetics Education 75
nuclear power   146

nurse practitioners   340
Nussbaum, M.   191

obesity
    childhood   111, 263
    chronic illness and   79, 81, 85
    health and cost impacts   311–14
    health expenditure   312
    ischemic heart disease   83
    as risk factor   185
    stigma   249
    type 2 diabetes   52
occupational health
    and safety   127, 156, 309, 328
Office of the High Commissioner for
    Human Rights   291–2
older adults   93
    see also ageing
old-old population   93–4
    see also ageing
opportunity cost   303, 305
oral disease   78, 233
O'Shaughnessy, M.   259
osteoporosis   78, 309
Ottawa Charter for Health
    Promotion (WHO)   3, 88, 108–9,
                                                   112–14, 149, 279
outbreaks of disease   47
Oxley, H.   330

palliative care   224
Palmore, Erdman   94
pandemic   47
pandemic influenza   182
parasites   24, 31–3
Parent's Jury, The   264
Parker, R.   252, 254
Parry, Y.K.   333
pathogens   23–31
    bacteria   25–7
    fungi   25
    viruses   27–30
Patient Admission Transport Scheme   335
People's Health Movement (PHM)   17, 301
Perkins, F.   206
Perry, L.   200
person-in-context approach   71
Peterson, C.L.   77, 81
Peterson, M.   199
pets   209
phagocytes   34

phenotype   61
physical inactivity   81, 83, 101, 156, 160
Pickett, K.E.   189, 192, 329
pinworms (Enterobius vermicularis,
    E. vermicularis)   31
Piotrow, P.T.   270
plague (the 'Black Death')   143
Planning and Environment Act 1987 (Vic.)   157
Plasmodium   32–3
polio   39
Pollard, C.M.   266
pollution   155–6
polygenic genetic disorders   85
Ponder, M.   68
population attributable risk (PAR)   311
population density   128
population health
    ACE-Prevention study   319
    approach to health care   122
    census data   55
    definition   111–12
    epidemiology and   47
    individual health and   185–6
Population Media Center   277
positive economics   304, 306
post-traumatic stress disorder   240, 261
poverty   79–80, 288
Power, C.   223
prediction in health economics   315–17
predictive genetic tests   63–5, 70–3
predictive genomic testing   65–6
Preston Curve   192–3
pre-symptomatic genetic tests   64–5, 70–1, 73
prevalence   49
Preventing chronic disease: A strategic framework
    (National Public Health Partnership)   78
prevention of disease   145
primary care   338–9
Primary Care Partnerships   169
Primary Healthcare Research and
    Information Centre   343
primary prevention   145
prions   25, 30
prisoners   247
prokaryotes   25
prostate cancer   309
protozoa   24–5
psychological determinants
    of health   10, 12, 72, 94, 96–7, 100
psychosocial determinants of health   129–30

psychosocial models of ageing 96–7
Psychosocial Stages of Development
(Erikson) 217–18
public health
advocacy 279, 293–5
history 181–5
human rights 297–300
legislation 181–2
Ottawa Charter for Health
Promotion 3
rights limitations 285
social justice 279
Public Health Advocacy Institute of WA 277
Public Health Agency of Canada 212
*Public Health and Wellbeing
Act 2008* (Vic.) 150, 157
Public Health Association of Australia 264
public health communication 264, 273–5
public health genomics 65
Public Health Information
Development Unit 343
public policies 328, 330
pyrogens 34–5

Q-fever 156
quality-adjusted life years
(QALYs/DALYs) 317–18

race
as health determinant 12–13
as 'tribal identity' 247
Ramazzini, Bernadino 45
Rasanathan, K. 298
Rawls, John 279
Rees, S. 299
Reeve, P. 98
Regan, S. 338
relative risk 311
religion
as health determinant 178
human rights and 281, 283–4, 289–90
social skeleton 203–4
stigmatisation 248
as 'tribal identity' 247
reproductive health 298
resilience 94, 96, 100
respiratory disease 80, 82, 118, 224
Rett syndrome 62
Rice, Thomas 307–8
Richards, M. 68, 72

Rift Valley Fever 143
risk
definitions 50–1
genetic risk 62, 71
relative risk 50
risk factors 50, 185
Riso, L.P. 83
Robinson, Mary 286
Rogers, M. 270–1
role substitution 340
Ross River Fever 143–4
Rowe, J. 96, 98
Rubella 39–40
Rumbold, Bruce 228
rural and remote healthcare 273–4, 305, 335,
337, 339
Rural Conservation Zones 164
Rutter, N. 219

Sabido, Miguel 270
safety and security 209
Saggers, S. 15
Salmonella outbreaks 53–4, 156, 158–9
Salmonella typhi (S. typhi) 27
Samson, C. 67
Sapir-Whorf hypothesis 231
Satariano, W.A. 93
Scali, E. 183, 185
Scambler, G. 250
Schneiderman, N. 83
secondary prevention 145
Seeman, T.E. 97
self-direction in work 188
self-esteem 97, 188, 249
Semenza, J.C. 148
semiotics 262
Sen, A. 191, 279
sense of community 210
separation rates 336–7
sex-linked genetic mutations 62
Shape of Water, The [documentary] 16
Shisana, O. 83
sick building syndrome 128–9
Singh, J.A. 295
Singhal, A. 270–1
single-gene disorders 62, 85
Siracusa principles 284–6
smallpox 22, 47
Smart Growth 155, 161, 163–4

smoking   54, 80–1, 83, 101, 184–5, 245, 320
    see also anti-tobacco media advocacy;
        tobacco advertising
Snow, John   45–6
social accumulation   225
social activism   253
social capital   82, 130, 156, 188
social class *see* socio-economic status
social construction of health   198
social determinants of health
    addiction   180, 247
    ageing   96–7, 100–2
    chronic illness and   77, 79–81, 87
    definition   13, 179
    deviance and stigma   242–55
    early life experiences   180
    equity   116–17, 190
    ethnicity   14
    food   180
    gender   14, 202
    health promotion and   109–11
    health sociology   201
    healthcare system   327–34
    human rights   280, 298–9
    income inequality   189–90, 202–3, 288
    individual risk factors   185
    life expectancy   15, 93, 202
    mass media   258
    social class   14
    social ecological model   208–10
    social exclusion   180, 190–1
    social gradient   180, 186–8, 223–5
    social model of health   198–201
    Social Skeleton   203–5
    social support   180
    socio-economic status   13–14, 79–81, 87, 187,
            189–90, 202–3, 207–9, 223–5, 320–1,
                            327, 336, 338
    stress   79, 81, 83, 100, 180, 199
    transport   13, 155, 163, 169–70,
                    180, 208–10, 328, 352
    unemployment   110, 180, 190, 202,
                            288, 306, 328
    vulnerability   142
    work stress   180, 188
    World Health Organization   178
    see also intermediary determinants of health;
        socio-economic status; structural
            determinants of health

Social determinants of health: The solid facts
    (Wilkinson & Marmot eds)   180
social ecological model   206–7
social epidemiology   182
social exclusion   180, 190–2, 210, 247–50
social gradient   180, 186–8, 223–5
social inclusion   190–1, 196
Social Inclusion initiative   130
social justice   206, 278–300
social justice approaches to health   15
social marketing   264–72, 277
social media   262
social mobility   225
social model of health   198–201
social norms   243–4
social protection   225
Social Skeleton model   203–5, 211
social support   180, 188, 290
Society for Longitudinal and Life
        Course Studies   227
socio-economic status
    access to services   336
    chronic illness and   79–81
    as health determinant   13–14, 87, 321
    health insurance   338
    income inequality   202–3
    life course   223–5
    life expectancy   320
    morbidity   321, 327
    mortality   320–1, 327
    social ecological model   207–9
    social gradient   187, 189–90
sociolinguistics   231–2
Solar, O.   327
solar power   146
solar ultraviolet radiation (UVR)   158
Sontag, S.   247
Soul City   271–2
Southern Grampians and Glenelg
        Primary Care Partnership   114
Spanish flu   28, 182
Special Collaborative Centre 186:
    Status Passages and Risks in the
        Life Course   228
spillover effects   307
Spirit Level, The (Wilkinson & Pickett) 329
spirituality   100
Stack, S.   261
Stadler, J.M.   259

Stafford, J. 268
stereotyping 249
stigma 243, 247–56
Stoppard, M. 79
Strasburger, V.C. 260
stress 79, 81, 83, 180, 199
    allostatic load 100
stroke 78, 81, 96–7, 309
structural determinants of health 327–30, 335
structure/agency debate 203–5, 223
Sudak, D.M. 261
Sudak, H.S. 261
suicide 224, 261, 309
Super Size Me [film] 275
supply-induced demand 307
Sustainability Victoria 153
Swinburn, B. 11
swine flu 22
Syme, S.L. 188

T cells 29, 35–6
Taket, A. 281, 297
Talbot, L. 148–9
Tamlyn, J.A. 78
Tannahill, A. 115
Tanner Stages of Puberty 221
tapeworms 24, 31–2
Tarantola, D. 251, 280, 296
Taylor, S.D. 70, 198, 200
Tay-Sachs disease 62
technical efficiency 303
telomeres 95
Temple-Smith, M. 202
tetanus (Clostridium tetani) 26–7, 43, 156
    immunisation 39
Thai health concepts 6
Thai women living with HIV/AIDS 252–4
thalassaemia 62
thalassaemia minor 61
Thomas, S. 100
Tilley, J.J. 284
tobacco advertising 261–2
town planning 155, 159
    see also urbanisation
trajectories 218
Transit Oriented Development (TOD) 163, 173
transitions 216–18
transport 13, 155, 163, 169–70, 180, 208–10, 328, 352

travel, international 131–2
tuberculosis 133–4
turning points 219
type A behaviour pattern 239
typhoid 27
'Typhoid Mary' 27

UN Human Rights Committee 298
UNAIDS 271
unemployment 110, 180, 190, 202, 288, 306, 328
United Nations Charter 281
United Nations Children's Fund (UNICEF) 297
United Nations Environment Program (UNEP) 17
United Nations Population Fund (UNFPA) 297
United Nations Programme on Ageing 105
Universal Declaration on Human Rights
    (United Nations) 279, 281–2, 284, 286, 288–91, 301
unprotected sex 81, 185
Unwin, N. 80
urban sprawl 159–63
urbanisation 128–9, 132–3, 155–6, 159–64
    see also new Urbanism; town planning
Usdin, Shereen 271–2
Using policy to promote mental health and
    well-being: An introduction for policy
    makers (Victorian Dept. Health) 200

vaccination 38–41
vaccine-preventable diseases (VPDs) 39
Varicella zoster 47
Varmus, Harold 86
Vaughan, C. 11
vector-borne diseases 131, 143–4, 149–50, 156
Venkatapuram, S. 279, 298
Verrinder, G. 148–9
Victorian Burden of Disease Study 168
Victorian Charter of Human Rights and
    Responsibilities 301
Victorian Health Promotion Foundation
    (VicHealth) 4, 124, 170
Vietnamese concepts of health 199
vital statistics 56

Wakefield, M. 268
Walker, A. 104
Walker, C. 77
Walker, N. 269
Walker, R. 144, 149

walking 161, 163, 173
Wan, N. 94
water quality and supply 12–13, 37, 46,
 82, 132, 143, 147–50, 155–6, 181, 288
water-borne diseases 143, 147, 149–50
Watson, James 58–9, 84
Weber, Max 223
welfare state 328
well-being 4–6
West Nile Virus 131, 143
White, K. 201–2
Whitehall Studies 187, 189
Whitehead, E. 249
whooping cough (pertussis) 39
Wilkinson, R.G. 80–1, 180–1, 189,
 192, 199, 203, 329
Willis, E. 66–7
wind power 146
Winsten, J. A. 271
Wong, S. 338
work stress 180, 188
workers' compensation 127, 133
workplace rage 130
World Health Organization
 ageing 103–4, 106
 chronic illnesses 77
 climate change 135, 153
 Closing the gap in a generation 192

Commission on Social Determinants
 of Health 17, 79, 116–17, 179, 192,
 196, 227, 279, 298, 327, 332
definition of health 2, 4
emerging diseases 131, 135
environmental health 13
epidemic monitoring 55
HIV 43
human rights 298, 301
infectious diseases 43
influenza vaccines 28–9
malaria 43
Milestones in Health Promotion 183
Millennium Development Goals 192, 196
Millennium Ecosystem Assessment 153
recognition of Soul City 272
right to health 286–7
social determinants of health 88, 123, 178–9
urbanisation 128
World health report 2008c 192
World health report 2008c (WHO) 192
Worm, I. 295
worms (helminths) 31–2

Yellow Fever 143
Yuill, C. 199–200, 210

zoonoses 126–7, 156